SECOND EDITION

AMERICAN CANCER SOCIETY

COMPLETE GUIDE TO

Nutrition for Cancer Survivors

SECOND EDITION

AMERICAN CANCER SOCIETY

COMPLETE GUIDE TO

Nutrition for
Cancer Survivors

Eating Well, Staying Well During and After Cancer

Barbara L. Grant, MS, RD, CSO, LD
Abby S. Bloch, PhD, RD
Kathryn K. Hamilton, MA, RD, CSO, CDN
Cynthia A. Thomson, PhD, RD, CSO

Published by the American Cancer Society / Health Promotions
250 Williams Street NW, Atlanta, Georgia 30303-1002

Printed in the United States of America
Design and composition by LaShae V. Ortiz
Indexing by Bob Land

7 8 9   16 17 18

Library of Congress Cataloging-in-Publication Data
American Cancer Society complete guide to nutrition for cancer survivors : eating well, staying well during and after cancer / Barbara Grant ... [et al].—2nd ed.
       p. cm.
    Rev. ed. of: Eating well, staying well during and after cancer. c2004.
    Includes bibliographical references and index.
    ISBN-13: 978-0-944235-78-2 (pbk. : alk. paper)
    ISBN-10: 0-944235-78-6 (pbk. : alk. paper)
1. Cancer—Nutritional aspects. 2. Cancer—Diet therapy.
I. Grant, Barbara (Barbara L.), 1958-
II. American Cancer Society.
III. Eating well, staying well during and after cancer.
IV. Title: Complete guide to nutrition for cancer survivors.
    RC268.45.E285 2010
    616.99'40654—dc22   2009050656

AMERICAN CANCER SOCIETY

Quantity discounts on bulk purchases of this book are available. Book excerpts can also be created to fit specific needs. For information, please contact the American Cancer Society, Health Promotions Publishing, 250 Williams Street NW, Atlanta, GA 30303-1002, or send an e-mail to **trade.sales@cancer.org**.

A NOTE TO THE READER

The treatment information in this book is not official policy of the American Cancer Society and is not intended as medical advice to replace the expertise and judgment of your cancer care team. It is intended to help you and your family make informed decisions, together with your doctor.

For more information about cancer, contact your American Cancer Society at **800-227-2345** or **cancer.org**.

CONTENTS

American Cancer Society

INTRODUCTION

A cancer diagnosis affects everything—your priorities, your family, your work, your outlook on life. The time after diagnosis can be stressful and difficult, a time filled with challenges and change. You and your family will be learning about your illness, your cancer treatment choices, and how to deal with work and family needs. What to eat may be the furthest thing from your mind. But eating well is more important than ever when you are preparing for, undergoing, or recovering from cancer treatment.

Nutrition and Cancer

Eating a healthy diet before, during, and after your treatment can help you in many ways:

- to feel better
- to reserve your strength and energy
- to maintain a healthy weight and your body's store of nutrients
- to tolerate treatment-related side effects
- to maximize the benefits of treatment
- to decrease your risk of infection and maintain a healthy immune system
- to heal and recover quickly

During your treatment, you will be concentrating on fighting cancer. Eating well will help keep you strong and supply you with the nutrients your body needs. Maintaining good nutrition will help you feel better and stay strong. Eating as well as you can during your treatment and your recovery is an important part of taking care of yourself. There are no hard and fast rules about how to eat during cancer treatment. Eat as well as possible—the importance of this cannot be overstated.

During active cancer treatment, your overall nutritional goal should be to eat a variety of foods that provide the nutrients needed to maintain health while fighting cancer. Studies show that patients who eat well during cancer treatment are better able to tolerate chemotherapy, radiation therapy, surgery, or biotherapy and their side effects. People who meet their nutritional needs during cancer treatment may even be able to tolerate higher doses of treatments. Proper nutrition continues to be essential during recovery from treatment and in life after cancer, as well as for those living with advanced cancer.

No one can predict how cancer treatment will affect you. Not everyone experiences side effects, and for those who do, not everyone experiences the same side effects or experiences them in the same way. People with cancer have unique nutritional needs and issues related to eating; what's more, these needs may change throughout the cancer experience. Your appetite may change from day to day. Foods may not taste or smell the way they did before treatment.

You may be surprised by some of the foods that appeal to you during your treatment. Cancer and cancer treatments can also cause side effects that can affect what and how you eat. People going through treatment may have to deal with weight loss or weight gain. No matter what side effects you may experience, nutrition is an essential part of dealing with cancer and cancer treatment.

Cancer Nutrition Information

Advice about what to eat when you have cancer is everywhere—which foods help or hinder cancer treatment, diets that are presented as cancer cures, and how to eat if you are experiencing side effects from treatment. You may already have heard and read all kinds of information from fellow cancer patients, friends, on the Internet, and in books. Some information—such as advice you receive from your doctor—is likely to be accurate and helpful; other suggestions may not help and may even be confusing or dangerous. How do you know where to start?

The search for information about cancer nutrition can be a challenge. At times, even respected sources offer conflicting information. There may not be solid evidence about a particular issue, which confuses matters. The *American Cancer Society Complete Guide to Nutrition for Cancer Survivors, Second Edition*, will explore many of the important issues and facts about nutrition, diet, and cancer. Your health care team—your doctor, registered dietitian, and nurse—can evaluate your situation and help you decide which eating plan may work best for you.

Rely on Your Health Care Team or Other Reliable Resources

Each person's body, cancer, and reactions to treatment will be different. Members of your health care team are invaluable resources and can help you navigate the often confusing maze of information about nutrition. They can help you put together an eating plan that takes into account your cancer diagnosis, your treatment plan, any side effects you experience, and your immune status and overall nutritional needs. Listening to your body and paying attention to what it's telling you will also help shape your nutrition plan to maximize your quality of life and your health.

Your health care team may also be able to provide referrals to other experts or researchers if you want additional opinions or nutritional advice. You may be considering integrating supplements or complementary therapies into your treatment. Seek the advice of your health care team and let them know if you plan to use any supplements or complementary therapies so they can determine any interactions that could possibly interfere with your cancer treatment. Using alternative treatments instead of standard cancer treatments is not recommended; make sure to discuss any plan to use alternative therapies in the place of standard treatments with your doctor. Chapter 14 also lists many resources for reliable information for people with cancer and their families or caregivers.

How This Book Is Organized

This book is designed for people with cancer and their families and other caregivers. It is organized so you can browse through it and read the sections that fit your current situation. Later you can read other sections as you need them. If you experience eating-related side effects during or after cancer treatment, you may first want to read the sections explaining how to cope with them. If you currently have no side effects or only mild side effects, you may find that the chapters about nutrition before treatment, particular foods of interest, dietary supplements, diets promoted as cures for cancer, and nutrition after treatment and for long-term wellness will be most useful.

Chapter 1. Healthy Eating

This chapter explains the components of a balanced diet and can help you learn the language needed to understand information about nutrition and cancer. Eating a healthy diet, maintaining a healthy weight, and being physically active are all essential aspects of maintaining well-being before, during, and after cancer treatment. Nutritional needs are often different for people with cancer, and this chapter discusses the importance of setting goals in preparation for cancer treatment and beyond.

Chapter 2. Making Informed Decisions

This chapter can help you navigate your way through the abundance of information about cancer and nutrition—how to research claims, understand study types, distinguish between complementary and alternative therapies, and interpret information about nutrition and cancer.

Chapter 3. Hot Topics in Cancer and Nutrition

This chapter discusses many foods of special interest to people with cancer. Topics include coffee, flaxseed, green tea, soy, sugar, alcohol, and many others that may get attention in the media for their possible links to cancer or better health. This chapter explores the claims made about certain foods and the evidence available about which foods may be helpful for those in cancer treatment or those hoping to reduce cancer risk.

Chapter 4. How Food Is Grown and Treated

This chapter provides information about the food you eat. Topics include genetically modified foods, irradiated foods, organic foods, pesticides, food additives, and how they affect people with cancer and those who have had cancer.

Chapter 5. Dietary Supplements: Vitamins, Minerals, and Herbs

This chapter defines dietary supplements and explores how to research them and talk about them with your doctor, how they are regulated and manufactured, and how to understand the claims and labels attached to dietary supplements. The potential risks for drug interactions are discussed, as well as the powerful effects of vitamins and minerals on your health, especially during cancer treatment.

Chapter 6. Diet and Nutrition Therapies Promoted as Treatments and Cures

This chapter explores various diets presented as curative or helpful for those with cancer. The potential risks and benefits associated with these diets will be discussed and you will be provided clear, evidence-based information about which diets may be helpful for those in cancer treatment or for people wanting to reduce cancer risk.

Chapter 7. Preparing for Cancer Treatment

This chapter offers suggestions for meal preparation, grocery shopping, ways that friends or family can help, and nutrition suggestions for people undergoing surgery, radiation therapy, chemotherapy, biotherapy, or hormonal therapy. Each treatment and its associated eating-related side effects are discussed briefly, along with some effective coping strategies.

Chapter 8. Maintaining a Healthy Body Weight

This chapter discusses the importance of body weight and why you might experience weight loss or weight gain during cancer treatment. Tools to evaluate your weight and coping strategies to deal with weight loss or weight gain are provided.

Chapter 9. Coping with Treatment-Related Fatigue

This chapter explains the causes of fatigue associated with cancer treatment, outlines coping strategies, and provides additional ways to boost your strength and energy.

Chapter 10. Strengthening Your Immune System

This chapter discusses how specific cancer treatments, including surgery, chemotherapy, biotherapy, and radiation therapy, can impact the immune system and how an altered immune system may affect your health during treatment. Coping strategies are provided, including tips about food preparation and storage safety.

Chapter 11. Staying Hydrated

This chapter stresses the importance of proper hydration during cancer treatment, outlining healthy fluid choices, causes of dehydration during therapy, and how to remain well hydrated, including daily fluid needs and suggestions. Water safety guidelines are also included.

American Cancer Society

Chapter 12. Coping with Changes in Eating and Digestion

Each person reacts differently to cancer treatment. This chapter covers potential treatment side effects, such as nausea and vomiting, diarrhea, constipation, lactose intolerance, changes in taste or smell, loss of appetite, sore mouth and throat, dry mouth or thick oral secretions, and difficulty eating and swallowing. Experts provide coping strategies to minimize discomfort and improve quality of life for those experiencing these treatment-related side effects.

Chapter 13. Lifestyle Choices to Enhance Health for Cancer Survivorship

This chapter provides suggestions for how cancer survivors can get back into healthy eating and physical activity. It also discusses the importance of good nutrition and being active in a healthful lifestyle and the effects of a healthy lifestyle on cancer recurrence.

Chapter 14. Resource Guide

This chapter lists various organizations and resources that provide reliable information and services for people dealing with cancer.

Other Sections

- **Appendix: Special Diets.** This section includes information on special diets that may be recommended for people experiencing eating- or digestion-related side effects of treatment.
- **Glossary.** Key terms and definitions related to nutrition and living well both during and after cancer are defined here.

Whether you need help dealing with treatment-related side effects or simply want to learn more about nutrition to maintain your health, we hope the *American Cancer Society Complete Guide to Nutrition for Cancer Survivors, Second Edition* can help make this time a little bit easier for everyone. Each person is different, and your cancer experience is unique. As mentioned earlier, there are no hard and fast rules about how to eat during cancer treatment. With trial and error, you can learn what works best for you.

For more information about cancer, nutrition, and managing the side effects of treatment, contact the American Cancer Society at **800-227-2345** or visit our Web site at **cancer.org**.

References

Doyle C, Kushi LH, Byers T, Courneya KS, Demark-Wahnefried W, Grant B, McTiernan A, Rock CL, Thompson C, Gansler T, Andrews KS; 2006 Nutrition, Physical Activity and Cancer Survivorship Advisory Committee; American Cancer Society. Nutrition and physical activity during and after cancer treatment: a guide for informed choices by cancer survivors. *CA Cancer J Clin.* 2006;56(6):323-353.

University of Michigan Comprehensive Cancer Center. Managing eating problems. University of Michigan Comprehensive Cancer Center Web site. http://www.cancer.med.umich.edu/support/managing_eating_problems.shtml. Accessed August 25, 2009.

Chapter One

Healthy Eating

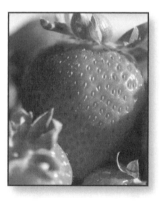

EATING WELL IS AN IMPORTANT PART OF A HEALTHY LIFESTYLE. But what is meant by "eating well"? Eating well is simply eating a balance of foods to help optimize your health. Along with avoiding tobacco, keeping a healthy weight, being physically active, and limiting the alcohol you drink, eating well helps your body stay strong before, during, and after cancer treatment.

Eating well is essential for people with cancer. Getting the foods and nutrients you need will help you be in the best health as you face the challenge of cancer and cancer treatment. In fact, several nutrients may actually slow the growth of some types of cancer. Cancer treatment lowers the body's immune response and can put you at greater risk for infection. Good nutrition can counteract these effects by boosting immune response and helping maintain healthful tissues and cells. Getting the nutrients you need also will help your body heal after the stress of therapy. More people are living long lives after cancer treatment, and eating a balanced, healthy diet and being physically active helps provide a solid foundation for a healthy life.

What Is a Healthy Diet?

Before treatment, your goal is to stay strong so treatment can have the most positive effects possible. As you prepare for treatment, talk to your health care team about whether and how your diet will need to change. The best place to start is to follow established guidelines for overall good health. The American Cancer Society publishes guidelines on nutrition and physical activity for cancer prevention to advise health care professionals and the public about making positive choices for their health (see page 4). These guidelines are consistent with those of the American Heart Association and the American Diabetes Association for the prevention of coronary heart disease and diabetes, as well as for general health promotion. They represent the most current scientific evidence related to dietary and activity patterns and cancer risk. These principles are also cited by the American Cancer Society Expert Committee report, *Nutrition and Physical Activity During and After Cancer Treatment: A Guide for Informed Choices.*

WHAT IS A SURVIVOR?
The word "survivor" can have many different meanings. Some people use the word to refer to anyone who has received a cancer diagnosis. Some people use it when referring to a person who has completed cancer treatment. And still others call a person a survivor if he or she has lived several years past a cancer diagnosis. The American Cancer Society believes that each individual has the right to define his or her own cancer experience, and considers a cancer survivor to be any person who chooses to define himself or herself that way.

American Cancer Society Guidelines for Cancer Prevention

- **Maintain a healthy weight throughout life.**
  - Balance caloric intake with physical activity.
  - Avoid excessive weight gain throughout the life cycle.
  - Achieve and maintain a healthy weight if currently overweight or obese.
- **Adopt a physically active lifestyle.**
  - Adults: Engage in at least thirty minutes of moderate-to-vigorous physical activity, above usual activities, on five or more days of the week. Forty-five to sixty minutes of intentional physical activity is preferable.
  - Children and adolescents: Engage in at least sixty minutes of moderate-to-vigorous physical activity at least five days per week.
- **Consume a healthy diet, with an emphasis on plant sources.**
  - Choose foods and beverages in amounts that help achieve and maintain a healthy weight.
  - Eat at least five servings of a variety of vegetables and fruits each day.
  - Choose whole grains in preference to processed (refined) grains.
  - Limit consumption of processed and red meats.
- **If you drink alcoholic beverages, limit consumption.**
  - Drink no more than one drink per day for women or two per day for men.

In general, these guidelines can be the basis for a nourishing diet throughout the cancer experience, with the counsel of your health care team. Remember, however, that your needs and abilities may be different during cancer treatment. For example, during cancer treatment you may need to consult with a registered dietitian to reach your goal weight. Your goal weight during treatment may be different from your goal after treatment. Staying active during treatment may be different from what one would expect after treatment. To meet activity goals, you might consider participating in planned exercise programs such as exercise and yoga classes, as well as adding physical activity into your daily life. Try to move more, sit less, go up and down stairs, and do household chores and yard work.

Maintaining a Healthy Weight

The way to achieve and maintain a healthy body weight is to balance food and drink intake with physical activity. Being overweight or obese is clearly linked with an increased risk for several types of cancer, such as breast, endometrial, prostate, pancreatic, and colorectal cancer. Some studies have shown a link between losing weight and lowering the risk for certain types of cancer, such as breast, endometrial, prostate, pancreatic, and colorectal cancer.

However, it is difficult to generalize about maintaining weight during cancer treatment. During treatment, goals for nutrition and weight are based on your specific needs or weight management issues. For example, if you are under-weight and preparing for an intensive type of cancer treatment (such as chemotherapy and radiation therapy given at the same time), you may be more likely to experience significant treatment-related weight loss. People receiving this type of treatment will most likely be advised by their health care team to gain weight by eating high-pro-tein, nutrient- and calorie-dense foods.

Most people are advised to main-tain their current body weight during cancer treatment. There is some evi-dence that gaining weight during cancer treatment can have unfavorable effects on cancer outcomes. And weight gain during or after treatment can contribute to the risk of cancer, as well as other obesity-related problems such as dia-betes, hypertension, or heart disease. If

YOUR HEALTH CARE TEAM

The term "health care team" can represent different things to different people. Depending on where you live or where you seek medical care, your "team" may be quite different from the care providers your family or friends may have had at different cancer treatment facilities. For example, if you are undergoing cancer treatment at a large metropolitan medical center or a community cancer center, your care may be provided by a large "team" of health care professionals such as doctors (e.g., surgeons, medical oncologists, and radiation oncologists), nurse practitioners, nurses, registered dietitians, pharmacists, social workers, therapists, and counselors. If you are receiving cancer treatment in a doctor's office or clinic, however, your "team" may be made up of only your doctor and a nurse. Throughout your cancer treatment, be sure to talk to your health care team about your questions and concerns.

you are overweight or obese, your doctor may advise you to lose weight before surgery—if there is time for you to do so safely. See chapter 8 for specific tips and suggestions for maintaining a healthy body weight before, during, and after your cancer treatment.

Adopting a Physically Active Lifestyle

Scientific evidence indicates that physical activity can decrease the risk for several types of can-cer. Taking part in physical activity can also be a great opportunity to spend time with a friend, spouse, or child. There is also evidence that physical activity is safe and possible while you are undergoing cancer treatment, and in some cases, can help to alleviate some of the side effects of treatment. Studies have shown that regular physical activity can reduce anxiety and depression, improve mood, boost self-esteem, and lessen nausea and pain. While most people who are fatigued do not feel like being physically active, current studies show this is exactly what is needed—people undergoing cancer treatment who are fatigued and get more physical activity can actually reduce their fatigue substantially.

Even among breast cancer survivors who are at risk for or who have been diagnosed with treatment-related lymphedema, new studies show that engaging in physical activity is not a problem and may actually lessen lymphedema symptoms. Exercise during treatment is discussed further in chapters 8, 9, 10, and 13. Talk to your health care team about the level of activity that is right for you.

Types of Physical Activity		
	WHAT'S INVOLVED	**EXAMPLES**
GENERAL PHYSICAL ACTIVITY	Muscle movement that uses energy, including exercise and daily activities	Swimming, dancing, mowing the lawn, walking the dog
AEROBIC ACTIVITY	Improving cardiovascular fitness	Jogging, bicycling, jumping rope, boxing
RESISTANCE TRAINING	Strengthening muscles and protecting joints	Lifting weights or using resistance training equipment, pushups, carrying, and lifting
FLEXIBILITY TRAINING	Stretching muscles to improve range of motion, balance, and stability	Stretching, yoga, bar work, Pilates

Consuming a Healthy Diet

Vegetables and Fruits

It is reasonable for most people with cancer to follow dietary recommendations for eating five or more servings of vegetables and fruits daily. Many vegetables and fruits, such as baby carrots, grapes, cherry tomatoes, and bananas, can be eaten on the spot, with minimal preparation. Fresh produce should always be well washed with water before eating to remove any surface dirt and bacteria, especially if you are going to eat the skin. The skin of vegetables and fruits contains fiber and is rich in healthy compounds known as phytochemicals (see page 68). In addition, for most vegetables and fruits, the nutrients are better preserved if the produce is fresh and raw. Purchasing produce twice a week and using local farmer's markets can help to ensure freshness, or you could be adventurous and plant a small garden. In addition, cooking can reduce nutrient content, as some vitamins are leached into cooking water; when you do cook vegetables, minimize the amount of water used and the cooking time as much as possible.

Whole Grains

A whole grain contains the germ (the sprout of a new plant), endosperm (the seed's source of energy), and bran (the outer layer) of a grain or seed. Whole grains provide complex carbohydrates (starches), which help provide energy, fiber (the part of plant foods that the body cannot digest), and vitamins and minerals such as folate. Whole grain foods differ in nutrient content, but all whole grain foods provide more vitamins, minerals, fiber, and other protective substances than refined grains. Refined grains such as bleached (white) flour have the bran and germ removed during milling and therefore lack many of the nutrients found in whole grains, including B vitamins, iron, zinc, phytochemicals, vitamin E, and fiber. A regular intake of fiber-rich foods such as whole grains (as well as many vegetables and fruits) helps maintain proper bowel function.

Whole grains provide foods with darker, richer color and heavier weight and texture. In the United States, people eat on average only half a serving of whole grains a day, which means we miss out on much of the folate, selenium, and other nutrients in them. Brown rice, millet, quinoa, kasha (buckwheat), barley, whole wheat pasta, and bulgur are good sources of whole grains. Between 15 and 20 percent of cereals contain whole grain as a main ingredient.

Dietary fiber includes a wide variety of plant carbohydrates that are not digested by humans. Fiber can be *soluble* (dissolvable in water), such as oat bran, or *insoluble* (not dissolvable in water), such as wheat bran or cellulose. Soluble fiber helps reduce blood cholesterol, thereby lowering the risk of coronary heart disease. Good sources of fiber are beans, vegetables, whole grains, and fruits.

WHAT COUNTS AS A SERVING?

Here's how the United States Department of Agriculture (USDA) defines a serving of fruit or vegetables:

- 1 medium piece of fruit or ½ cup fruit
- ½ cup of 100 percent juice
- ¼ cup dried fruit
- ½ cup raw non-leafy or cooked vegetables
- 1 cup raw leafy vegetables (such as lettuce)
- ½ cup cooked beans or peas (such as lentils, pinto beans, and kidney beans)

There is no solid scientific evidence that eating fiber reduces the risk of developing cancer, but eating fiber-rich whole grains is still recommended because they contain other substances beyond fiber alone that may help prevent cancer and because they have other health benefits.

WHAT IS FIBER?

Fiber refers to the parts of plant foods that the body cannot digest. Fiber is most abundant in whole grains and gives them their dark color, heavy feel, and great nutrient content. Fiber can also be found in vegetables, fruits, nuts, seeds, and beans. The amount of whole grains and fiber you need depends on your age, gender, and amount of physical activity. Currently, the recommendation is that healthy adults should try to eat at least twenty-five grams of fiber daily. One way to increase fiber is buying whole grain products whenever possible, such as brown rice instead of white rice, whole grain pasta instead of egg noodles, and old-fashioned rolled oats instead of instant oatmeal. Most people will need to work up to this level slowly over time because gas or bloating can occur with abrupt increases in fiber intake. A supplement such as Beano that contains natural enzymes can help to decrease the digestive problems that can occur after eating these foods.

Fiber is classified as either soluble or insoluble, which refers to whether it dissolves in water (is soluble) or not. Both types are important to health. Soluble fiber is found in oats, legumes, barley, apples, berries, and carrots, and it helps reduce the amount of cholesterol in your blood and may help control blood sugar and insulin levels. Insoluble fiber is found in whole grains, bran, some vegetables and fruits, and seeds, and it promotes normal, regular bowel movements.

Fiber also can be consumed as a supplement, but food sources are considered the best sources for fiber. Fiber supplements are known as functional fibers and are generally manufactured from dietary sources (for example, chitin from crab and lobster shells, fructans from chicory and onions, beta glucans from oats and barley, guar gum from guar beans, and psyllium from psyllium seed). Whereas supplements are considered an easy way to get adequate fiber each day, there is little data on the role of supplemental fiber products in cancer prevention. Fiber is best obtained from beans, whole grains, vegetables, and fruits, rather than from supplements.

Benefits of Whole Grains

Many of the carbohydrates eaten in the United States are sugars and refined starches, which have little to no fiber and do not do the body much good. Whole grains, however, contain many more nutrients than refined grains and provide several health benefits:

- They help maintain a healthy body and weight. The high fiber content of many whole grains may help you feel full with fewer calories.
- Fiber-containing foods, when eaten with adequate water or other fluids, promote proper bowel function.
- These foods may help you live a longer life. A study of thirty-five thousand women showed that those who ate at least one serving of whole grains a day lived longer than women who ate few or no whole grains.

There are some simple ways to incorporate more whole grains into your diet:

- Eat whole grain bread, bagels, and English muffins instead of white, and choose plain oatmeal over low-fiber, sugary cereals.
- Add whole grains such as barley or whole wheat pasta to your soup.
- Try whole grain crackers (such as wheat, rye, pumpernickel, etc.) as a snack.
- Choose whole wheat flour over refined white flour. (Whole wheat flour contains nutrients that can spoil and should be stored in the refrigerator.)
- Experiment with bulgur, millet, quinoa, and pearl barley.

Look for foods with whole grain listed as the first ingredient, and try to choose unprocessed foods—foods that have not been altered from their original states. Processed foods include frozen dinners, many canned or boxed "convenience" foods, processed meats (such as lunch meats, bologna, hot dogs, and sausage), and packaged cakes, cookies, and snack foods.

Also note the following when selecting foods:

- "Multigrain," "seven grain," and "made with whole grain" labels do not mean a food is whole grain. Only whole grain foods may be labeled as "whole grain."
- The Nutrition Facts panel lists how much fiber a serving of food contains. Although two grams or more of fiber per serving qualifies a food as whole grain, selecting foods with more than four grams per serving is advised.
- A claim can be made that a food is a "good source" of fiber if it provides 10 percent (two and a half grams) of the Daily Value (twenty-five grams) of fiber per serving. Foods can be called "high in fiber," "rich in fiber," or an "excellent source of fiber" if they contain 20 percent (five grams) of the Daily Value of fiber per serving.

- Whole grain foods contain 51 percent or more whole grain ingredients by weight and are labeled as "100 percent whole grain" or may carry the claim that "diets rich in whole grain foods and other plant foods low in total fat, saturated fat, and cholesterol may reduce the risk of heart disease and certain cancers."
- Dark breads are not necessarily whole grain. They may be made with refined white flour and darkening agents such as molasses.

Limiting Red Meat and Processed Meats

Red meat contains protein, iron, and other important vitamins and minerals, but it also contains saturated fat and cholesterol. People with health concerns such as heart disease and diabetes may have been asked by their doctor to limit their intake of red meat. Consumption of red and processed meats over time are associated with an increased risk of colon cancer. If you do eat red meat, choose small portion sizes and lean cuts of meat (look for "loin" on the label). A moderate amount of lean red meat can be included in a balanced diet along with fish, chicken, fruits, vegetables, whole grains, and healthy sources of fat. Generally speaking, a "moderate amount" would reflect servings of two to three ounces eaten fewer than three times a week. More importantly, intake of processed meat has been linked to increased cancer risk. Intake should be occasional at the most (less than once a week). Baking, broiling, or poaching meat is healthier than frying or charbroiling. Other ways to cut down on your intake of excessive calories from meat include making meat a side dish rather than the main course and trimming the fats from meat prior to cooking. In studies that have examined red meat and processed meat separately, the data suggest that the risk for colon cancer is slightly higher for processed meat. Consumption of both should be limited.

WHAT IS PROCESSED MEAT?

Examples of processed meat include hot dogs, salami, pepperoni, bologna, bacon, and luncheon meat, as well as frozen products such as breakfast meats, chicken patties, or chicken nuggets. These foods tend to be higher in salt, fat, and nitrites.

Limiting Alcohol

If people drink alcohol, they should limit their intake to no more than two drinks per day for men and one drink per day for women. Excessive intake of alcoholic beverages is known to cause cancers of the mouth, pharynx, larynx, esophagus, liver, and breast. Alcohol also contributes extra calories, which may lead to weight gain. A general guideline is that one serving of alcohol equals 12 ounces of beer, 5 ounces of wine, or 1.5 ounces of spirits. Alcohol is discussed further in chapter 3.

The Components of a Balanced Diet

Your body uses the energy from food (calories) as fuel to nourish itself. Food contains nutrients that are needed for health, to fight infection, and to heal and repair body tissues. Calorie-containing nutrients include protein, carbohydrate, and fat.

- *Protein* helps build and repair cells and maintain a healthy immune system. Protein is found in animal food sources such as meat, poultry, fish, dairy products, and eggs. Protein also is found in plant food sources such as beans, peas, lentils, nuts, nut butters, soy products, and grains.
- *Carbohydrates* provide quick sources of energy to fuel the body. Carbohydrates are found in whole grains, cereals, bread products, and fruits and vegetables.
- *Fat* helps build new cells, provides energy, and assists with important bodily functions. Fat comes from vegetable oil, butter, margarine, animal foods (such as meat, fish, poultry, dairy products, and eggs), nuts, and seeds.

Other vital nutrients found in food are vitamins, minerals, phytonutrients, and, of course, water.

- *Vitamins* and *minerals* are very small, organic compounds that are needed by the body to use the energy from food and to assist in bodily functions.
- *Phytonutrients*, *phytochemicals, or bioactive compounds* (plant chemicals) are found in colorful fruits and vegetables and are powerful cancer fighters and health promoters.
- *Water* is essential to keep your body hydrated.

Eating a diverse diet is the easiest way to make sure you are getting all the nutrients you need from the food you eat each day. Keep in mind that there is a real difference between getting the nutrition you need through food and taking dietary supplements. Whereas dietary supplements can be an easy-to-obtain concentrated source of micronutrients (vitamins and minerals), there is concern among many health experts that these products may have different chemical make-ups or may lack important substances necessary for health compared with vitamins and minerals found naturally in food. Why is this important? Because different chemical forms can act differently in the body and may even be absorbed differently. Of concern is the fact that several studies using dietary supplements rather than whole foods to study the effects of micronutrients on cancer have actually increased cancer risk in some people. There is also concern that certain dietary supplements—for example, vitamins C and E and folic acid—may interfere with the effectiveness of certain chemotherapy agents or with radiation therapy. This area of research needs more study before any clear recommendations can be made.

For now, most health care professionals advise people to learn which foods contain important micronutrients that promote health, to eat more of these foods, and to exercise caution in their use of dietary supplements, especially during therapy, until more is known. Be sure to talk to your health care team about any supplements you may be taking. Remember that when you eat food, you are eating a variety of micronutrients together. It is likely that the combination of micronutrients in certain foods promotes health by working together to provide benefit to the body. You'll find tips for incorporating healthy food into your diet in chapters 7 and 8. For more information about dietary supplements, see chapter 5.

Protein

Protein provides the body with amino acids, which allow for growth, repair of body tissue, and maintenance of a healthy immune system. Protein also helps build cells and create hormones and enzymes. Without enough protein, the body takes longer to recover from illness and lowers its resistance to infection.

People undergoing cancer treatment often need more protein than usual. Taking in additional protein before and after surgery and during and after chemotherapy or radiation therapy helps heal tissues and prevent infection.

Good sources of protein include animal foods such as lean meat, fish, poultry, eggs, and dairy products. Some plant foods, such as nuts, dried beans, peas, lentils, and soy foods, can provide important sources of protein as well. In fact, there is some evidence that protein found in plants, compared to protein from animal sources, is more beneficial for people who have poor kidney function.

Eating a higher-protein diet, as many people with cancer are advised to do during treatment, requires that one also consume adequate fluids to help keep kidney function optimal. For the amount of water that is right for you, consult with a registered dietitian or your health care team. See chapter 11 for tips to stay hydrated.

How Much Protein Do I Need?

People undergoing cancer treatment tend to need more protein than healthy people. Most healthy people need to consume 0.4 grams of protein for every pound of body weight (or 0.8 grams of protein for every kilogram of body weight). Generally this means at least fifty grams for women and sixty or more for men. However, most people in treatment need at least 0.5 grams of protein for every pound of body weight. Some people will need to increase the amount of protein in their diets before treatment to catch up if their stores are low. Work with a registered dietitian or your health care team to determine how much protein you need before, during, and after your cancer treatment. See chapter 8 for information on determining protein needs and how to add protein to your diet.

Carbohydrates

Carbohydrates supply the body with the majority of the calories it needs to function. The amount of carbohydrates each person needs depends on age, size, and level of physical activity.

Carbohydrates provide quick energy, which is needed during cancer treatment. Breads, pasta, grains, cereal products, dried beans, peas, lentils, fruits, and vegetables are all sources of carbohydrates. Carbohydrates that are rich in whole grains, rather than refined starches, are best.

Carbohydrates and the Glycemic Index

There are three types of carbohydrates: complex carbohydrates (vegetables, nuts, seeds, legumes [beans and peas], and whole grains), simple carbohydrates (white bread, white pasta, and other starches), and sugars (table sugar, honey, sugar-sweetened beverages, and candy). All carbohydrates are broken down into sugar when they are digested in the intestines. This sugar enters the blood and raises blood sugar levels. The body reacts by producing insulin, which helps the body's cells get energy from sugar and also regulates blood sugar levels. High insulin levels have been suggested to contribute to cancer risk.

Whereas all carbohydrates are broken down into sugar, that conversion happens at different rates, depending on the food. The glycemic index is one way of classifying carbohydrates. It is determined by measuring how quickly and how high blood sugar levels rise after eating a specified amount of a single food item. High-glycemic foods cause fast, significant increases in a person's blood sugar level. Highly processed carbohydrates, in which the bran and germ layers are removed, are high glycemic (they make blood sugar levels go up very quickly). Grains that are not processed as much are absorbed more slowly—which means that whole grain items are generally low glycemic.

The proteins and fats you eat with carbohydrates also affect the speed at which they enter the bloodstream and raise insulin levels. For example, adding butter to your bread will actually lower its glycemic level. Carbonated, sweetened beverages have a high glycemic response and are frequently consumed alone, causing more rapid increases in insulin levels. There is limited information available as to the glycemic response of whole meals.

The following high-glycemic foods, which contain refined or simple carbohydrates, are processed by the body quickly and rapidly raise blood sugar levels:

- potatoes
- white rice
- white bread
- pasta (not whole wheat)
- bananas
- sweetened soft drinks

- refined flour products
- sugar, honey, molasses, and other natural sweeteners

The following low-glycemic foods, which contain unrefined or complex carbohydrates, take longer to digest and raise blood sugar levels more slowly:

- whole grains (whole wheat, rye, oats, and bran)
- brown rice
- millet
- quinoa
- barley
- bulgur
- beans and most other legumes (pinto, black, kidney, garbanzo, navy)
- many whole fruits
- 100 percent whole grain breakfast cereals

While more research needs to be conducted, many health experts believe a diet with a low glycemic index (composed mainly of low-glycemic foods) may be better for the body, both for a healthy person and for a person with cancer. Choosing less-processed whole grains over highly processed products is one simple way to eat more healthfully. Eating fewer refined and simple sugars, including sweetened beverages, and selecting low-glycemic carbohydrates along with a variety of healthy proteins and fats can help balance your daily intake of foods. At times during cancer treatment, some people may need to limit or increase their intake of fiber-containing foods because of gastrointestinal discomfort. Be sure to consult your health care team if you have concerns.

Sugars like honey, molasses, syrups, and white or brown sugar are all sources of concentrated carbohydrates, whether they are eaten in their "raw" state or used as ingredients in prepared and processed foods such as soft drinks, cakes, cookies, jams, or frozen desserts. All of these foods add calories to your diet but offer very few nutrients. Foods high in refined (processed) sugars or carbohydrates also increase the glycemic index of the diet. Choosing whole grains (such as whole grain rice, bread, pasta, and cereals) over refined grains (like white bread and potatoes) and sugars (including pastries, sweetened cereals, soft drinks, and sugars) will give your body the carbohydrate energy it needs while also providing other nutrients and health benefits. Sugar's effect on cancer is discussed in chapter 3.

The American Heart Association recently released dietary guidelines that recommend that all Americans reduce their intake of beverages and foods containing sugar:

- Women should eat no more than 100 calories per day from added sugar.
- Men should eat no more than 150 calories per day from added sugar.

Fat

Fat provides the body with calories for physical activity as well as fatty acids that help the body grow, produce hormones, transport vitamins, and build new cells. Excess calories are stored as fat, which becomes reserve energy for times of need. Fat also makes food feel good in your mouth and on your tongue. If you are having difficulty with cancer-related weight loss or taste changes, including fat in your diet can help add needed calories for maintaining your body weight. However, for some people, eating too much fat can actually cause uncomfortable feelings of fullness because high-fat foods can take longer to digest and absorb. For people taking medications that cause increased appetite or whose level of physical activity has gone down because of fatigue or not feeling well, too much fat also can add unwanted calories. People with heart disease who are currently following a "heart-healthy diet" should be sure to talk to their doctor or a registered dietitian to see whether adding fat to their diets is right for them. See chapters 7 and 8 for other ideas on adding calories to your diet.

There are two general categories of fat: saturated fat (saturated fatty acids) and unsaturated fat (unsaturated fatty acids). Saturated fatty acids are mostly found in high-fat meats, animal fats such as lard and tallow, fat-containing dairy products, chocolate, and coconut oil, cottonseed oil, and palm kernel oil. Research shows that people eating diets containing large amounts of saturated fat are at increased risk for developing cardiovascular disease.

Unsaturated fatty acids can be classified as monounsaturated fat (monounsaturated fatty acids), polyunsaturated fat (polyunsaturated fatty acids), omega-3 fatty acids, omega-6 fatty

ON THE HORIZON: EARLY RESEARCH STUDIES OF INTEREST
Good Health Includes Weight Control
Several studies evaluating the diets and physical activity habits of children and teens are beginning to suggest that what we eat in those early years influences our risk for cancer later in life. One study of 121,000 women is reinforcing what researchers have long suspected: that a teen's diet may affect her adult risk of breast cancer. Other studies show that physical activity started in the teen years and continued throughout adulthood may offer the best protection against cancer risk.

Weight gain over adulthood has been repeatedly linked to breast cancer risk and likely plays a role in other hormone-associated cancers. Therefore, it is important as one enters adulthood to practice prevention. Even small increases in body weight or clothing size should be considered important. Evaluate how your weight has changed since age eighteen. If it has increased by even eight to ten pounds, be concerned and work to get those extra pounds off!

acids, and trans fat. Foods containing unsaturated fat include avocados, nuts, fish, seafood, and oils such as olive and canola. People who consume heart-healthy diets, limiting their intake of saturated fat and choosing unsaturated fats, have been shown be at decreased risk for developing cardiovascular disease.

Research shows that eating trans fat increases the risk of heart disease and cancer. Trans fatty acids and trans fat are found naturally in small amounts in meat and dairy products, but are primarily manufactured in the processing of margarines, vegetable shortenings, and packaged breads, cakes, cookies, and crackers to give these products longer shelf lives. Recent labeling requirements for trans fats have led food manufacturers to reduce or remove trans fats from many food products. Be aware, though, that a product can have up to 0.5 grams of trans fat per serving and still be labeled as having 0 grams of trans fat. It is a good idea to limit your intake of packaged foods such as those listed above.

It is best to balance the types of fat sources consumed, including selecting foods containing a greater concentration of monounsaturated fats, such as olive oil or other nut oils, and some polyunsaturated and saturated fats.

Much of the interest in the possible effects of dietary fat on the risk of developing cancer has focused on breast and colorectal cancers. The Women's Health Initiative (WHI) study of more than thirty-eight thousand postmenopausal women randomly assigned to a low-fat diet versus their usual diet showed no significant reduction in breast or colorectal cancers overall. However, there was a reduced risk for breast cancer among women who started out with a high fat intake and reduced it to the lower, recommended level. The low-fat diet reduced the risk for ovarian cancer but was not associated with reduced risk for other types of cancer.

What About Calories?

So how many calories do you need each day? Generally, eating twelve to fourteen calories per pound of body weight will be adequate to meet your needs during treatment without promoting undesirable weight gain. However, having a fever, infection, or high levels of stress can increase your caloric needs. Also, overweight or obese people may need to decrease the estimate somewhat, as a high body weight will falsely increase the calorie estimate. See chapter 8 for tips to help you add or cut back on calories.

Some doctors or registered dietitians have access to special equipment that can more accurately measure your body's energy needs. Regardless of whether they have equipment, ask a member of your health care team to help you calculate how many calories you need. Remember, caloric needs can change. As you age, your body generally needs fewer calories. Increased physical activity can increase your caloric requirements. During your cancer treatment and while you recover from treatment, your caloric needs can increase because of stress, fever, or infection. See chapter 7 for help in preparing for cancer treatment.

Vitamins and Minerals

Vitamins help the body use energy (calories) from carbohydrates, fats, and proteins. Vitamins are needed to maintain bone strength, vision, and skin, hair, and nails, whereas minerals spur on and regulate the body's processes and bone health. For example, iron carries oxygen to your cells. Calcium helps your bones and teeth stay strong. And potassium helps nerves and muscles function.

A balanced diet with sufficient calories and protein usually supplies the body with enough vitamins and minerals to maintain health. However, eating a balanced diet during cancer treatment can be challenging, particularly if side effects continue for an extended period. Cancer treatments such as surgery and chemotherapy can deplete the body's stores of vitamins and minerals. It may also be difficult for you to eat enough micronutrients, which are dietary elements essential in small quantities for growth and health. Taking a standard vitamin and mineral supplement that contains approximately 100 percent of the Daily Value of each vitamin and mineral is often recommended during and after cancer treatment. Talk to your registered dietitian or doctor about whether a daily multivitamin/mineral supplement is appropriate for your situation. See chapter 5 for more information about vitamin and mineral supplements.

Water

Water and fluids are vital to health. They make up one-half to two-thirds of your total body weight. Water regulates the body's temperature, transports nutrients to the parts of the body where they are needed, and removes waste.

If you do not take in enough fluids, or if you are vomiting or have diarrhea during cancer treatment, you may become dehydrated. Water is the best choice to help you maintain adequate hydration. Unless you are directed to do otherwise, try to drink as much water as you can each day. Ask your doctor or nurse how much fluid you need each day to prevent dehydration. Try to avoid sugar-sweetened beverages, as these can increase blood glucose levels, which can lead to increased urination and fluid imbalance. Caffeine-containing beverages can have similar fluid-losing effects. See chapter 11 for more information about staying hydrated.

RDAs, DRIs, AIs, and ULs: Learning the Language

For more than sixty years, the Recommended Dietary Allowances (RDAs) have been published by the Food and Nutrition Board of the National Academy of Sciences. Knowledge about nutrients and how nutrient levels affect individuals and groups has grown significantly since the RDAs were first established. The RDAs are gradually being replaced with Dietary Reference Intakes (DRIs).

You do not have to be a health expert to eat nutritiously. The information listed on the labels of food products and vitamin and mineral supplements is a guide for healthy eating and informed dietary supplement use. These values provide individuals with information about what they are eating and how they can make educated health choices when buying groceries and dietary supplements. The following information is provided to help you better understand the abbreviations and terms that are used by the food and supplement industries to describe the nutritional content of their products.

1. **Recommended Dietary Allowance (RDA).** The average daily dietary intake of a nutrient that meets the nutritional needs of nearly all (97 to 98 percent) healthy individuals in a population.

2. **Adequate Intake (AI).** The average intake for a nutrient as observed in a group of healthy people. When an RDA cannot be estimated for a nutrient, an AI is determined and serves as a guide. An AI is less precise than an RDA.

3. **Tolerable Upper Intake Level (UL).** The highest daily level of a nutrient that is likely to be safe for almost all individuals—that is, likely not to pose a risk of adverse health effects. The UL is not an ideal or a recommended intake level.

4. **Estimated Average Requirement (EAR).** The amount of a nutrient that meets the estimated nutrient needs of half of all healthy individuals in a population. EARs are used as a guide in the development of RDAs.

5. **Dietary Reference Intake (DRI).** A term used to describe four specific types of nutrient recommendations, including RDA, AI, UL, and EAR.

6. **Daily Value (DV).** A term used on food labels to help people choose a healthy diet.

Simply stated, these are the basics:

- RDAs or AIs can help you to evaluate your appropriate average daily nutrient intake.
- Use ULs as a guide to maximum safe intake levels for nutrients.
- Keep in mind that DRIs are nutrient estimates for healthy individuals. RDAs and AIs are average nutrient intake guidelines and may not be accurate recommendations for people with increased nutritional needs.

Most important, talk to your health care team about your specific nutrient needs throughout the different stages of your cancer and treatment.

Your Nutritional Goals—During and After Treatment

Nutritional needs vary from person to person. People with cancer—especially those in treatment—often have increased and specific nutritional needs. Before you begin cancer treatment, discuss with your health care team how to achieve optimal nutritional status. Your registered dietitian, doctor, and nurse can help tailor an eating plan to your health, your cancer type, the treatment you will receive, and the treatment's expected effects. They can help you identify nutritional goals and plan detailed strategies to help you meet them. They can also guide you in maintaining nutritional goals during your recovery from treatment and in life after cancer. (See page 20 for information about finding a registered dietitian.)

Getting Adequate Nutrients

When you are healthy, eating enough food to get the nutrients you need is usually not a problem. Most nutrition guidelines recommend eating lots of vegetables, fruits, and whole grain products and fiber; consuming adequate protein through lean meats, fish, and lower-fat dairy foods; and cutting back on polyunsaturated and trans fats, sugar, refined carbohydrates, salt, and alcohol.

During and after cancer treatment, however, getting enough nutrients may become a challenge, especially if you experience side effects or simply do not feel well. Cancer and cancer treatment may affect your metabolism (the breaking down of food to make energy for the body), your appetite, and your body's ability to tolerate certain foods and use nutrients. As a result, you may have to change your diet to help build up strength and withstand the effects of cancer and its treatment.

The basics of optimal nutrition for people with cancer may not be what

EVALUATE YOUR DIET

If you are concerned about getting enough nutrients or are curious about whether your meals are balanced, talk to your registered dietitian about using nutrient analysis computer programs to track your intake of nutrients. These programs can even track trace minerals and amino acids, calculate recommended daily intakes, and show your eating and nutrient patterns over time.

Many programs can be downloaded for free online or can be purchased from computer retailers. One option is on the USDA's www.mypyramid.gov Web site. Here you can input the types and amounts of food you eat, and the program will evaluate the nutrients in your diet and show you the shape of your own pyramid. You can also save the information and follow your dietary patterns over time to see if changes you make to improve your diet are having the effects you desire. Another option is the web site www.nutritiondata.com. Not only can you determine the nutritional content of the foods you eat, you can keep track of and log the nutrient value of the snacks and meals you eat each day.

When setting goals for healthy eating, it is a good idea to get advice from a registered dietitian in your area.

FINDING A NUTRITION EXPERT

- Survivors should ask their oncologist for a referral to see a registered dietitian.
- If a dietitian does not work in the clinic or medical center where they receive their treatment, an appointment with a registered dietitian associated with their primary care clinic can be arranged.
- Survivors and providers can also consult the American Dietetic Association's Web site (www.eatright.org), using the "Find a Nutritional Professional" feature and putting "Oncology Nutrition" in the expertise/specialty tab. Alternately, you can call the American Dietetic Association at 800-877-1600 to find a dietitian in your area.

you expect. Many people going through cancer treatment or recovery need extra calories and protein to stay strong. In such cases, eating frequent, small meals rich in calories and protein and adding some fat is often recommended. In contrast, people being treated for some types of cancer, such as breast, prostate, or even early-stage colorectal cancer, may be more likely to gain weight during treatment. They will want to work with their registered dietitian or health care team on developing healthy eating and physical activity habits, rather than emphasizing the intake of extra calories.

If you lose too much weight, your registered dietitian or health care team may advise you to boost calories by eating high-protein foods. Examples of these foods include milk, cheese, cottage cheese, meats, fish, beans, and egg whites. You can also try adding some healthy fats such as olive oil or nuts and nut butters to your meals and snacks. Refer to chapter 8 for ideas for maintaining a healthy body weight. Because fiber may cause early satiety or a full feeling during meals, your doctor or registered dietitian may also encourage you to eat fewer high-fiber foods. Increasing calories and protein without relying on refined sugar, refined starches, or high-glycemic carbohydrates is the healthiest approach.

While you are focusing on a plan to give your body what it needs, do not forget to take into account your enjoyment of life and basic health and nutritional priorities. In developing a nutrition plan, make sure to do the following:

- Include foods you like. If you cannot tolerate foods you normally like or if your appetite changes, do not be afraid to bend the rules of traditional meals and foods. It is okay to eat your usual lunch food at dinner time or your typical breakfast meal at dinner.
- Choose foods packed with nutrients. Nutrient-rich foods help the body function properly and are especially important during times of stress.

LOOKING FOR A FITNESS EXPERT?

The American College of Sports Medicine (ACSM) offers a certification for trainers who want to work specifically with people who have been affected by cancer. A Certified Cancer Exercise Trainer (CET) is able to develop exercise programs and train clients who are going through cancer diagnosis or treatment. Visit the ACSM Web site at www.acsm.org to find an ACSM-certified professional.

- Make physical activity a part of your plan. Take part in activities you enjoy. Being physically active can increase appetite, help regulate bowel movements, increase energy levels, and boost mood.
- Consult your health care team. Your registered dietitian, doctor, and nurse can all contribute information as you develop an individualized plan that takes into account your health, your body, your cancer, and your treatment. For example, you may be advised to eat more of certain types of food, avoid other foods, or increase your intake of water.

A diagnosis of cancer motivates some people to make positive lifestyle changes. The best plan for you may change over time. Your nutritional needs will be different as you prepare for, undergo, and recover from cancer treatment and as you maintain your long-term health. Reevaluate your nutrition needs as you enter new stages of treatment and recovery.

Staying Active

Evidence from a number of studies has shown that being active is possible, safe, and beneficial for people undergoing cancer treatment. Exercise can help to manage common side effects of cancer treatment, such as fatigue, pain, and nausea; improve physical, emotional, and functional well-being; and improve quality of life.

Studies looking at the role of physical activity in cancer prevention have shown that physical inactivity can lead to obesity, and obesity leads to increased risk for cancer of the colon, pancreas, gallbladder, endometrium, breast (among postmenopausal women), kidney, and other types of cancer. For colon cancer in particular, the risk seems to be highest for people with accumulated body fat in the abdomen. Physical inactivity itself contributes to increased risk for colon cancer, postmenopausal breast cancer, and endometrial cancer. There is also limited evidence that inactivity increases risk for cancer of the lung, ovaries, and pancreas, as well as risk for breast cancer among premenopausal women.

For people with cancer or cancer survivors who are trying to reduce the risk of cancer recurrence, no large-scale studies have explored the possible effects of exercise on cancer recurrence or cancer survival rates although one study of more than three thousand breast cancer survivors showed thirty minutes of walking six times per week, combined with a diet that included at least five servings of fruits and vegetables per day did reduce mortality. More research is necessary to determine whether exercise during treatment directly helps, harms, or has no effect on rates of recurrence and survival. However, evidence is growing that being overweight can increase the risk of recurrence for some types of cancer, and being active on a regular basis is important for weight control.

A good strategy for people undergoing cancer treatment or recovering after treatment is to be as active as your physical abilities allow. Choosing to be more active and maintaining some level of regular exercise can improve your sense of autonomy, which may have been negatively affected since your cancer diagnosis.

Light, regular exercise can improve appetite, aid digestion, prevent constipation, and boost energy levels. It also helps to maintain muscle mass and reduce stress. Making an attempt to get out every day and walk—even one hundred yards—early in your cancer treatment will help you stay physically active.

There are several simple ways of changing your routine to include more physical activity: take the stairs instead of the elevator, walk to lunch rather than drive, or stand while talking on the phone.

Keep the following issues in mind as you work physical activity into your treatment plan:

- If you are in bed because of your cancer or treatment, talk to your health care team about physical therapy in bed to keep up your strength and maintain range of motion. Physical activity can help lessen fatigue and depression often experienced by some people confined to bed.
- Because of fatigue, some people in chemotherapy may feel like waiting until finishing their chemotherapy before starting an exercise program. But it is generally better to try to include some level of activity throughout therapy. Exercise may be easier during early treatment if you are not experiencing fatigue. Establishing a habit of activity early on will make it easier to continue even if fatigue sets in. Talk to your health care team about your situation.
- Older people and those with conditions such as arthritis should pay careful attention to balance exercises that can help to prevent falls. A caregiver or exercise professional may be able to help those who need assistance.

References

Ahn J, Schatzkin A, Lacey JV Jr, Albanes D, Ballard-Barbash R, Adams KF, Kipnis V, Mouw T, Hollenbeck AR, Leitzmann MF. Adiposity, adult weight change, and postmenopausal breast cancer risk. *Arch Intern Med.* 2007;167(19):2091-2102.

American Cancer Society. *Good for You! Reducing Your Risk of Developing Cancer.* Atlanta, GA: American Cancer Society; 2002.

The American Cancer Society's skinny on trimming the fat. American Cancer Society Web site. http://www.cancer.org/docroot/MED/content/MED_2_1X_The_American_Cancer_Society_s_Skinny_on_Trimming_the_Fat.asp. Published February 24, 1998. Accessed December 4, 2009.

Benefits of good nutrition. American Cancer Society Web site. http://www.cancer.org/docroot/MBC/content/MBC_6_2X_Benefits_of_nutrition_during_treatment.asp. Updated February 4, 2008. Accessed December 4, 2009.

Beresford SA, Johnson KC, Ritenbaugh C, Lasser NL, Snetselaar LG, Black HR, Anderson GL, Assaf AR, Bassford T, Bowen D, Brunner RL, Brzyski RG, Caan B, Chlebowski RT, Gass M, Harrigan RC, Hays J, Heber D, Heiss G, Hendrix SL, Howard BV, Hsia J, Hubbell FA, Jackson RD, Kotchen JM, Kuller LH, LaCroix AZ, Lane DS, Langer RD, Lewis CE, Manson JE, Margolis KL, Mossavar-Rahmani Y, Ockene JK, Parker LM, Perri MG, Phillips L, Prentice RL, Robbins J, Rossouw JE, Sarto GE, Stefanick ML, Van Horn L, Vitolins MZ, Wactawski-Wende J, Wallace RB, Whitlock E. Low-fat dietary pattern and risk of colorectal cancer: the Women's Health Initiative Randomized Controlled Dietary Modification Trial. *JAMA.* 2006;295(6):643-654.

Brody JE. For unrefined healthfulness: refined grains. *The New York Times.* March 4, 2003: F5.

Carbohydrates. Harvard School of Public Health Web site. http://www.hsph.harvard.edu/nutritionsource/what-should-you-eat/carbohydrates/. Accessed December 4, 2009.

Doyle C, Kushi LH, Byers T, Courneya KS, Demark-Wahnefried W, Grant B, McTiernan A, Rock CL, Thompson C, Gansler T, Andrews KS; 2006 Nutrition, Physical Activity and Cancer Survivorship Advisory Committee; American Cancer Society. Nutrition and physical activity during and after cancer treatment: a guide for informed choices by cancer survivors. *CA Cancer J Clin.* 2006;56(6):323-353.

Fruit and vegetable benefits. Fruits and Veggies Matter Web site. http://www.fruitsandveggiesmatter.gov/benefits/index.html. Accessed December 4, 2009.

Ghosh K, Carson L, Cohen E. *Betty Crocker's Living with Cancer Cookbook: Easy Recipes and Tips through Treatment and Beyond.* New York: Hungry Minds; 2002.

Inside the pyramid: how many grain foods are needed daily? United States Department of Agriculture Web site. http://www.mypyramid.gov/pyramid/grains_amount.aspx. Updated September 11, 2008. Accessed November 20, 2009.

Johnson RK, Appel LJ, Brands M, Howard BV, Lefevre M, Lustig RH, Sacks F, Steffen LM, Wylie-Rosett J; American Heart Association Nutrition Committee of the Council on Nutrition, Physical Activity, and Metabolism and the Council on Epidemiology and Prevention. Dietary sugars intake and cardiovascular health: a scientific statement from the American Heart Association. *Circulation.* 2009;120(11):1011-1020.

Kantor LS, Variyam JN, Allshouse JE, Putnam JJ, Lin BH. Choose a variety of grains daily, especially whole grains: a challenge for consumers. *J Nutr.* 2001;131(2S-1):473S-486S.

Kushi LH, Byers T, Doyle C, Bandera EV, McCullough M, McTiernan A, Gansler T, Andrews KS, Thun MJ; American Cancer Society 2006 Nutrition and Physical Activity Guidelines Advisory Committee. American Cancer Society Guidelines on Nutrition and Physical Activity for cancer prevention: reducing the risk of cancer with healthy food choices and physical activity. *CA Cancer J Clin.* 2006;56(5):254-281; quiz 313-314.

Lajous M, Willett W, Lazcano-Ponce E, Sanchez-Zamorano LM, Hernandez-Avila M, Romieu I. Glycemic load, glycemic index, and the risk of breast cancer among Mexican women. *Cancer Causes Control.* 2005;16(10):1165-1169.

Margie JD, Bloch AS. *Nutrition and the Cancer Patient.* Radnor, PA: Chilton Publishing; 1984. Out of print.

Mayfield E. A consumer's guide to fats. *FDA Consumer Magazine.* US Food and Drug Administration Web site. http://vm.cfsan.fda.gov/~dms/fdfats.html. Published May 1994. Revised January 1999. Accessed May 1, 2009. Content no longer available.

McCullough ML, Feskanich D, Stampfer MJ, Rosner BA, Hu FB, Hunter DJ, Variyam JN, Colditz GA, Willett WC. Adherence to US dietary guidelines and risk of major chronic disease in women. *Am J Clin Nutr.* 2000;72(5):1214-1222.

National Cancer Institute. Eating hints: before, during, and after cancer treatment. National Cancer Institute Web site. http://www.cancer.gov/cancerinfo/eatinghints. Published September 2009. Accessed November 20, 2009.

The nutrition source: shining the spotlight on trans fats. Harvard School of Public Health Web site. http://www.hsph.harvard.edu/nutritionsource/nutrition-news/transfats/. Accessed December 4, 2009.

Penland JG. Dietary Reference Intakes (DRIs): new dietary guidelines really are new! United States Department of Agriculture, Agricultural Research Service Web site. http://www.ars.usda.gov/News/docs.htm?docid=10870. Updated October 23, 2006. Accessed December 4, 2009.

Phend C. Exercise eases lymphedema symptoms. MedPage Today Web site. http://www.medpagetoday.com/HematologyOncology/BreastCancer/15498. Accessed November 20, 2009.

Prentice RL, Caan B, Chlebowski RT, Patterson R, Kuller LH, Ockene JK, Margolis KL, Limacher MC, Manson JE, Parker LM, Paskett E, Phillips L, Robbins J, Rossouw JE, Sarto GE, Shikany JM, Stefanick ML, Thomson CA, Van Horn L, Vitolins MZ, Wactawski-Wende J, Wallace RB, Wassertheil-Smoller S, Whitlock E, Yano K, Adams-Campbell L, Anderson GL, Assaf AR, Beresford SA, Black HR, Brunner RL, Brzyski RG, Ford L, Gass M, Hays J, Heber D, Heiss G, Hendrix SL, Hsia J, Hubbell FA, Jackson RD, Johnson KC, Kotchen JM, LaCroix AZ, Lane DS, Langer RD, Lasser NL, Henderson MM. Low-fat dietary pattern and risk of invasive breast cancer: the Women's Health Initiative Randomized Controlled Dietary Modification Trial. *JAMA.* 2006;295(6):629-642.

Prentice RL, Thomson CA, Caan B, Hubbell FA, Anderson GL, Beresford SA, Pettinger M, Lane DS, Lessin L, Yasmeen S, Singh B, Khandekar J, Shikany JM, Satterfield S, Chlebowski RT. Low-fat dietary pattern and cancer incidence in the Women's Health Initiative Dietary Modification Randomized Controlled Trial. *J Natl Cancer Inst.* 2007;99(20):1534-1543.

Sabatino SA, Coates RJ, Uhler RJ, Pollack LA, Alley LG, Zauderer LJ. Provider counseling about health behaviors among cancer survivors in the United States. *J Clin Oncol.* 2007;25(15):2100-2106.

Stephenson TJ, Setchell KD, Kendall CW, Jenkins DJ, Anderson JW, Fanti P. Effect of soy protein-rich diet on renal function in young adults with insulin-dependent diabetes mellitus. *Clin Nephrol.* 2005;64(1):1-11.

Survivors guide: understanding the diet-cancer connection. American Institute of Cancer Research Web site. http://www.aicr.org/survivor. Content no longer available.

Uauy R, Solomons N. Diet, nutrition, and the life-course approach to cancer prevention. *J Nutr.* 2005;135(12 Suppl):2934S-2945S.

United States Department of Agriculture. Common questions. United States Department of Agriculture Web site. http://fnic.nal.usda.gov/nal_display/index.php?info_center=4&tax_level=3&tax_subject=358&topic_id=1614&level 3_id=5944&level4_id=0&level5_id=0&placement_default=0. Updated August 3, 2009. Accessed August 20, 2009. Content no longer available.

US Department of Health and Human Services and United States Department of Agriculture. Dietary Guidelines for Americans, 2005. US Department of Health and Human Services Web site. http://www.health.gov/ dietaryguidelines/dga2005/document/default.htm. Published January 2005. Accessed December 4, 2009.

US Department of Health and Human Services, Office of the Surgeon General. Overweight and obesity: at a glance. The Surgeon General's call to action to prevent and decrease overweight and obesity. Office of the Surgeon General Web site. http://www.surgeongeneral.gov/topics/obesity/calltoaction/fact_glance.htm. Accessed November 20, 2009.

US Food and Drug Administration. How to understand and use the nutrition facts label. US Food and Drug Administration Web site. http://www.fda.gov/Food/LabelingNutrition/ConsumerInformation/ucm078889.htm. Published June 2000. Updated November 2004. Accessed December 4, 2009.

What are oils? United States Department of Agriculture. MyPyramid.gov Web site. www.mypyramid.gov/oils.html. Accessed December 22, 2009.

Chapter Two

Making Informed Decisions

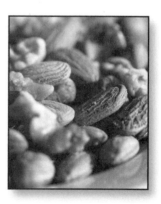

NO FOOD OR DIET ALONE CAN CURE CANCER, but good nutrition can help lessen the side effects of your treatment and help your body to heal and recover as quickly as possible. Sensible, healthy eating and keeping your body weight stable are common sense goals to help improve your feeling of well-being, reduce your risk of infection, and preserve your body's nutrition stores.

In the course of your treatment, you most likely will hear about many different cancer-fighting dietary supplements, foods, and diets. How can you tell which of these foods and diets are best? How can you tell whether dietary supplements are helpful or even harmful? Will they make you stronger and really fight your cancer? Or could these products be dangerous and interfere with your treatment and recovery? The information in this chapter can help you separate fact from fiction.

Talk to the Experts

If you have a question about how a food or diet relates to you, your cancer, or your treatment, ask your registered dietitian or your health care team for more detailed information. Taking the following actions before you speak with your health care team can ensure that you have a productive conversation:

- Do your own research before appointments and gather information from unbiased and trustworthy information sources. The most reliable sources are often voluntary health organizations staffed or backed by health experts; accredited cancer centers; medical, nursing, and registered dietitians' professional organizations; and government agencies—such as those listed in the resources section of this book.
- Write down questions as they occur to you so that you can discuss them with your health care team. Explain why you want to know about certain topics.
- Bring relevant information to appointments. Be sure to note the source of your information so your medical team can determine its reliability.
- Bring any dietary supplements or a complete list of any supplements you are taking for review by your health care team.
- Keep a diary where you write down what you eat and your activities for three or four days. Bring the diary with you to the appointment for review by your health care team.
- Ask a friend or family member to accompany you to appointments to ensure that your questions are clear and that you get complete answers.

In addition to your doctor or nurse, a registered dietitian can be a great source of information about diet and can provide more information on the topics in this book. A registered dietitian is an expert in food and diet, has at least a bachelor's degree, and has passed a national competency exam. In contrast, there are often no educational requirements associated with the title of nutritionist.

For more information or for a referral to a registered dietitian, contact the American Dietetic Association (ADA) at 800-877-1600 or www.eatright.org. The ADA helps people locate registered dietitians, including dietitians specializing in oncology nutrition, in their area. The ADA Web site contains information on diet and nutrition and a registered dietitian locator service.

So you don't have ready access to nutrition professionals?

Not every person diagnosed with cancer or their family members have access to a nutrition professional to answer their questions. But there are other ways to find the help you need. For example, the American Cancer Society National Cancer Information Center (800-227-2345) is a nationwide help line—open twenty-four hours a day, seven days a week—to answer calls about cancer-related issues. Cancer Information Specialists and Oncology Nurse Information Specialists can provide information on issues such as treatments, side effects of treatments, testing, and nutrition. In addition, here are some other resources that could be helpful:

- Contact your local American Cancer Society office.
- Visit the Web for reliable sites, such as www.fruitsandveggiesmatter.gov (see chapter 14 for more resources).
- Visit your local hospitals' Web sites or the National Cancer Institute Web site (www.cancer.gov).
- Go to www.mypyramid.gov on the Web and learn about improving your diet.
- Contact local colleges and universities to determine whether they have a nutrition or dietetics department that can provide assistance.
- Contact your local Cooperative Extension office staff for information and resources (see page 90 for more information).
- Take an online nutrition course through a university or community college.
- Call the American Institute for Cancer Research's Nutrition Hotline at 800-843-8114 or go online to www.aicr.org to ask a registered dietitian a question.

Getting the Facts: Reliable Research

Before pinning your hopes on a nutrition strategy, get the facts. Getting solid information and consulting your health care team can help you determine whether a food, supplement, or dietary regimen may help or harm your health. When you are looking into something that sounds promising, consider whether its claims are likely valid by keeping in mind the following information.

Understand the Study Types

Scientific discoveries are the result of experiments and studies. But some studies are more comprehensive and more reliable than others. Understanding the different types of studies can help you better evaluate their implications.

Before a drug or other treatment can be used regularly to treat people, it is studied and tested carefully, first in the laboratory and then in animals. Laboratory studies, or test tube studies, are often the first step. Researchers test substances on bacteria, animal, or human cells grown in laboratory dishes or test tubes. Animal studies are typically the next step. Animal research helps researchers learn more about a substance's effects on a whole organism in a controlled environment. After these studies are completed and the therapy is found safe and promising, it is tested to see whether it can help people.

Epidemiologic studies look at the factors that influence the way diseases occur in human populations. The two general categories of epidemiologic studies are observational studies and intervention studies:

- *Observational studies* follow real people going about their normal lives, without any intervention from researchers. For example, in an observational study of nutrition and cancer, researchers might ask people questions about their diets and look for associations with their cancer prognoses. In an observational study, no attempt is made to affect the outcome.
- *Intervention studies* explore whether a given intervention (such as a diet or physical activity) that results in a change in behavior or nutritional status is related to the risk of a disease. For example, researchers might suggest that study participants eat a specified amount of certain foods or take certain dietary supplements. Then researchers might look for potential effects on cancer risk, prognosis, or recurrence. A clinical trial is an intervention study.

Randomized controlled clinical trials are intervention studies in which people are randomly assigned to one group or another and a factor is intentionally kept different between the two. Randomized controlled clinical trials are considered to be the most reliable and conclusive type of study. Unfortunately, they are less commonly undertaken by researchers because they are very expensive and require much time to conduct.

While there are several advantages, enrolling in a study means you are committing to additional clinic visits, bloodwork, and demands on your schedule. The decision to take part in a clinical trial needs to be considered carefully and should be discussed with others, including family members, health care providers, and maybe even employers, based on the additional demands on your time. Refer to the Web sites www.cancer.org and www.clinicaltrials.gov for more information on clinical trials.

Study the Claims

When you hear a dietary supplement, diet, or other drug called a "breakthrough," "cure for all cancers," or "miracle cure," it is probably safe to assume that it has not been through traditional routes of testing for safety and effectiveness. Promises of "miracle cures" or quick-fix wonder drugs are red flags. Your body and its processes are intricate, and cancer, a group of more than one hundred diseases, does not have one cause or one treatment. As you evaluate a product or diet, consider the claims made for the treatment: To cure cancer? To enable the evidence-based treatment to work better? Or to relieve symptoms or side effects? If it sounds too good to be true, it probably is.

Get the Whole Story

News reports often do not have enough space or time to delve into the background of promising studies. Simplified

---

SHOULD I ENROLL IN A CLINICAL TRIAL?

Research is crucial to the advancement of knowledge and understanding of cancer and its risks. Many cancer patients question whether they should enroll in clinical trials. Specifically, for this book we are addressing trials that evaluate diet and/or physical activity. So why might you enroll? Here are some common reasons cited by participants in studies addressing diet or physical activity and cancer:

- The trial provides diet and/or lifestyle counseling free-of-charge.
- Participating in a trial is like having your own support group.
- It may help you embrace healthier lifestyle choices, particularly if you have been challenged to do this on your own.
- You may receive information about your health status, such as information on body composition, bone health, blood pressure, or blood glucose or lipid levels, etc.
- It's a great way to meet other cancer survivors.
- The knowledge gained may reduce cancer risk for future generations.

versions of the facts may sound more definitive than the evidence actually is. When you see a headline touting a research finding, look to the comments from experts in the field—do they also support what the headline is saying? Results that indicate true scientific progress usually build upon conclusions from earlier studies; one study with results out of the norm could be flawed and not indicative of typical effects. When evaluating the results of a study, consider the following:

- Who conducted the study? For example, was the study conducted by researchers at leading universities or with grants from the National Cancer Institute?
- What type of study was it? Animal or laboratory studies are conducted early on and are not always relevant to humans. Human studies are more likely to prove or disprove relevance.
- Who sponsored the study? Sometimes there can be bias if a study is funded by a group that would benefit from the findings. This is not always so, because companies often seek out expert scientists and doctors to perform their research. Such experts, however, become well-respected by demonstrating a highly ethical and rigorous approach to research.
- How long did the study last? How large was it? Generally, studies affecting medical policy or guidelines are the result of years of research examining a large number of people.
- Do other studies back up the findings? It usually takes a number of studies with similar results before results are considered definitive.

Read Carefully

Products or diets that count on user testimonials to prove their effectiveness are not likely to be based on scientific evidence. Promising discoveries lead to medications or treatments only through testing and evaluation. Trustworthy ideas are usually backed by scientific data that was collected over a period of time and published in respected, peer-reviewed journals. When considering a new treatment, ask yourself the following:

- What are the credentials of the people supporting the treatment? Are they recognized experts in cancer treatment? Have they published their findings in peer-reviewed, respected journals? If you are unsure, check with your health care team.
- Is the product or method widely available for use within the health care community, or is it controlled, with limited access to its use? Legitimate treatments should not be available at only one clinic or require you to travel to a specific country.
- Is the product or treatment promoted for use in place of standard therapies or clinical trials? If purveyors advocate that you discontinue use of the accepted therapy, be wary.
- Is the treatment or drug a "secret" that only certain providers can give? No tested, proven therapy will be secretive or restricted to a select few providers.

TERMS TO KNOW

You may have heard the terms "alternative" or "complementary" used to refer to methods of diagnosing, preventing, or treating cancer and wondered exactly what they mean. How can you know if these approaches are safe and if they are likely to help you?

A **proven treatment** is an evidence-based, medical treatment that has been tested following a strict set of guidelines and found to be safe and effective. The results of studies testing the drug or treatment have been published in peer-reviewed journals—journals reviewed by other doctors or scientists in the field. The treatment has been approved by the U.S. Food and Drug Administration (FDA) and is accepted as "mainstream" medicine.

Investigational treatments are therapies being studied in clinical trials. Clinical trials determine whether a new treatment is effective and safe for humans. If this careful testing shows that the drug or other treatment is safe and effective, the FDA may approve it for regular use. Only then does the treatment become part of the standard proven therapies used to treat disease in human beings.

Complementary therapies or integrative therapies are those that patients use *along with* conventional medicine. Examples might include meditation to reduce stress or ginger tea for nausea. Complementary methods are not used to cure disease, but they may help control symptoms and improve quality of life. Some methods, such as massage therapy, yoga, and meditation, are now categorized as complementary but were referred to as supportive care in the past.

Alternative therapies are treatments that patients use *instead of* conventional therapy in an attempt to prevent, lessen, or cure disease. Alternative therapies are considered unproven either because they have not been scientifically tested using rigorous, scientifically designed studies that include comparison to standard therapies or because they were tested and found to be ineffective. Regardless, adequate scientific evidence is not available to support the use of such treatments. Using an alternative therapy instead of evidence-based treatment can be dangerous—either because it delays access to helpful treatment or because the alternative treatment itself is harmful.

Turn to Trustworthy Sources

Information about cancer and its treatment reported through radio, TV, newspapers, magazines, and the Internet can be both exciting and confusing. Respected health information sources collect, assess, and share established information and can help you tell the difference between preliminary or unfounded findings and established developments you might want to pursue. Keep in mind that evidence-based methods will be promoted in scientific journals and not only in the mass media (books, magazines, and TV and radio talk shows). The sources in chapter 14 are a good place to start your research.

References

American Cancer Society. *American Cancer Society Complete Guide to Complementary and Alternative Cancer Therapies*. 2nd ed. Atlanta, GA: American Cancer Society; 2009.

Be an informed consumer. National Center for Complementary and Alternative Medicine Web site. http://nccam.nih.gov/health/decisions/. Accessed December 4, 2009.

Clinical trials. National Cancer Institute Web Site. http://www.cancer.gov/clinicaltrials. Accessed December 5, 2009.

Frazier AL, Ryan CT, Rockett H, Willett WC, Colditz GA. Adolescent diet and risk of breast cancer. *Breast Cancer Res*. 2003;5(2):R59-R64.

Making informed decisions. American Cancer Society Web site. http://www.cancer.org/docroot/MBC/content/MBC_4_1X_Making_Informed_Decisions.asp. Accessed December 4, 2009.

Chapter Three

Hot Topics in Nutrition and Cancer

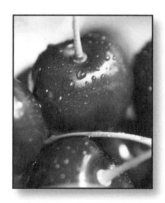

THERE ARE CLAIMS THAT CERTAIN FOODS CAN CAUSE CANCER, prevent it, keep it from recurring, or cause its return. The claims are as numerous as the foods themselves. Understandably, this is a topic of great interest for many cancer survivors. Because many foods have been associated with cancer—either its occurrence or prevention—many cancer survivors are interested in the proof surrounding these claims.

In this chapter, the claims and the available scientific evidence surrounding some foods, nutrients, and dietary supplements that are controversial or often-discussed in the cancer community will be examined. Some foods are recognized as having protective properties. Others could potentially aid cancer treatment. Some appear to have no effect on cancer outcomes. And still others are considered harmful.

In this chapter, "foods" are defined as substances that are consumed in the forms in which they are typically sold through grocery stores (for example, soy foods can be found as soybeans, soy milk, tofu, and other forms; green tea is the liquid from brewed, dried tea leaves). Some of the substances in the foods discussed here are also available in supplement form. The substances in supplements are often more concentrated than they naturally are in foods; therefore, supplements may cause different effects on the body than would the foods themselves when eaten in moderate amounts as part of a balanced diet. Food sources naturally contain a variety of healthy ingredients that may act together to affect cancer risk; supplements do not. Dietary supplements are discussed in more detail in chapter 5.

Keep in mind that even if one particular food has health benefits, relying on that food alone is not a sound nutritional strategy. Eating a diet that contains a wide variety of healthy foods—including five or more servings a day of vegetables and fruits, along with a variety of whole grain products: lean poultry, meat, and fish; low-fat dairy; and beans—is the best way to eat well before, during, and after cancer treatment.

Evaluating Foods as Part of the Overall Diet

The anticancer effects of any single food cannot be completely understood without evaluating the food as part of the overall diet. The many healthy compounds found in vegetables, fruits, and whole grains most likely work in combination to exert their health-promoting benefits. Many of the health benefits gained by eating whole foods cannot be replicated by taking dietary supplements. For example, glucosinolates, phytochemicals found in broccoli, appear to have less benefit when consumed as a supplement than when consumed in broccoli. It seems the vitamin C, beta carotene, folate, and glucosinolates in broccoli all work together in the right quantities to improve health.

The way foods affect the body—and especially how they affect the body of a person with an illness like cancer—is complex. It is very difficult to establish how a particular food relates to the cancer process. It is even more difficult when the food in question is typically consumed in small amounts. In this chapter, a selection of foods and substances of interest will be discussed: coffee, flaxseed, garlic, ginger, green tea, omega-3 fatty acids, soy, broccoli, shiitake mushrooms, tomatoes, noni plant, berries, sugar, and alcohol. For each of these, the information provided includes what each substance contains that has the potential to help or harm, what has been proven and what is not scientifically determined, and how to evaluate the role of these foods or substances in a balanced diet.

In some cases, evidence about a food's effects on reducing cancer risk is limited to results from animal studies. Animal studies, while informative, are generally completed in the very early stages of evidence building. Controlled clinical studies in humans, in which specific food components, whole foods, or whole diets are fed to a group of individuals, are needed to prove the usefulness of foods in cancer treatment and prevention.

Please note: Some of the information presented in this chapter is also available in a more comprehensive form in the American Cancer Society Complete Guide to Complementary and Alternative Cancer Therapies, Second Edition. *Please refer to this publication for further reading on foods, nutrients, and dietary supplements of interest for people with cancer.*

COFFEE

Coffee is made from the seeds of tropical African shrubs or trees from the genus *Coffea*, particulary *Coffea arabica*. The seeds are dried, roasted, and ground and are used to prepare a drink. Coffee contains caffeine, a mild stimulant also found in many soft drinks and some teas.

The Claim

Drinking coffee causes cancer.

The Evidence

At this time, there is no evidence that coffee, or the caffeine in it, causes cancer. The possible link between coffee and pancreatic cancer, which received a lot of attention in the past, is controversial and has not been confirmed in recent studies. Most studies have shown no substantial association, and evidence indicates that coffee is not significantly related to pancreatic cancer risk or may not be related at all.

A phytochemical called methylxanthine, which is found in coffee, can cause painful breast lumps, a symptom of fibrocystic breast disease (a type of benign breast disease) in some women. At this time, there is no evidence that coffee increases the risk for breast or other types of cancer.

One study showed that caffeine had a weak protective effect against breast cancer in post-menopausal women.

One small study investigated whether adding caffeine during chemotherapy increased survival in patients with sarcomas. The study did not include a control group, but results did suggest that caffeine improved survival. More research is needed to investigate the potential benefit of combining caffeine with chemotherapy drugs in cancer treatment.

Possible Problems or Complications

The caffeine in coffee has a diuretic effect on the body that lasts for a couple of hours after it is consumed, so drinking many cups of coffee may contribute to dehydration. In addition, patients who need more calories will not get any from coffee alone, though adding creamers will help. Consuming large amounts of caffeinated beverages may also contribute to stomach upset and irritability.

Bottom Line

Although several large-scale studies have been conducted to determine whether there is an association between coffee intake and cancer risk, most have not found an increased incidence of cancer among people who drink coffee.

FLAXSEED

Flax is an annual plant cultivated for its fiber, which is used in making linen. Flaxseed and its oil are used in herbal remedies. Flaxseed is available in flour, meal, and seed form and is found in some multigrain breads, cereals, breakfast bars, and muffins. The toasted seeds are sometimes mixed into bread dough or sprinkled over salads, yogurt, or cereal. Flaxseed oil is available in many health food stores in liquid form and is sometimes mixed into cottage cheese or other foods. The oil is also available in softgel capsules. Ground flaxseeds should be stored in the freezer to prevent them from spoiling.

Flaxseed—also called linseed—and its oil have been promoted since the 1950s as dietary nutrients with anticancer properties. Only recently has there been some clinical evidence suggesting that flaxseed supplements, along with a diet low in fat, may be useful in men with early-stage prostate cancer. Controlled clinical studies are needed to determine its usefulness in preventing or treating cancer in humans.

The Claim

Taking flaxseed dietary supplements or adding ground flaxseed or flaxseed oil to food can prevent or cure cancer.

The Evidence

Flaxseed oil is high in alpha-linolenic acid, an omega-3 fatty acid that is thought to have beneficial effects against cancer when consumed.

Recently, attention has also focused on the flaxseed itself, which is a rich source of lignans, compounds that can act as anti-estrogens or as weak estrogens. It is thought that lignans may play a role in preventing estrogen-dependent cancers, such as breast cancer. Lignans may also function as antioxidants and, through mechanisms that are not yet fully understood, may slow cell growth. When flaxseeds are consumed, the lignans are activated by bacteria in the intestine.

Most of the evidence for the anticancer effects of flaxseed and flaxseed oil comes from research using laboratory animals or cells grown in laboratory dishes. In one cell culture study, flaxseed lignans reduced stickiness and movement of breast cancer cells, both properties related to the cancer's ability to spread, or metastasize. Researchers have also found that a diet supplemented with flaxseed may reduce the formation, growth, or spread of prostate cancer, breast cancer, and melanoma in mice. Flaxseed reduced the formation of precancerous colon polyps in one study of rats but in another study had no effect on the formation of intestinal cancer in mice. In a 2007 report, flaxseed reduced growth of breast cancer cells in mice and enhanced the effectiveness of tamoxifen, a conventional drug for hormonal therapy.

There have been some small studies of the effects of flaxseed in humans. A small study of fifteen men found that a low-fat diet supplemented with flaxseed lowered blood prostate-specific antigen (PSA) levels and slowed the growth of benign prostate cells, suggesting that it might be useful in reducing risk for prostate cancer. Another study of twenty-five men with prostate cancer found that a low-fat diet along with ground flaxseed reduced serum testosterone, slowed the growth rate of cancer cells, and increased the death rate of cancer cells.

Possible Problems or Complications

The immature pods of flaxseed are poisonous and should never be used. Flaxseed and flaxseed oil can spoil if they are not kept refrigerated. They should be protected from light, heat, air, and moisture. Since the substances in flaxseeds are concentrated in flaxseed oil, the potential for side effects is greater when the oil is used.

Some possible side effects of ingesting flaxseed include diarrhea, gas, and nausea. Flaxseed oil should not be used with other laxatives or stool softeners. Flaxseed seems to interact with tamoxifen and, until more is understood about this interaction, women taking tamoxifen should not consume significant amounts of flaxseed.

Bottom Line

While research has yielded some promising results, additional research is needed to determine the usefulness of flaxseed in cancer treatment and prevention. Randomized clinical trials are needed to study whether taking flaxseed could affect cancer development in humans. Be sure to tell your doctor or health care team if you are currently taking or if you are thinking about using flaxseed-containing dietary supplements or eating large amounts of flaxseed or flaxseed oil.

GARLIC

Garlic (*Allium sativum*) is a member of the lily family and is closely related to onions, leeks, shallots, scallions, and chives. Extracts and oils made from garlic are sometimes used as herbal remedies.

The Claim

Garlic and garlic supplements can prevent or cure cancer.

The Evidence

Garlic is currently under study for its ability to reduce cancer risk. While there is some evidence that suggests garlic may reduce the risk of some types of cancer, there is not enough evidence at this time to support eating large amounts of garlic or taking garlic supplements for cancer prevention. It is reasonable to include garlic as part of a balanced diet, unless one has a particular health problem or is taking medication that has been shown to be adversely affected by garlic.

Several compounds in garlic may have anticancer properties, but compounds of one type in particular—the allyl sulfur compounds—are thought to play a major role. These compounds reportedly help the body get rid of cancer-causing chemicals and help cause cancer cells to die naturally, a process called apoptosis. There have also been claims that garlic has immune-boosting properties that may reduce cancer cell growth and help the body fight off diseases such as colds or the flu. These claims are currently being studied.

There is considerable debate as to which preparations and amounts of garlic could influence health. For example, cooking garlic reduces the potency of its active ingredients. Therefore, it may be best to simply mince garlic and eat it raw or to add it to foods near the end of the cooking time. However, this topic is still under consideration.

Many laboratory studies done in cell cultures and animals suggest garlic may help reduce tumor growth. Cell culture studies have shown garlic can help cancer cells die off normally. Other studies in cell cultures have found that substances in garlic seem to be able to act as antioxidants.

Several studies from around the world have found that people who eat more garlic seem to be at lower risk for certain types of cancer. In particular, large human studies that looked at diet and cancer have suggested that people who eat more garlic are at lower risk for stomach, prostate,

HERBS WITH BENEFITS
Increasingly, the scientific community is looking at culinary herbs and spices for their ability to improve health and possibly reduce cancer risk. Several herbs, including parsley, mint, and oregano, show antioxidant capacity. Some spices, such as turmeric, capsaicin (red pepper), cumin, and curry, seem to reduce inflammation in the body. Garlic and clove seem to reduce cholesterol levels, fenugreek reduces blood glucose, and ginger has been shown to reduce chemotherapy-related nausea in some people undergoing chemotherapy.

mouth, throat, kidney, and colorectal cancer. A recent review of available evidence suggested that diets high in garlic reduce colorectal cancer risk by as much as 30 percent. The evidence is limited to a small number of studies but does suggest garlic and other *Allium* vegetables should be investigated further for cancer-protective effects. The effect on risk for breast, bladder, ovarian, and lung cancers is less clear. As always with observational studies, other factors could account for the differences in cancer risk. The few human studies that have looked at garlic supplements have not found them to be helpful against cancer.

Possible Problems or Complications

Consumption of large amounts of garlic may lead to irritation of the gastrointestinal tract, causing stomach pain, gas, and vomiting. One study suggests that the use of garlic may increase the risk of bleeding because it has anti–blood clotting properties. People who are undergoing surgery should avoid garlic, especially if they have been given blood thinners or if postoperative bleeding is a concern.

Garlic seems to affect enzymes in the liver that help remove certain drugs from the body. This may result in reduced levels of some drugs in the body, which could be especially important in people undergoing chemotherapy. This effect is currently under study, but people thinking about taking garlic supplements should speak with their doctor or health care team first.

Bottom Line

Although results of some observational studies are encouraging, randomized clinical trials in which people receive either garlic or an inactive control substance are needed to obtain more reliable information. Very few studies of this type have studied garlic and cancer risk. Be sure to tell your doctor or health care team if you are currently taking (or thinking about taking) garlic-containing dietary supplements or eating large amounts of garlic.

GINGER

Ginger is a plant native to Southeast Asia that is now also grown in the United States, China, India, and various tropical regions. The root is usually the part of the plant used in herbal remedies.

The Claim

Eating ginger or taking ginger supplements can prevent nausea for people undergoing chemotherapy.

The Evidence

Ginger has been used to control or prevent nausea, vomiting, and motion sickness. It has also been used as an anti-inflammatory (a drug that reduces pain and swelling, as occurs with arthritis), a cold remedy, an aid to digestion, a remedy for intestinal gas, and to help relieve nausea in cancer patients who are undergoing chemotherapy. Some proponents have also claimed ginger can keep tumors from developing, even though available scientific evidence does not support this claim.

According to some, but not all, controlled studies in humans, ginger reduces nausea. Most studies also show that ginger reduces motion sickness and severe vomiting in early pregnancy. Although some clinicians warn that using ginger during pregnancy or breastfeeding (at doses that are higher than the amount eaten in foods) might cause harmful effects, there is no objective evidence of harm to the mother, fetus, or infant.

The chemotherapy drug cisplatin can cause significant nausea and vomiting and delay emptying of the stomach. In one study, researchers found that extracts from ginger helped to speed up stomach emptying in dogs and rats that were given cisplatin chemotherapy. However, extracted chemicals or substances are different from the raw plant. Thus, study results of extracts will not necessarily have the same result as studies using the raw plant. In a clinical trial of patients receiving cisplatin, addition of ginger to standard drugs for nausea did not reduce this symptom.

New research showed taking a ginger supplement just before and during chemotherapy treatment (involving various agents, not just cisplatin) helped reduce treatment-related nausea in some people. Ask a registered dietitian or your doctor whether a ginger supplement is right for you.

Studies of ginger's ability to reduce nausea and vomiting associated with surgery have had mixed results. At least three studies found ginger had no effect on nausea and vomiting after surgery, while other studies have found a significant decrease in nausea and vomiting when ginger was given before the operation. These inconsistencies may be due to the difficulty in measuring symptoms of nausea.

Possible Problems or Complications

The taste and aroma of ginger is calming for some individuals. In rare cases, people have experienced an allergic reaction to ginger or mild upset stomach. While ginger supplements may be effective in treating nausea and vomiting associated with some cancer treatments, it may also interfere with blood clotting. This side effect could be harmful for some people undergoing cancer treatment and receiving anticoagulation therapy (blood-thinning agents). Talk with your doctor or health care team before using ginger supplements.

Bottom Line

Given ginger's potential benefits and limited evidence of harm, integrating ginger into your diet may help to promote health. The best way get ginger's beneficial properties is to eat fresh ginger root. Some brands of ginger snaps, ginger ale, and ginger candy contain real ginger, but the amount is minimal and these foods may add extra undesired calories to the diet. Tea made from ginger root may be a good alternative as well. Be sure to tell your doctor or health care team if you are currently taking (or thinking about taking) ginger dietary supplements or eating large amounts of ginger.

GREEN TEA

Green tea is a drink made from the steamed and dried leaves of the *Camellia sinensis* plant, a shrub native to Asia. Black tea is also made from this plant, but unlike green tea, black tea is made from leaves that have been fermented. In contrast, herbal teas are made from fruit and spices instead of tea leaves and therefore do not contain the antioxidants found in actual teas. An antioxidant is a compound that blocks the action of activated oxygen molecules, known as free radicals, which can damage cells.

The Claim

Drinking green tea or taking green tea dietary supplements can prevent or cure cancer.

The Evidence

Some researchers believe green tea may have a protective effect because it contains chemicals known as polyphenols, which have antioxidant properties. The major group of polyphenols in green tea are called catechins, and the most important catechin seems to be epigallocatechin-3-gallate (EGCG). EGCG may cause cancer cells to die in much the same way that normal cells do. This effect is important because cancer cells are different from normal cells in that they do not die when they should—they continue to grow and spread.

DOES SUGAR FEED CANCER CELLS?

Some people believe that cancer thrives on sugar and recommend that people with cancer stop eating sugar. Sugar intake has not been shown to directly increase cancer risk, nor does it hasten the growth of cancer cells. Individuals who consume large amounts of sugar generally do not eat adequate amounts of cancer-protective vegetables and fruits. Instead, they tend to consume more high-fat foods, processed foods, and fast foods. These factors—rather than sugar intake—may account for any increase in cancer risk. In addition, excess sugar intake can lead to higher blood insulin levels, particularly in older people. The higher insulin levels may increase risk of some cancers, suggesting that high sugar intake may indirectly influence cancer risk.

Highly refined or highly sugared foods, which are typically low in nutrients, low in fiber, and high in carbohydrates, contribute calories but little else to the diet. Foods high in refined sugars or carbohydrates may also increase insulin resistance. It is not known whether insulin resistance influences chances of surviving cancer, but it is likely to increase the likelihood of obesity, diabetes, and cardiovascular disease. Researchers are increasingly interested in whether refined carbohydrates and foods high in sugar indirectly increase the risk of certain cancers, such as breast, colorectal, or pancreatic cancer.

Studies evaluating the effects of consuming concentrated sources of sugar, such as sweetened beverages, on cancer risk are limited and have produced mixed results. There is some indication that consuming concentrated sources of sugar increases pancreatic cancer risk, especially among women with borderline insulin resistance. A study among Mexican women showed a significant increase in breast cancer risk among those who consumed higher amounts of sugared beverages. More research is needed to determine whether these risks only apply to people with underlying insulin resistance.

During treatment, your goal may be to take in enough calories and keep up your energy. To help you meet these goals, your health care team may advise you to include high-calorie foods in your diet, but this can be done without consuming excessive amounts of highly refined or highly sugared foods. Emphasize a well-balanced selection of foods, including complex carbohydrates, proteins, and fats.

Although tea is consumed in a variety of ways and varies in its chemical makeup, one study has shown that steeping green or black tea for about five minutes releases more than 80 percent of its catechins into the water. (Instant iced tea contains almost no catechins.)

Some laboratory studies have indicated that green tea may help prevent the growth of certain cancers, including cancer of the skin, lung, breast, bladder, liver, prostate, colon, and esophagus. Test tube studies have suggested that compounds in the tea may help stop new blood vessels from forming, thereby cutting off the supply of blood to cancer cells. It is tempting to think that it would therefore prevent cancer in humans, but results of studies in humans have been mixed. Most human studies have been observational epidemiologic studies in East Asia, in which researchers compared tea drinkers with non–tea drinkers while trying to account for other lifestyle differences. It is difficult to draw firm conclusions from these types of studies. A meta-analysis of several studies that analyzed whether green tea can prevent gastric cancer found no protective effect.

Large observational epidemiologic studies in East Asia generally have not found that green tea drinkers are at a lower risk for breast, stomach, or colon cancer than non–tea drinkers. One study found that Asian American women who drink green tea regularly have a lower risk of breast cancer than those who do not. A Chinese study found that green tea drinking was linked to fewer cancers of the esophagus for people who did not smoke. On the other hand, a 2006 Japanese study showed that those with cancer of the esophagus were more likely to be green tea drinkers than those who did not have the cancer. Other studies of green tea's ability to prevent or treat lung, prostate, bladder, or other types of cancer have yielded similarly mixed results.

Possible Problems or Complications

Green tea is generally considered safe. A daily cup or two of green tea is not known to be at all harmful. However, some people may develop allergic reactions to the tea, and they should stop drinking it. In addition, there have been increasing reports of acute (but reversible) liver failure among people who took green tea extracts. These cases suggest that people should drink the tea rather than take green tea supplements.

If you are taking warfarin (Coumadin) or other blood thinners, do not drink large amounts of green tea. Drinking large amounts of green tea—a half gallon to a full gallon a day—could reduce the effectiveness of these drugs.

In addition, drinking large amounts of tea may cause nutritional and other problems. Green tea contains caffeine, and high doses of caffeine can contribute to dehydration. The tannins in tea may reduce the body's absorption of iron. Individuals with cancer who are having problems with eating and maintaining weight might need to replace tea with higher-calorie liquids.

Bottom Line

While the results of laboratory studies have been promising, at this time the available scientific evidence does not support claims that green tea can help prevent or treat any specific type of cancer in humans. Controlled, randomized clinical trials are needed to determine its effectiveness. Several studies are currently under way. Be sure to tell your doctor or health care team if you are currently taking (or thinking about taking) green tea dietary supplements or drinking large amounts of green tea.

OMEGA-3 FATTY ACIDS (FISH, FISH OIL, AND LEGUMES)

Omega-3 fatty acids are important nutrients that are involved in many bodily processes. The body cannot make these fatty acids and must obtain them from food sources or from supplements. Three fatty acids compose the omega-3 family: alpha-linolenic acid, eicosapentaenoic acid, and docosa-hexaenoic acid. Alpha-linolenic acid (ALA) is found in English walnuts, in some types of beans, and in canola, soybean, flaxseed/linseed, and olive oils. The other two, eicosapentaenoic acid (EPA) and docosahexaenoic acid (DHA), are found in fish, including fish oil and supplements.

The Claims

- Taking omega-3 fatty acid dietary supplements or eating foods rich in omega-3 fatty acids can prevent or cure cancer.
- Taking fish oil supplements containing omega-3 fatty acids can prevent cancer-related weight loss.
- One should avoid eating fish as a way to get omega-3 fatty acids because it could contain unsafe amounts of mercury (not a cancer-related claim, but very common).

The Evidence

Some people believe that omega-3 fatty acids protect against the spread of solid-tumor cancers (those that form solid masses) that are related to hormone production, particularly breast cancer. Some also believe that omega-3 fatty acids inhibit the growth of colon, pancreatic, and prostate cancer. Some people and groups advocate use of omega-3 fatty acids to protect against cardio-vascular disease and fatal heart attacks. Others believe that omega-3 fatty acids help rheumatoid arthritis, Crohn's disease, eczema, asthma, kidney failure, depression, and more. Omega-3 fatty acids may reduce the physical wasting and malnourishment that can occur during later stages of some cancers. Some registered dietitians recommend eating a diet rich in fish containing omega-3 fatty acids or eating one to two teaspoons of flaxseed oil daily.

Studies in animals have found that fish rich in omega-3 fatty acids suppress cancer formation and reduce inflammation. The evidence from the few studies on humans published in peer-reviewed medical journals is mixed. Some studies even show an increase in disease when omega-3 supplements are used. The strongest evidence for the health benefits of fatty acids from fish is in the area of heart disease and its risk factors, such as high blood pressure (hypertension).

In 2006, researchers reviewed thirty-eight studies conducted over the past forty years on the effects of omega-3 fatty acid supplementation on cancer risk. Researchers looked at studies that showed positive effects, no effects, and negative effects of omega-3 fatty acids on the development of cancer. In the final analysis, it appeared that there was no effect overall. Researchers concluded that omega-3 supplements are unlikely to prevent cancer.

ALCOHOL AND CANCER

Current recommendations suggest that people who drink alcoholic beverages should limit their intake to no more than two drinks per day for men and one drink a day for women. The recommended limit is lower for women because of their smaller body size and slower metabolism of alcohol. Alcohol consumption is an established cause of cancer of the mouth, pharynx, larynx, esophagus, and liver. For each of these cancers, risk increases substantially with intake of more than two drinks per day. Evidence also implicates alcohol consumption as a cause of breast cancer and probably colon and rectal cancer as well. Regular consumption of more than one drink per day has been associated with an increased risk of breast cancer in women. Although alcohol intake has been linked with an increase in the risk for breast cancer, there is limited evidence at this time of a relationship between alcohol intake and the risk for recurrence and survival.

People who have a decreased appetite during cancer treatment may be able to stimulate appetite by drinking a *small serving* of an alcoholic beverage before meals, such as a small glass of wine. Alcoholic beverages provide calories but not many nutrients, however, and it is especially important for people with cancer to avoid replacing nutrient-rich foods with alcohol.

Complicating the recommendation for alcohol and cancer risk is the fact that low to moderate intake of alcoholic beverages, particularly red wine, has been associated with decreased risk for cardiovascular disease. There is no compelling reason for adults who currently do not consume alcoholic beverages to start consuming alcohol to reduce their risk for heart disease, as cardiovascular risk can be reduced by other means, such as avoiding smoking, consuming a diet low in total fat and trans fats, maintaining a healthy weight, staying physically active on a regular basis, and controlling blood pressure and lipids.

There is growing interest in the role of omega-3 fatty acid supplements for people with cachexia, a problem of severe weight loss and wasting that occurs with some types of advanced cancer. A clinical study published in the journal *Cancer* concluded that omega-3 fatty acids seemed to prolong the survival of cancer patients who were also severely malnourished. An earlier small study looked at patients with advanced pancreatic cancer and severe weight loss. It compared use of EPA mixed with a high-protein, high-calorie supplement to use of the supplement without EPA. After eight weeks, the study found that EPA did not help the patients gain weight. A more recent review of all research on the use of EPA for cancer-related weight loss found only five studies. The reviewers concluded that there was not enough information to determine whether EPA helped people with cancer-related weight loss.

Studies have shown that the fatty acids in fish oil help protect against heart disease and reduce risk factors such as high blood levels of triglycerides. In one study, fish oils appeared to help improve heart rhythm problems. However, they may also increase cholesterol and reduce blood clotting. ALA, the omega-3 fatty acid from vegetable oils, has not shown as strong an effect in studies to date, although it may reduce risk of fatal heart disease. There appears to be more evidence of health-promoting effects for ALA from nuts, such as walnuts and pecans, although studies remain limited in number and are generally focused on benefits specific to heart disease.

Research is also focusing on the role of omega-3 fatty acids in relation to omega-6 fatty acids. Omega-6 is another type of essential fatty acid that is found in many vegetable oils (such as corn, safflower, and sunflower oils), cereals, snack foods, and baked goods. Unlike omega-3s, omega-6s are plentiful in the typical American diet. Some researchers believe one cause of Americans' high rates of cardiovascular disease may be an imbalance in the ratio of omega-3 to omega-6 fatty acids. Ideally, the ratio of omega-3 to omega-6 fatty acids in the human body is 1-to-1. However, the typical American diet is low in omega-3s and high in omega-6s. Many people have ten to twenty times more omega-6 fatty acids than omega-3 fatty acids in their systems.

A large study followed more than thirty-four thousand women from 1980 to 1998, observing their fish intake and the ratio of fish fatty acids to omega-6 fatty acids in their diets to determine how the ratio affected their colorectal cancer risk. Women who took in more omega-3 fatty acids did not have a lower colorectal cancer risk, but they had fewer large benign colorectal tumors, or adenomas. This study suggests that omega-3 fatty acids may not reduce colorectal cancer risk but may slow growth of benign tumors. More research is needed.

Possible Problems or Complications

Omega-3 fatty acids may increase total blood cholesterol and inhibit blood clotting. People who take blood-thinning medications (anticoagulants) or aspirin should not take extra omega-3 because of the risk of excessive bleeding.

The source of some omega-3 fatty acids may also be a health concern. Many large predatory fish contain toxic chemicals absorbed from pollution. Swordfish, shark, and tilefish (golden bass or golden snapper), for instance, are high in omega-3 fatty acids but may also contain high levels of mercury. King mackerel, a lesser source of omega-3s, may also have high mercury levels. Grouper, red snapper, and fresh or frozen tuna may have more moderate amounts of mercury. Other large fish, such as tuna and salmon, may contain other chemicals such as dioxin and polychlorinated biphenyls or PCBs, although fresh or frozen salmon usually has low mercury levels and large amounts of omega-3 fatty acids. Some studies have shown that farm-raised fish may carry more toxins than fish caught in the wild. Unfortunately, there is no way for a consumer to know what might be present in any particular fish, although some fish are inclined to have higher levels of contamination than others.

The precise risks and benefits of eating these fish are not known at this time. Experts recommend that adults vary the type of fish they eat as part of a healthy, balanced diet to reduce the chances of getting too many contaminants. Mercury poses the greatest risk to young children and unborn babies. Women who are pregnant, trying to get pregnant, or nursing, as well as young children, should avoid eating fish likely to be highly contaminated. They should also limit their intake of moderately contaminated fish.

Prolonged use of fish oil supplements can cause vitamin E deficiency, which is why vitamin E is added to many supplements. Fish liver oils (such as cod liver oil) can cause toxic levels of vitamins A and D if overused. Supplements may also cause fishy breath odor, belching, or abdominal bloating. They may also increase a tendency toward anemia in menstruating women. Women who are pregnant or breastfeeding should talk to their doctor before adding extra omega-3 supplements or fish to their diets.

People who are allergic to fish may have serious reactions to fish oil or supplements made from fish and should avoid them. People who are allergic to nuts should avoid supplements that are made from nuts to which they react.

Bottom Line

At this time, not enough is known about omega-3 fatty acid supplements to determine whether they are safe when taken in large quantities or when taken with other drugs, including cancer treatments. In addition, evidence is mixed as to whether taking fish oil supplements containing omega-3 fatty acids improves cancer-related weight loss. If you are taking or if you are thinking about taking omega-3 fatty acid supplements, be sure to talk to your doctor or health care team for guidance about whether supplements are right for you.

For men and middle-aged or older women (after menopause), the benefits of eating fish may outweigh the risks of mercury or other contaminants. Even so, most experts suggest that all Americans should limit intake of the most-contaminated fish to one serving per week. Most refined fish oil supplements have little or none of these contaminants.

SOY

The soybean plant is an annual plant native to Southeast Asia. Soybeans are legumes, a member of the pea family, and are a source of good-quality protein. Soy can be consumed in many forms, such as tofu, miso, soybeans (edamame), soy milk, texturized soy protein, and soy powder.

The Claims

- Eating soybean products or soy-containing foods can prevent cancer.
- People with some kinds of breast cancer should not eat soy or soy-containing foods because they can cause cancer to come back.

The Evidence

Soybean products are promoted for their protective properties against breast, prostate, colon, and lung cancer. The anticancer effects of soy are thought to be due to phytochemical substances called isoflavones, although other substances may also contribute. Isoflavones are sometimes called plant estrogens or phytoestrogens because they mimic (although weakly) estrogen that is produced in humans and animals. Genistein, daidzein, and glycitein are isoflavones that are present in small amounts in other foods but are most abundant in soy.

Soy is also a good source of low-fat protein. As a protein source, soybean products are promoted as a healthier alternative to meat and as an aid to weight loss. Soybean products are also used to lower cholesterol and blood pressure and to relieve symptoms of menopause and osteoporosis. Proponents also suggest that including soy protein as part of a diet low in saturated fat and cholesterol may help reduce the risk for heart disease.

Researchers believe that the isoflavones in soy, such as genistein, daidzein, and glycitein, may play a role in reducing cancer risk. A number of laboratory and animal experiments and human observational studies have found that soy isoflavones may reduce the risk for several types of cancer, including breast, prostate, and colon cancer. However, these results have not yet been reflected in human clinical trials, so no definite conclusions can be made.

There is enough evidence, scientists believe, for phytoestrogens to be studied in clinical trials as an addition to conventional breast or prostate cancer treatment. Human studies sponsored by the National Cancer Institute are under way. Large studies that looked at groups of women with a high soy intake showed a lower risk for breast cancer and endometrial cancer, but there are many possible explanations other than the soy. People who eat soybean products have a tendency to eat healthier in general. Further studies that control for these factors are needed. It is also possible that the weak estrogen-like effect of soy might be helpful in prostate cancer prevention, but large human studies are needed.

Some studies have suggested that the effect of soy foods on breast cancer risk depends on the age at which they are consumed. It is thought that high soy intake by young women at a time when breast tissue is developing and estrogen levels are relatively high may offer some protection. However, it is unclear whether soy intake after menopause, when estrogen levels are naturally low, is of any benefit or could even be harmful.

Several clinical studies of women with breast cancer have been done to determine whether soy capsules help with symptoms of menopause. The results have not shown any consistent improvement in menopausal symptoms such as hot flashes.

Several studies of men with prostate cancer have suggested that soybean products and/or supplements may reduce levels of prostate-specific antigen (PSA), a substance that typically increases as prostate cancer grows. In another study, while PSA levels did not decrease during soy treatment, they increased less rapidly than they had before the study began. Although these results are encouraging, further research is needed to learn whether soybean products help men with prostate cancer live longer.

Soybeans and soybean products have been shown in clinical trials to lower cholesterol and reduce blood pressure.

Possible Problems or Complications

For the population at large, eating soybean products is generally considered safe for those who are not allergic to them. Side effects are rare, but may include occasional gastrointestinal problems such as stomach pain, loose stools, and diarrhea.

The isoflavones in soy have weak estrogen-like activity, yet recent studies do not suggest soy affects the growth of estrogen responsive cancers, including breast, ovarian, and endometrial cancer. Researchers suggest they may act as anti-estrogens and reduce cancer growth. Some doctors caution people (female and male breast cancer survivors) with a diagnosis of estrogen receptor–positive breast cancer to limit their intake of soy and soy-containing foods and products because of concern that tamoxifen and other drugs taken for estrogen receptor–positive breast cancer might not be as effective. However, a recent prospective study of more than nineteen hundred female breast cancer survivors showed tamoxifen levels did not drop when soy foods were eaten. The study also found that including moderate amounts of soy foods in the diet may even reduce the risk for breast cancer recurrence. Until more studies are conducted, people with estrogen receptor–positive breast cancer, after consulting with their doctors, should feel comfortable eating one to three servings of soy foods as part of a healthy, plant-based diet. Just as for all healthy eating recommendations, it is better to focus on eating whole soy foods such as edamame, tofu, tempeh, or soy milk, rather than concentrated sources of soy such as soy-containing pills, powders, or supplements containing high amounts of isoflavones.

With the exception of female survivors of hormone-sensitive cancers, current evidence indicates that most people can safely take soy isoflavone-containing supplements. A few people are allergic to soy proteins and may have serious or life-threatening reactions to soy-containing foods. These people should avoid all forms of soy and supplements made from it. Soy ingredients may also be listed as soya.

Bottom Line

Eating soy and soy-containing foods as part of a healthy diet has not been shown to be harmful for people with cancer. If you do have concerns, be sure to talk with your doctor and your health care team. As with any dietary supplementation, tell your doctor if you are taking supplements containing soy or soy isoflavones.

PROBIOTICS

Probiotics are foods and supplements that contain potentially beneficial live bacteria or yeasts. Lactic acid bacteria, such as *Lactobacillus* and *Bifidobacterium*, are the most common type of microbes used as probiotics. Lactic acid bacteria convert sugars and other carbohydrates into lactic acid and have been used in the food industry for many years. Probiotic bacterial cultures are believed to assist the body in reestablishing naturally occurring gut flora. Doctors and registered dietitians sometimes recommend using probiotic cultures after a course of antibiotics or as part of the care of diarrhea.

The most common sources of probiotics are yogurt-based products, acidophilus milk, or probiotic-fortified foods. Tablets, capsules, powders, and sachets containing the bacteria in freeze-dried form are also available. Some fermented products also contain lactic acid bacteria, which has also been promoted for health. These include pickled vegetables*; fermented bean products such as tempeh, miso, and doenjang*; kefir; sauerkraut*; and soy sauce.*

* **Caution:** These foods are high in sodium and would not be a good choice for people who have high blood pressure.

Vegetables and Fruits

Vegetables and fruits are excellent sources of vitamins and provide ample fiber, the part of plant foods that helps move food waste out of the body quickly. Also keep in mind that beneficial nutrients are generally more concentrated in vegetables than in fruit. Vegetables and fruits also contain other beneficial phytochemicals, called nutraceuticals or phytonutrients, which are also found in beans, grains, and other plant foods, that seem to benefit the body and may even fight cancer. In the majority of observational studies, eating more vegetables, fruits, or both has been associated with a lower risk for cancers of the lung, mouth, pharynx/larynx, esophagus, and possibly colon. Also keep in mind that since each food has different phytochemicals that may act in different ways to reduce cancer risk, eating fruits and vegetables in a variety of colors provides the broadest benefit.

A diet high in vegetables and fruits might help improve the likelihood of surviving cancer, but there have been only a few studies of this issue. One study of breast cancer survivors found that those who ate more than five servings of vegetables and fruit daily and performed moderate exercise (thirty minutes of walking five to six times per week) were at lower risk for a recurrence of breast cancer. While the studies are limited, it is sensible for most people with cancer to follow the general nutrition recommendations issued by the American Cancer Society and many other public health and medical organizations (as outlined in chapter 1) for eating at least five servings of vegetables and fruits a day.

BROCCOLI (AND OTHER CRUCIFEROUS VEGETABLES)

Broccoli is a cruciferous vegetable (a plant that often has four flowers resembling a cross) that belongs to the cabbage family, which also includes arugula, cauliflower, collards, bok choy, kale, mustard greens, radishes, turnips, watercress, rutabaga, and Brussels sprouts.

The Claim
Eating broccoli and other cruciferous vegetables can prevent or cure cancer.

The Evidence
Broccoli contains certain chemicals that may reduce the risk for colorectal or other types of cancer, although it is not clear which individual compounds may be responsible for the protective effects. Broccoli is considered a good source of nutrients because it is rich in vitamin C, carotenoids (vitamin A–like substances), fiber, calcium, and folate. Broccoli is also a source of many substances called phytochemicals, or plant chemicals, which may have anticancer properties. For example, broccoli contains several compounds called isothiocyanates, including sul-

foraphane and indole-3-carbinol (I3C), which have been touted as possible anti-cancer agents in recent years. Early studies have shown these substances may act as antioxidants and may boost detoxifying enzymes in the body. Some studies have also suggested they may alter the levels of estrogen in the body, which might affect breast cancer risk.

Raw broccoli may have a slightly bitter taste, but cooking broccoli reduces the bitterness. The bitter taste has actually been traced to higher levels of the same chemicals thought to provide cancer protection. Scientists have developed different types of cruciferous vegetables, such as green cauliflower and broccolini, a cross between broccoli and Chinese kale, which looks more like asparagus and tastes sweeter than broccoli. Cooking broccoli and other cruciferous vegetables destroys myrosinase, the active enzyme in the plant that releases the protective compounds. The gut also contains these enzymes, which compensates for their loss in cooking. However, it would be best to eat more raw or lightly cooked cruciferae for the most benefit. Younger plants such as broccolini and broccoli sprouts also have higher concentrations of the protective phytochemicals.

The chemical composition of broccoli and other cruciferous vegetables is complex, which makes it hard to determine which compound or combination of compounds may provide protection

RAW VS. COOKED PRODUCE: THE NUTRIENT DEBATE

Fresh produce is usually considered to have more nutritional value than cooked produce. Generally, the less produce is cooked, the more nutrients it retains. Boiling vegetables, especially for long periods, can leach out B and C vitamins and other nutrients that are water soluble. Water-soluble nutrients dissolve easily in water and your body does not store them, so daily intake is important. Microwaving and steaming may be the best ways to preserve the nutritional content of vegetables, as long as the amount of cooking water and cooking time are limited. One method that works well to optimize nutrient content is to microwave vegetables in a dish with a wet paper towel covering the vegetable. Not only will nutrients be retained, but the vegetables will be colorful and appealing to eat!

Frozen vegetables and fruits may be more nutritious than canned and even fresh foods because they are often picked ripe and quickly frozen. The high heat involved in the canning process can reduce heat-sensitive and water-soluble nutrients, such as vitamin C and B vitamins. Always be aware that some fruits are packed in heavy syrup (which contains a lot of added sugar), and some canned vegetables are high in sodium.

The important thing to remember is to EAT YOUR VEGETABLES!

against cancer. Eating a wide variety of plant-based foods may be the best way to get the necessary components.

Diets high in cruciferous vegetables appear to be linked with a lower risk for certain types of cancer. Studies investigating the role of cruciferous vegetables in reducing cancer risk seem to indicate that these vegetables are more likely to reduce risk for hormone-related cancers such as endometrial, prostate, or breast, as well as colorectal and bladder cancers, but the data are not consistent. Intake of these vegetables is relatively low in most populations, making it difficult to ascertain whether higher levels of intake might be more protective. An observational epidemiologic study found that those who ate diets high in lutein, a vitamin A–like chemical obtained from vegetables such as broccoli, spinach, and lettuce, had fewer cases of colon cancer. A similar study suggested that those who ate cruciferous vegetables seemed to have a lower risk of bladder cancer, but a similar study of smokers found no such benefit. Recent studies suggest that the effect of broccoli and related cruciferous vegetables on cancer risk may partly depend on an inherited variation in certain metabolic enzymes. For example, when people with certain glutathione S-transferase types eat a diet high in cruciferous vegetables, their risk for lung cancer is lower. Randomized clinical trials are needed to clarify these results.

Laboratory and animal studies have suggested that certain compounds in broccoli may have anticancer properties. These types of studies can suggest possible helpful effects, but they do not provide proof that such effects can be achieved in humans. Further studies are needed to find out whether possible anticancer properties could benefit humans. Some research has suggested that sulforaphane, a substance that is present at much higher levels in broccoli sprouts than in the mature vegetable, may be a powerful cancer-preventing agent. Some researchers have suggested that eating small amounts of broccoli sprouts may protect against the risk of cancer as effectively as much larger amounts of the mature vegetable. To date, there do not appear to have been any clinical studies in humans to verify this claim. Sulforaphane is thought to prompt the body to make higher levels of enzymes that protect against cancer-causing chemicals. One study showed that breast tumor development was significantly reduced in laboratory animals that ate sulforaphane. Other laboratory studies have shown that sulforaphane may help protect against prostate, colon, pancreatic, and other types of cancer. Some studies have also suggested that the compound may help treat some types of cancer. More research in animals and humans will be needed to confirm these findings.

The substance I3C seems to alter estrogen levels and may also raise levels of protective enzymes in the body. Several studies of cancer cells growing in laboratory dishes or flasks have shown it may slow or stop the growth of breast, prostate, and other cancer cells. Some early studies in animals have shown similar results. Small studies in humans have found it may prevent the development of precancerous growths in the cervix, as well as growths called papillomas in the throat. Again, larger studies are needed to find out what benefits I3C may have against cancer. Importantly, growing evidence suggests that diindolylmethane—a metabolite of I3C—may be even more important to cancer risk reduction than I3C. Active clinical trials funded by the National Institutes of Health are under way using this phytochemical to determine its role in cancer.

Scientists caution that while broccoli appears promising as an excellent food for preventing cancer, the results of such studies cannot be considered by themselves. The anticancer effects of any single food cannot be completely understood without looking at it as part of a bigger dietary picture. It is still unclear, for example, whether the phytochemicals in broccoli have benefit on their own or whether it is the vitamin C, beta carotene, folate, and other compounds working together and in the right quantities that might protect people against cancer.

Possible Problems or Complications

Cruciferous vegetables eaten in large amounts may cause gas for some people. Taking anti-gas medication may help to improve tolerance and promote greater intake. Also, gradually increasing intake over time will help increase tolerance. If you are taking warfarin (Coumadin) or other blood thinners, do not eat large amounts of green-colored cruciferous vegetables or other green-colored vegetables and fruits such as spinach, collard greens, green beans, honeydew melon, and kiwi fruit. Typically, these foods are high in vitamin K, and eating too much of them can reduce the effectiveness of blood-thinning agents. Most doctors managing blood coagulation disorders advise people on these medications to eat a consistent amount of vitamin K–containing foods every day and to limit portion sizes for the best blood control. Talk with your doctor if you have any concerns.

Bottom Line

While research in this area continues, the best advice at this time to reduce cancer risk is to eat a wide variety of vegetables, including broccoli and other cruciferous vegetables, as part of a healthy, balanced diet.

SHIITAKE MUSHROOMS

A wide variety of mushrooms have been proposed to reduce cancer risk because of their potential to enhance immune response. Shiitake mushrooms, edible fungi native to Asia and grown in forests, are the second most commonly cultivated edible mushrooms in the world and have been of particular interest. Natural shiitake mushrooms are widely available in grocery stores.

The Claim

Eating shiitake mushrooms or taking shiitake mushroom supplements can prevent or cure cancer.

The Evidence

Shiitake mushrooms are promoted to fight the development and progression of cancer by boosting the body's immune system. These mushrooms are also said to help prevent heart disease by lowering cholesterol levels and to help treat infections such as hepatitis by producing interferon, a group of natural proteins that stop viruses from multiplying. Promoters claim that shiitake mushrooms contain several compounds with health benefits. A compound called lentinan is believed to stop or slow tumor growth. Another component, activated hexose-containing compound (also known as 1,3-beta glucan), is said to reduce tumor activity and lessen the side effects of cancer treatment. The mushrooms also contain the compound eritadenine, which is thought to lower cholesterol by blocking the way cholesterol is absorbed into the bloodstream. These claims are currently being studied.

Animal studies have shown some positive results regarding the antitumor, cholesterol-lowering, and virus-inhibiting effects of several active compounds in shiitake mushrooms. There have been some studies in humans. At least one randomized clinical trial of lentinan has shown it to prolong life of patients with advanced and recurrent gastrointestinal cancer who were also given chemotherapy. Lentinan is a beta glucan (sometimes called beta glycan) that is found in several mushrooms, yeasts, and other foods. Beta glucan is a polysaccharide, a large and complex molecule made up of smaller sugar molecules. The beta glucan polysaccharide is believed to stimulate the immune system and activate certain cells and proteins that attack cancer, including macrophages, T-cells, and natural killer cells. In laboratory studies, beta glucan appears to slow the growth of cancer in some cell cultures.

Several potential cancer-fighting substances have been found in shiitake mushrooms, and purified forms of these compounds are being studied as treatment for gastrointestinal cancer. It is not known whether any of these results will apply to the mushrooms bought in supermarkets or the extracts that are sold as supplements. One nonrandomized study published in 2002 looked at use of shiitake mushroom extract by men with prostate cancer but did not find any positive effect. Sixty-two men took the extract three times a day. After six months, they did not have any significant decrease in their level of prostate-specific antigen (PSA), a protein in the body that typically increases as prostate cancer grows, and nearly a quarter of them had increases in their PSA levels. More human clinical trials are under way to understand which, if any, compounds in shiitake mushrooms may be effective for which types of cancers.

Possible Problems or Complications

There are rare, isolated reports of some individuals experiencing diarrhea and bloating after eating shiitake mushrooms. In some people, allergic reactions have developed, affecting the skin, nose, throat, or lungs.

Bottom Line
Shiitake mushrooms and their extracts are generally considered safe.

TOMATOES AND LYCOPENE

Lycopene is the compound that gives tomatoes and other vegetables and fruits a red color. It is one of the major carotenoids in the diet of North Americans. Carotenoids are pigments that give yellow, red, and orange vegetables and fruits their color. The body uses some types of carotenoids (but not lycopene) to make vitamin A.

Dietary lycopene comes primarily from tomatoes, although apricots, guava, watermelon, papaya, and pink grapefruit are also significant sources. When processed tomatoes such as canned tomatoes or those in tomato sauce or tomato juice are eaten along with oil or fat (in tomato sauce or paste, for example), they provide a more readily absorbed source of lycopene than raw tomatoes. During processing, the heating action evaporates much of the water in the tomatoes, leaving the more easily absorbed pulp that contains the lycopene. Also, since lycopene is a fat-soluble nutrient, the oil found in tomato sauces is thought to help promote its absorption.

The Claim
Eating tomatoes or taking lycopene supplements can prevent or cure cancer.

The Evidence
Studies suggest that diets rich in tomatoes are associated with a lower risk of oral, pharynx/larynx, and prostate cancer. Higher intake of carotenoids in general also appears to have a protective benefit against a number of additional cancers, including cancer of the lung, stomach, cervix, breast, pancreas, colon, rectum, and esophagus. However, a direct relationship between tomatoes and protection against these cancers has not yet been proved. And the protective effect associated with lycopene may be caused at least in part by other compounds in tomatoes that could act either alone or with lycopene.

Observational epidemiologic studies in many countries have shown that the risk for some types of cancer is lower in people who have diets high in tomato products or who have higher levels of lycopene in their blood. Studies suggest that diets rich in tomatoes may account for this reduction in risk. Evidence is strongest for lycopene's protective effect against cancer of the lung, stomach, and prostate. It may also help protect against cancer of the cervix, breast, mouth, pancreas, esophagus, colon, and rectum.

Some observational epidemiologic studies have found that a diet high in lycopene from tomato-based foods was linked with a lower risk for prostate cancer. Other studies, however,

IT'S ALL IN THE LABEL

How can you determine the nutritional value of vegetables and fruits? For frozen and canned items, you can look at the Nutrition Facts panel on the side or back label. For fresh vegetables and fruits, your market may display posters created by the U.S. Food and Drug Administration (FDA), giving nutritional information for these foods. The FDA also makes this information available on its Web site (www.fda.gov). This information may appear on the labels of packaged fresh vegetables and fruits or on posters or brochures in the produce area.

The nutrition information lists the kinds and amounts of important nutrients in a serving of a vegetable or fruit and gives the Percent Daily Value, which shows how much those amounts contribute to the daily diet. Some information is required: such as the amount of fat, fiber, vitamins A and C, iron and calcium. Some labels will carry additional information, such as the amount of folic acid and iron.

You can quickly find vegetables and fruits that provide the nutrients you need by looking for short descriptive terms on the front, side, or back of the food label. For example, an orange juice label may say "provides 100 percent of the Daily Value for vitamin C." (Do not confuse this statement with "100 percent fruit juice." A product can contain 100 percent of the Daily Value for vitamin C and not be 100 percent juice.) These claims refer to the contents of one serving.

Less frequently, you may see longer claims describing the relationship between the food or a nutrient in the food to a certain disease or medical condition.

Only claims approved by the FDA can be used in food labeling. These approved health claims pertain to vegetables and fruits:

- Vegetables and fruits may help lower the risk of some cancers.
- Fruits, vegetables, and grain products that contain fiber, particularly soluble fiber, may help reduce the risk of coronary heart disease.

In addition, in the spring of 1996, the FDA approved a claim stating that a diet with adequate folic acid may reduce the risk of certain birth defects. This claim might appear, for example, on labels of orange juice, Brussels sprouts, asparagus, tomato juice, and dried beans—foods that are excellent or good sources of folic acid.

found no link between tomato products or other lycopene-rich foods and prostate cancer. A recent study suggested that variation in a particular gene (known as XRCC1) that helps repair damaged DNA can influence whether lycopene intake will affect a man's prostate cancer risk.

Since tomatoes also contain vitamins, potassium, and other carotenoids and antioxidants, it is possible that other compounds in tomatoes, either alone or in combination with lycopene, may be responsible for some of the protective effects attributed to lycopene in some studies. When researchers look at large groups with different lifestyles and habits, their findings also may be explained by other factors that were not examined.

A 2004 review of twenty-one observational studies concluded that tomato products appear to have a weak protective effect against prostate cancer. This review did not include lycopene supplements, only tomato and tomato-based foods. Some of the individual studies, however, did consider lycopene levels in the blood. The analysis noted that the protective effect was slightly stronger for cooked tomato products and that small amounts of added fat improved lycopene absorption. On the other hand, two studies from 2007, one of about fifteen hundred men and the second of more than twenty-eight thousand men, found no difference in blood lycopene levels between those in whom prostate cancer later developed and those in whom it did not.

There have been several experimental studies on the role of lycopene in preventing or treating cancer. One animal study found that lycopene treatment reduced the growth of brain tumors. Another animal study showed that frequent intake of lycopene over a long period considerably suppressed breast tumor growth in mice. However, breast cancer in humans is very different from breast cancer in mice, and those results may not apply to the disease in humans. In laboratory studies, lycopene has also been shown to interfere with the growth of many different types of human cancer cells growing in test tubes or petri dishes, especially those that grow in response to insulin-like growth factor I. Laboratory and animal studies can suggest possible helpful effects, but they do not provide proof that such effects can be achieved in humans. Further studies are needed to find out if possible anticancer properties could benefit humans.

To test whether lycopene is the main cancer-fighting substance in tomatoes, one animal study compared lycopene supplements with powdered tomatoes. Groups of rats who were fed tomato powder were compared with rats given lycopene. The rats that received tomato powder had a much lower cancer risk, whereas the rats receiving lycopene supplements did not differ significantly from the group that received no special supplements.

A few controlled studies on the affects of lycopene in humans have recently been published, and additional studies are under way. More clinical information is needed, however, to determine whether lycopene-rich foods can be helpful in preventing or treating cancer. All of the clinical trials completed so far have reported relatively short-term effects on the level of prostate-specific antigen (PSA) in the blood, which is generally considered a good indicator of prostate cancer growth. Although these studies are an important step, they are not as valuable as long-term studies that determine whether a treatment actually helps patients live longer or relieves their symptoms.

One study assigned men at high risk for prostate cancer to take an ordinary multivitamin either with or without a lycopene supplement and found no difference in PSA levels between the two groups. A controlled study in a small group of men with prostate cancer found that lycopene supplements appeared to reduce the rapid growth of prostate cancer cells. However, a more recent study with men whose prostate cancer had stopped responding to hormonal therapy found that a tomato-based lycopene-containing supplement did not have a significant effect. One short-term study from 2006 reported that lycopene supplements were safe, but that they did not lower the PSA levels in men with recurrent prostate cancer. Another reported that the combination of lycopene and soy supplements prevented PSA levels from increasing in some men with prostate cancer.

Possible Problems or Complications

Lycopene, when obtained from eating fruits and vegetables, has no known side effects and is thought to be safe for humans. The potential side effects of lycopene supplements are not fully known. Patients in one study who took a lycopene-rich tomato supplement of fifteen milligrams twice a day had some intestinal side effects such as nausea, vomiting, diarrhea, indigestion, gas, and bloating. When consumed over a long period, very large amounts of tomato products can give the skin an orange color.

Bottom Line

Supplements containing antioxidants such as lycopene may interfere with radiation therapy and chemotherapy if taken during cancer treatment. Although studies have not been done in people undergoing treatment, antioxidants are known to help prevent the harmful effects of free radicals, which could interfere with one of the methods by which chemotherapy and radiation therapy destroy cancer cells. Eating fruits and vegetables high in antioxidants is still considered safe during cancer treatment. As with any dietary supplementation, tell your doctor if you are taking supplements containing lycopene or other antioxidants. If you have concerns, talk with your doctor and your health care team.

NONI PLANT

The noni or morinda plant is a tropical evergreen tree that grows in Tahiti and other Pacific Islands, as well as in parts of Asia, Australia, South America, and the Caribbean. The tree can grow to as tall as ten feet and bears a fruit about the size of a potato, which starts out green and ripens into yellow or white. The juice, fruit, bark, and leaves are used in herbal remedies and Polynesian folk medicine.

The Claim

Eating noni fruit or drinking noni juice can prevent or cure cancer.

The Evidence

Several animal and laboratory experiments have been done on different compounds taken from the noni plant. A group of Hawaiian researchers caused tumors to grow in mice and then injected specially prepared noni juice into their abdomens. Mice who received the treatment survived twice as long as the untreated mice. Other scientists studying freeze-dried extract from the roots of the plant found that the substance appeared to prevent pain and induce sleep in mice.

Another team of investigators reported that damnacanthal, a compound removed from the root of the noni plant, may inhibit a chemical process that turns normal cells into cancer cells. However, since extracted chemicals or substances are different from the raw plant, a study of an extract might not produce the same result as a study using the whole plant. In addition, while animal and laboratory studies may show a certain substance holds promise as a helpful treatment, further studies are necessary to learn whether the results apply to humans.

An early (phase I) clinical trial of freeze-dried noni fruit extract was done on twenty-nine patients at the University of Hawaii to learn about its actions and toxicities in people with cancer. This study found no toxic effects on patients even at daily doses of ten grams, but it also found that there was no significant effect on quality of life. It was noted, however, that those who got higher doses reported feeling somewhat better. In addition, researchers at Louisiana State University are working to isolate and purify any compounds in the juice that may be active in humans so that further testing can be done.

Possible Problems and Complications

The safety and long-term effects of noni juice and other noni products are not well known. A few cases of liver problems have been reported in people taking noni in European countries. One of these patients had previous liver damage and required a liver transplant, but the others recovered when noni was stopped. Three cases of acute liver inflammation (hepatitis) in people using noni products have been reported, although other herbal products they were using may have been responsible or may have interacted with noni ingredients. Further information is needed to find out the cause of these problems.

The juice has a significant amount of potassium, equivalent to a similar amount of tomato juice or orange juice, and it may pose problems for people with kidney disease and others who must restrict their potassium intake. Noni products are also high in sugar (natural fruit sugar and added sugar), which must be considered for people with diabetes and others restricting their calorie intake. Be aware that consumption of this juice may cause the urine to turn a pink or reddish color. Noni juice and supplements have not been studied in pregnant or breastfeeding women.

Bottom Line

To date, there is no reliable clinical evidence that noni juice or its fruit is effective in preventing or treating cancer or any other disease in humans. Although animal and laboratory studies have shown some positive effects, human studies are just beginning. Research is under way to isolate various compounds in the noni plant so that further testing can be done to learn whether they may be useful in humans. More research is needed before it can be determined what role, if any, noni plant compounds may play in the treatment of cancer or other health conditions.

BERRIES (ELLAGIC ACID)

Ellagic acid is a phytochemical, or plant chemical, found in raspberries, strawberries, cranberries, walnuts, pecans, pomegranates, and other plant foods. The highest levels of ellagic acid are found in raspberries, strawberries, and pomegranates, especially when they are freeze-dried. Extracts from red raspberry leaves or seeds, pomegranates, or other sources are said to contain high levels of ellagic acid and are available as dietary supplements in capsule, powder, or liquid form. The best dose of these preparations is not known.

The Claim

Eating berries or using ellagic acid can prevent or cure cancer.

The Evidence

Ellagic acid seems to have some anticancer properties. It can act as an antioxidant and has been found to cause cell death in cancer cells in the laboratory. In other laboratory studies, ellagic acid seems to reduce the effect of estrogen in promoting growth of breast cancer cells in tissue cultures. There are also reports that it may help the liver break down or remove some cancer-causing substances from the blood.

Some supporters have claimed these results mean that ellagic acid can prevent or treat cancer in humans. This claim has not been proved. Unfortunately, many substances that show promise against cancer in laboratory and animal studies are not found to be useful in people. Ellagic acid has also been said to reduce heart disease, birth defects, liver problems, and to promote wound healing.

Almost all studies conducted on ellagic acid have been done in cell cultures or laboratory animals. Several animal studies have found that ellagic acid can inhibit the growth of tumors of the skin, esophagus, and lung, as well as other tumors caused by carcinogens. Other studies have also found positive effects. A recent study in cell cultures found that ellagic acid may act against substances that help tumors form new blood vessels (angiogenesis). Further studies are needed to determine whether these results apply to humans.

In the only study reported thus far in humans, Italian researchers found that ellagic acid seemed to reduce the side effects of chemotherapy in men with advanced prostate cancer, although it did not slow disease progression or improve survival. The researchers cautioned that more research would be needed to confirm these results.

The interaction between phytochemicals like ellagic acid and other compounds in foods is not well understood, but it is unlikely that any single compound offers the best protection against cancer. A balanced diet that includes five or more servings a day of fruits and vegetables, along with foods from a variety of other plant sources such as nuts, seeds, whole grain cereals, and beans is likely to be more effective in reducing cancer risk than eating one particular food in large amounts. However, some studies suggest that foods high in ellagic acid might be useful additions to a balanced diet. For example, one nonrandomized clinical study of men with prostate cancer reported that pomegranate juice slowed the increase in blood levels of prostate-specific antigen, a substance that is routinely measured to estimate growth of prostate cancer.

BERRY AND CHERRY GOODNESS
Researchers have discovered, that cranberries, black currants, lingonberries (related to cranberries), bilberries (which are like blueberries), and sweet and sour cherries contain high levels of a flavonoid called quercetin as well as anthocyanins that may fight cancer. Onions, green beans, lettuce, and rhubarb (as well as red wine) are other sources of quercetin. In laboratory studies, quercetin and the anthocyanins that give berries and cherries their intense color have been shown to be powerful antioxidants. Berries also contain fiber, vitamin C, other flavonoids, and other compounds that may inhibit the growth of certain types of human tumors. Many of the antioxidants in berries are destroyed when they are cooked, although cooked berries are still rich in other nutrients.

Possible Problems or Complications

Ellagic acid is available in supplement form. Some reports indicate that it may affect certain enzymes in the liver, which could alter the way in which some drugs are absorbed in the body. For this reason, people taking medicines or other dietary supplements should talk with their doctors or pharmacists about all their medicines and supplements before taking ellagic acid. The raspberry leaf, or preparations made from it, should be used with caution during pregnancy because it may initiate labor.

Bottom Line

Eating berries or other natural sources of ellagic acid is generally considered safe. These foods should be part of a balanced diet that includes several servings of vegetables and fruits each day. As with any dietary supplementation, tell your doctor if you are taking supplements containing ellagic acid. If you have concerns, talk with your doctor and your health care team.

Phytochemical Power

The term phytochemicals refers to a wide variety of compounds found naturally in fruits, vegetables, beans, grains, and other plants. Scientists have identified thousands of phytochemicals. Some of the more commonly known phytochemicals include carotenoids, vitamin C, folic acid, and anthocyanins. Recently, there has been a movement to rename these phytochemicals "bioactive food compounds" to place more emphasis on their health-promoting activities in the body rather than their chemical structure.

There is growing evidence that phytochemicals may help prevent the formation of potential cancer-causing substances, block the action of carcinogens on their target organs or tissue, or act on cells to suppress cancer development. Some scientists estimate that people can reduce their risk of cancer by 30 to 40 percent simply by eating more vegetables and other plant foods that are rich in these compounds.

Much of the evidence about the powerful effects of phytochemicals comes from observations of cultures where the diet consists mainly of plant sources and where there are noticeably lower rates of certain types of cancer and heart disease. Some of the associations between individual phytochemicals and cancer risk are very compelling and make a very strong case for additional investigation. To date, none of the findings are conclusive, and it remains to be determined which of the numerous compounds in vegetables and fruits actively help the body fight disease. Until conclusive research findings emerge, most health care professionals advise a balanced diet with emphasis on a wide variety of vegetables, fruits, legumes, and whole grains.

Phytochemicals are present in almost every vegetable, fruit, legume, or whole grain we eat, but they are most concentrated in brightly colored plant foods. For instance, a carrot contains more than one hundred different phytochemicals. According to one estimate, more than four thousand phytochemicals have been identified, but only about one hundred fifty have been studied in detail. The information below outlines a few of the phytochemicals researchers have studied.

There is no evidence that taking phytochemical supplements is as beneficial as consuming the vegetables, fruits, beans, and grains from which they are isolated.

Polyphenols, Flavonoids, and Phytoestrogens

There are several major groups of phytochemicals. One group, the polyphenols, includes a sub-group of chemicals called flavonoids. These plant chemicals are found in a range of grains, vegetables, and fruits. The flavonoids found in soy products, chickpeas, licorice, and tea may mimic the actions of estrogen (a female sex hormone linked to the growth of some cancers, such as some types of breast cancer). Estrogen-like substances from these plant sources are called phytoestrogens. Most phytoestrogens are present in foods in small amounts and are relatively weak, and not all flavonoids are phytoestrogens. Flavonoids are being studied to determine whether they can prevent chronic diseases such as cancer and heart disease.

Antioxidants

Antioxidants protect the body's cells against free radicals (byproducts of the body's normal processes), which can damage a cell's DNA and are thought to trigger some forms of cancer and other diseases.

Antioxidants such as vitamin C, indoles, and carotenoids are found in broccoli, Brussels sprouts, cabbage, cauliflower, tomatoes, carrots, mangoes, sweet potatoes, soybeans, cantaloupe, oranges, spinach, nuts, leafy lettuce, fish oil, seeds, grains, and black and green tea. A good way to take in more antioxidants is to eat a variety of richly colored vegetables and fruits, which, in general, contain higher levels of antioxidants and other phytochemicals than less colorful ones.

Carotenoids and Anthocyanins

Carotenoids give carrots, yams, cantaloupe, butternut squash, and apricots their orange color and also are promoted as anticancer agents. Tomatoes, red peppers, and red grapefruit contain the carotenoid lycopene, which is a powerful antioxidant (see the Tomatoes section on page 61 for more information about lycopene).

Grapes, eggplant, red cabbage, and radishes all contain anthocyanins—phytochemicals that protect against cancer and heart disease. Ellagic acid, found in raspberries, blackberries, cranberries, strawberries, and walnuts, also is said to have anticancer effects. Plant growers are currently developing a number of vegetables and fruits to help promote higher intake of phytochemicals, including tomatoes that are higher in lycopene, purple carrots that are rich in carotenoids and anthocyanins, and purple potatoes that are rich in anthocyanins.

Sulfides

A group of phytochemicals called sulfides are found in garlic and onions. Sulfides may reduce the risk for stomach and colorectal cancers, lower blood pressure, and strengthen the immune system.

References

About herbs, botanicals, & other products, Memorial Sloan-Kettering Information Resource Database. Memorial Sloan-Kettering Cancer Center Web site. http://www.mskcc.org/aboutherbs. Accessed December 4, 2009.

Ahn D, Putt D, Kresty L, Stoner GD, Fromm D, Hollenberg PF. The effects of dietary ellagic acid on rat hepatic and esophageal mucosal cytochromes P450 and phase II enzymes. *Carcinogenesis.* 1996;17(4):821-828.

Allred CD, Allred KF, Ju YH, Virant SM, Helferich WG. Soy diets containing varying amounts of genistein stimulate growth of estrogen-dependent (MCF-7) tumors in a dose-dependent manner. *Cancer Res.* 2001;61(13):5045-5050.

American Cancer Society. *American Cancer Society Complete Guide to Complementary and Alternative Cancer Therapies.* 2nd ed. Atlanta, GA: American Cancer Society; 2009.

Anderson J, Deskins B. *The Nutrition Bible: A Comprehensive, No-Nonsense Guide to Foods, Nutrients, Additives, Preservatives, Pollutants and Everything Else We Eat and Drink.* New York: William Morrow and Company, Inc; 1995.

Attorneys general curb claims for "tahitian noni." Quackwatch Web site. http://www.quackwatch.org/04ConsumerEducation/News/noni.html. Updated September 12, 2002. Accessed December 4, 2009.

Bagga D, Capone S, Wang HJ, Heber D, Lill M, Chap L, Glaspy JA. Dietary modulation of omega-3/omega-6 polyunsaturated fatty acid ratios in patients with breast cancer. *J Natl Cancer Inst.* 1997;89(15):1123-1131.

Baliga MS, Meleth S, Katiyar SK. Growth inhibitory and antimetastatic effect of green tea polyphenols on metastasis-specific mouse mammary carcinoma 4T1 cells in vitro and in vivo systems. *Clin Cancer Res.* 2005;11(5):1918-1927.

Basch E, Bent S, Collins J, Dacey C, Hammerness P, Harrison M, Smith M, Szapary P, Ulbricht C, Vora M, Weissner W; Natural Standard Resource Collaboration. Flax and flaxseed oil (*Linum usitatissimum*): a review by the Natural Standard Research Collaboration. *J Soc Integr Oncol.* 2007;5(3):92-105.

Bell MC, Crowley-Nowick P, Bradlow HL, Sepkovic DW, Schmidt-Grimminger D, Howell P, Mayeaux EJ, Tucker A, Turbat-Herrera EA, Mathis JM. Placebo-controlled trial of indole-3-carbinol in the treatment of CIN. *Gynecol Oncol.* 2000;78(2):123-129.

Bergman Jungestrom M, Thompson LU, Dabrosin C. Flaxseed and its lignans inhibit estradiol-induced growth, angiogenesis, and secretion of vascular endothelial growth factor in human breast cancer xenografts in vivo. *Clin Cancer Res.* 2007;13(3):1061-1067.

Blumenthal M, ed. *The Complete German Commission E Monographs: Therapeutic Guide to Herbal Medicines.* Austin, TX: American Botanical Council; 1998.

Boileau TW, Liao Z, Kim S, Lemeshow S, Erdman JW Jr, Clinton SK. Prostate carcinogenesis in N-methyl-N-nitrosourea (NMU)-testosterone-treated rats fed tomato powder, lycopene, or energy-restricted diets. *J Natl Cancer Inst*. 2003;95(21):1578-1586.

Borchers AT, Keen CL, Gershwin ME. Mushrooms, tumors, and immunity: an update. *Exp Biol Med* (*Maywood*). 2004;229(5):393-406.

Borchers AT, Stern JS, Hackman RM, Keen CL, Gershwin ME. Mushrooms, tumors, and immunity. *Proc Soc Exp Biol Med*. 1999;221(4):281-293.

Borrelli F, Capasso R, Aviello G, Pittler MH, Izzo AA. Effectiveness and safety of ginger in the treatment of pregnancy-induced nausea and vomiting. *Obstet Gynecol*. 2005;105(4):849-856.

Brennan P, Hsu CC, Moullan N, Szeszenia-Dabrowska N, Lissowska J, Zaridze D, Rudnai P, Fabianova E, Mates D, Bencko V, Foretova L, Janout V, Gemignani F, Chabrier A, Hall J, Hung RJ, Boffetta P, Canzian F. Effect of cruciferous vegetables on lung cancer in patients stratified by genetic status: a mendelian randomisation approach. *Lancet*. 2005;366(9496):1558-1560.

Bunker CH, McDonald AC, Evans RW, de la Rosa N, Boumosleh JM, Patrick AL. A randomized trial of lycopene supplementation in Tobago men with high prostate cancer risk. *Nutr Cancer*. 2007;57(2):130-137.

Burns CP, Halabi S, Clamon G, Kaplan E, Hohl RJ, Atkins JN, Schwartz MA, Wagner BA, Paskett E. Phase II study of high-dose fish oil capsules for patients with cancer-related cachexia. *Cancer*. 2004;101(2):370-378.
    Comment in:
    Cancer. 2005;103(3):651-652.

Campbell JK, Canene-Adams K, Lindshield BL, Boileau TW, Clinton SK, Erdman JW Jr. Tomato phytochemicals and prostate cancer risk. *J Nutr*. 2004;134(12 Suppl):3486S-3492S.

Cao G, Booth SL, Sadowski JA, Prior RL. Increases in human plasma antioxidant capacity after consumption of controlled diets high in fruit and vegetables. *Am J Clin Nutr*. 1998;68(5):1081-1087.

Chen J, Hui E, Ip T, Thompson LU. Dietary flaxseed enhances the inhibitory effect of tamoxifen on the growth of estrogen-dependent human breast cancer (mcf-7) in nude mice. *Clin Cancer Res*. 2004;10(22):7703-7711.

Chen J, Power KA, Mann J, Cheng A, Thompson LU. Flaxseed alone or in combination with tamoxifen inhibits MCF-7 breast tumor growth in ovariectomized athymic mice with high circulating levels of estrogen. *Exp Biol Med* (*Maywood*). 2007;232(8):1071-1080.

Chen J, Stavro PM, Thompson LU. Dietary flaxseed inhibits human breast cancer growth and metastasis and downregulates expression of insulin-like growth factor and epidermal growth factor receptor. *Nutr Cancer*. 2002;43(2):187-192.

Chen J, Wang L, Thompson LU. Flaxseed and its components reduce metastasis after surgical excision of solid human breast tumor in nude mice. *Cancer Lett*. 2006;234(2):168-175.

Chen S, Oh SR, Phung S, Hur G, Ye JJ, Kwok SL, Shrode GE, Belury M, Adams LS, Williams D. Anti-aromatase activity of phytochemicals in white button mushrooms (*Agaricus bisporus*). *Cancer Res*. 2006;66(24):12026-12034.

Chihara G, Hamuro J, Maeda Y, Shiio T, Suga T, Takasuka N, Sasaki T. Antitumor and metastasis-inhibitory activities of lentinan as an immunomodulator: an overview. *Cancer Detect Prev Suppl.* 1987;1:423-443.

Chung R. Functional properties of edible mushrooms. *Nutr Rev.* 1996;54(11 Pt 2):S91-S93.

Clark PE, Hall MC, Borden LS Jr, Miller AA, Hu JJ, Lee WR, Stindt D, D'Agostino R Jr, Lovato J, Harmon M, Torti FM. Phase I-II prospective dose-escalating trial of lycopene in patients with biochemical relapse of prostate cancer after definitive local therapy. *Urology.* 2006;67(6):1257-1261.

Colomer R, Moreno-Nogueira JM, García-Luna PP, García-Peris P, García-de-Lorenzo A, Zarazaga A, Quecedo L, del Llano J, Usán L, Casimiro C. N-3 fatty acids, cancer and cachexia: a systematic review of the literature. *Br J Nutr.* 2007;97(5):823-831.

Cover CM, Hsieh SJ, Tran SH, Hallden G, Kim GS, Bjeldanes LF, Firestone GL. Indole-3-carbinol inhibits the expression of cyclin-dependent kinase-6 and induces a G1 cell cycle arrest of human breast cancer cells independent of estrogen receptor signaling. *J Biol Chem.* 1998;273(7):3838-3847.

Covington MB. Omega-3 fatty acids. *Am Fam Physician.* 2004;70(1):133-140.

Cunningham-Rundles S, Lin H, Cassileth B. Are botanical glucans effective in enhancing tumoricidal cell activity? American Society for Nutrition. *J Nutr.* 2005;135:2919S.

Cyber letters. US Food and Drug Administration Web site. http://www.fda.gov/Drugs/GuidanceCompliance RegulatoryInformation/EnforcementActivitiesbyFDA/CyberLetters/default.htm Accessed December 5, 2009.

Dalais FS, Meliala A, Wattanapenpaiboon N, Frydenberg M, Suter DA, Thomson WK, Wahlqvist ML. Effects of a diet rich in phytoestrogens on prostate-specific antigen and sex hormones in men diagnosed with prostate cancer. *Urology.* 2004;64(3):510-515.

Davis CD, Swanson CA, Ziegler RG, Clevidence B, Dwyer JT, Milner JA. Executive Summary Report: Promises and Perils of Lycopene/Tomato Supplementation and Cancer Prevention. Conference proceedings. Division of Cancer Epidemiology and Genetics. National Cancer Institute Web site. http://dceg.cancer.gov/pdfs/davis1352014s2005.pdf. Accessed December 5, 2009.

de Lorgeril M, Salen P, Martin JL, Monjaud I, Boucher P, Mamelle N. Mediterranean dietary pattern in a randomized trial: prolonged survival and possible reduced cancer rate. *Arch Intern Med.* 1998;158(11):1181-1187.

Demark-Wahnefried W, Price DT, Polascik TJ, Robertson CN, Anderson EE, Paulson DF, Walther PJ, Gannon M, Vollmer RT. Pilot study of dietary fat restriction and flaxseed supplementation in men with prostate cancer before surgery: exploring the effects on hormonal levels, prostate-specific antigen, and histopathologic features. *Urology.* 2001;58(1):47-52.

Demark-Wahnefried W, Robertson CN, Walther PJ, Polascik TJ, Paulson DF, Vollmer RT. Pilot study to explore effects of low-fat, flaxseed-supplemented diet on proliferation of benign prostatic epithelium and prostate-specific antigen. *Urology.* 2004;63(5):900-904.

deVere White RW, Hackman RM, Soares SE, Beckett LA, Sun B. Effects of a mushroom mycelium extract on the treatment of prostate cancer. *Urology.* 2002;60(4):640-644.

Dewey A, Baughan C, Dean T, Higgins B, Johnson I. Eicosapentaenoic acid (EPA, an omega-3 fatty acid from fish oils) for the treatment of cancer cachexia. *Cochrane Database Syst Rev.* 2007;(1):CD004597.

Dorant E, van den Brandt PA, Goldbohm RA. Allium vegetable consumption, garlic supplement intake, and female breast carcinoma incidence. *Breast Cancer Res Treat.* 1995;33(2):163-170.

Doyle C, Kushi LH, Byers T, Courneya KS, Demark-Wahnefried W, Grant B, McTiernan A, Rock CL, Thompson C, Gansler T, Andrews KS; The 2006 Nutrition, Physical Activity and Cancer Survivorship Advisory Committee; American Cancer Society. Nutrition and physical activity during and after cancer treatment: an American Cancer Society guide for informed choices. *CA Cancer J Clin.* 2006;56(6):323-353.

Ellagic acid. Memorial Sloan-Kettering Cancer Center Web site. http://www.mskcc.org/mskcc/html/11571.cfm? RecordID=644&tab=HC. Accessed December 5, 2009.

Erlund I, Marniemi J, Hakala P, Alfthan G, Meririnne E, Aro A. Consumption of black currants, lingonberries and bilberries increases serum quercetin concentrations. *Eur J Clin Nutr.* 2003;57(1):37-42.

Etminan M, Takkouche B, Caamaño-Isorna F. The role of tomato products and lycopene in the prevention of prostate cancer: a meta-analysis of observational studies. *Cancer Epidemiol Biomarkers Prev.* 2004;13(3):340-345.

Fahey JW, Zhang Y, Talalay P. Broccoli sprouts: an exceptionally rich source of inducers of enzymes that protect against chemical carcinogens. *Proc Natl Acad Sci U S A.* 1997;94(19):10367-10372.

Falsaperla M, Morgia G, Tartarone A, Ardito R, Romano G. Support ellagic acid therapy in patients with hormone refractory prostate cancer (HRPC) on standard chemotherapy using vinorelbine and estramustine phosphate. *Eur Urol.* 2005;47(4):449-454; discussion 454-455.

Fang N, Li Q, Yu S, Zhang J, He L, Ronis MJ, Badger TM. Inhibition of growth and induction of apoptosis in human cancer cell lines by an ethyl acetate fraction from shiitake mushrooms. *J Altern Complement Med.* 2006;12(2):125-132.

Fish and omega-3 fatty acids. American Heart Association Web site. http://www.americanheart.org/presenter. jhtml?identifier=4632. Accessed December 5, 2009.

Fish, levels of mercury and omega-3 fatty acids. American Heart Association Web site. http://www.americanheart. org/presenter.jhtml?identifier=3013797. Accessed December 5, 2009.

Flaxseed. Memorial Sloan-Kettering Cancer Center Web site. http://www.mskcc.org/mskcc/html/69220.cfm. Accessed December 5, 2009.

Fleischauer AT, Arab L. Garlic and cancer: a critical review of the epidemiologic literature. *J Nutr.* 2001;131(3s):1032S-1040S.

Fournier DB, Erdman JW Jr, Gordon GB. Soy, its components, and cancer prevention: a review of the in vitro, animal, and human data. *Cancer Epidemiol Biomarkers Prev.* 1998;7(11):1055-1065.

Fruit and vegetable benefits. Fruits and Veggies Matter Web site. http://www.fruitsandveggiesmatter.gov/ benefits/index.html. Accessed December 4, 2009.

Galeone C, Pelucchi C, Levi F, Negri E, Franceschi S, Talamini R, Giacosa A, La Vecchia C. Onion and garlic use and human cancer. *Am J Clin Nutr*. 2006;84(5):1027-1032.

Ganmaa D, Willett WC, Li TY, Feskanich D, van Dam RM, Lopez-Garcia E, Hunter DJ, Holmes MD. Coffee, tea, caffeine and risk of breast cancer: a 22-year follow-up. *Int J Cancer*. 2008;122(9):2071-2076.

Gao YT, McLaughlin JK, Blot WJ, Ji BT, Dai Q, Fraumeni JF Jr. Reduced risk of esophageal cancer associated with green tea consumption. *J Natl Cancer Inst*. 1994;86(11):855-858.

Gardner CD, Lawson LD, Block E, Chatterjee LM, Kiazand A, Balise RR, Kraemer HC. Effect of raw garlic vs commercial garlic supplements on plasma lipid concentrations in adults with moderate hypercholesterolemia: a randomized clinical trial. *Arch Intern Med*. 2007;167(4):346-353.

Garlic. Memorial Sloan-Kettering Cancer Center Web site. http://www.mskcc.org/mskcc/html/69230.cfm. Accessed December 5, 2009.

Garlic. National Center for Complementary and Alternative Medicine Web site. http://nccam.nih.gov/health/garlic/. Accessed December 5, 2009.

Garlic. PDRhealth Web site. http://www.pdrhealth.com/drug_info/nmdrugprofiles/herbaldrugs/101190.shtml. Accessed December 5, 2009.

Geelen A, Schouten JM, Kamphuis C, Stam BE, Burema J, Renkema JM, Bakker EJ, van't Veer P, Kampman E. Fish consumption, n-3 fatty acids, and colorectal cancer: a meta-analysis of prospective cohort studies. *Am J Epidemiol*. 2007;166(10):1116-1125.

Gerster H. The potential role of lycopene for human health. *J Am Coll Nutr*. 1997;16(2):109-126.

Ginger. Memorial Sloan-Kettering Cancer Center Web site. http://www.mskcc.org/mskcc/html/69234.cfm. Accessed December 5, 2009.

Giovannucci E. Tomatoes, tomato-based products, lycopene, and cancer: review of the epidemiologic literature. *J Natl Cancer Inst*. 1999;91(4):317-331.

Godley PA, Campbell MK, Gallagher P, Martinson FE, Mohler JL, Sandler RS. Biomarkers of essential fatty acid consumption and risk of prostatic carcinoma. *Cancer Epidemiol Biomarkers Prev*. 1996;5(11):889-895.

Gogos CA, Ginopoulos P, Salsa B, Apostolidou E, Zoumbos NC, Kalfarentzos F. Dietary omega-3 polyunsaturated fatty acids plus vitamin E restore immunodeficiency and prolong survival for severely ill patients with generalized malignancy. *Cancer*. 1998;82(2):395-402.

González CA, Pera G, Agudo A, Bueno-de-Mesquita HB, Ceroti M, Boeing H, Schultz M, Del Giudice G, Plebani M, Carneiro F, Berrino F, Sacerdote C, Tumino R, Panico S, Berglund G, Simán H, Hallmans G, Stenling R, Martinez C, Dorronsoro M, Barricarte A, Navarro C, Quiros JR, Allen N, Key TJ, Bingham S, Day NE, Linseisen J, Nagel G, Overad K, Jensen MK, Olsen A, Tjønneland A, Büchner FL, Peeters PH, Numans ME, Clavel-Chapelon F, Boutron-Ruault MC, Roukos D, Trichopoulou A, Psaltopoulou T, Lund E, Casagrande C, Slimani N, Jenab M, Riboli E. Fruit and vegetable intake and the risk of stomach and oesophagus adenocarcinoma in the European Prospective Investigation into Cancer and Nutrition (EPIC-EURGAST). *Int J Cancer*. 2006;118(10):2559-2566.

Goodman M, Bostick RM, Ward KC, Terry PD, van Gils CH, Taylor JA, Mandel JS. Lycopene intake and prostate cancer risk: effect modification by plasma antioxidants and the XRCC1 genotype. *Nutr Cancer.* 2006;55(1):13-20.

Green tea. Memorial Sloan-Kettering Cancer Center Web site. http://www.mskcc.org/mskcc/html/69247.cfm. Updated October 21, 2009. Accessed December 5, 2009.

Gruenwald J, Brendler T, Jaenicke C, eds. *PDR for Herbal Medicines.* 4th ed. Montvale, NJ: Thomson Healthcare; 2007.

Guha N, Kwan ML, Quesenberry CP Jr, Weltzien EK, Castillo AL, Caan BJ. Soy isoflavones and risk of cancer recurrence in a cohort of breast cancer survivors: the Life After Cancer Epidemiology study [published online ahead of print February 17, 2009]. *Breast Cancer Res Treat.*

Haggans CJ, Hutchins AM, Olson BA, Thomas W, Martini MC, Slavin JL. Effect of flaxseed consumption on urinary estrogen metabolites in postmenopausal women. *Nutr Cancer.* 1999;33(2):188-195.

Harttig U, Hendricks JD, Stoner GD, Bailey GS. Organ specific, protocol dependent modulation of 7,12-dimethylbenz-[a]anthracene carcinogenesis in rainbow trout (Oncorhyncus mykiss) by dietary ellagic acid. *Carcinogenesis.* 1996;17(11):2403-2409.

Henkel J. Soy: health claims for soy protein, questions about other components. *FDA Consumer Magazine.* May-June 2000. US Food and Drug Administration Web site. http://www.fda.gov/fdac/features/2000/300_soy.html. Accessed June 10, 2008. Content no longer available.

Hiramatsu T, Imoto M, Koyano T, Umezawa K. Induction of normal phenotypes in ras-transformed cells by damnacanthal from Morinda citrifolia. *Cancer Lett.* 1993;73(2-3):161-166.

Hirazumi A, Furusawa E. An immunomodulatory polysaccha-ride-rich substance from the fruit juice of Morinda citrifolia (noni) with antitumor activity. *Phytother Res.* 1999;13(5):380-387.

Hirazumi A, Furusawa E, Chou SC, Hokama Y. Anticancer activity of Morinda citrifolia (noni) on intraperitoneally implanted Lewis lung carcinoma in syngeneic mice. *Proc West Pharmacol Soc.* 1994;37:145-146.

Hites RA, Foran JA, Carpenter DO, Hamilton MC, Knuth BA, Schwager SJ. Global assessment of organic contaminants in farmed salmon. *Science.* 2004;303(5655):226-229.

Hong SA, Kim K, Nam SJ, Kong G, Kim MK. A case-control study on the dietary intake of mushrooms and breast cancer risk among Korean women. *Int J Cancer.* 2008;122(4):919-923.

Hsing AW, Chokkalingam AP, Gao YT, Madigan MP, Deng J, Gridley G, Fraumeni JF Jr. Allium vegetables and risk of prostate cancer: a population-based study. *J Natl Cancer Inst.* 2002;94(21):1648-1651.

Huang YC, Jessup JM, Forse RA, Flickner S, Pleskow D, Anastopoulos HT, Ritter V, Blackburn GL. n-3 fatty acids decrease colonic epithelial cell proliferation in high-risk bowel mucosa. *Lipids.* 1996;31 Suppl:S313-S317.

Ikekawa T, Uehara N, Maeda Y, Nakanishi M, Fukuoka F. Antitumor activity of aqueous extracts of edible mushrooms. *Cancer Res.* 1969;29(3):734-735.

Indole-3-Carbinol. PDRhealth Web site. http://www.pdrhealth.com/drug_info/nmdrugprofiles/nutsupdrugs/ind_0315.shtml. Accessed December 5, 2009.

International Food Information Council Foundation. Functional foods fact sheet: antioxidants. Food Insight Web site. http://www.foodinsight.org/Resources/Detail.aspx?topic=Functional_Foods_Fact_Sheet_Antioxidants. Updated March 2006. Accessed December 5, 2009.

Ishikawa A, Kuriyama S, Tsubono Y, Fukao A, Takahashi H, Tachiya H, Tsuji I. Smoking, alcohol drinking, green tea consumption and the risk of esophageal cancer in Japanese men. *J Epidemiol.* 2006;16(5):185-192.

Issell BF, Gotay C, Pagano I, Franke A. Quality of life measures in a phase I trial of noni. *J Clin Oncol.* 2005 ASCO Annual Meeting Proceedings. Vol 23, No. 16S, Part I of II (June 1 Supplement), 2005:8217.

Jacobsen BK, Knutsen SF, Fraser GE. Does high soy milk intake reduce prostate cancer incidence? The Adventist Health Study (United States). *Cancer Causes Control.* 1998;9(6):553-557.

Janssen PL, Meyboom S, van Staveren WA, de Vegt F, Katan MB. Consumption of ginger (Zingiber officinale roscoe) does not affect ex vivo platelet thromboxane production in humans. *Eur J Clin Nutr.* 1996;50(11):772-774.

Jatoi A, Burch P, Hillman D, Vanyo JM, Dakhil S, Nikcevich D, Rowland K, Morton R, Flynn PJ, Young C, Tan W; North Central Cancer Treatment Group. A tomato-based, lycopene-containing intervention for androgen-independent prostate cancer: results of a Phase II study from the North Central Cancer Treatment Group. *Urology.* 2007;69(2):289-294.

Jatoi A, Ellison N, Burch PA, Sloan JA, Dakhil SR, Novotny P, Tan W, Fitch TR, Rowland KM, Young CY, Flynn PJ. A phase II trial of green tea in the treatment of patients with androgen independent metastatic prostate carcinoma. *Cancer.* 2003;97(6):1442-1446.

Ji BT, Chow WH, Hsing AW, McLaughlin JK, Dai Q, Goa YT, Fraumeni JF Jr. Green tea consumption and the risk of pancreatic and colorectal cancers. *Int J Cancer.* 1997;70(3):255-258.

Jian L, Xie LP, Lee AH, Binns CW. Protective effect of green tea against prostate cancer: a case-control study in southeast China. *Int J Cancer.* 2004;108(1):130-135.

Johansen R. The health food product Noni—does marketing harmonize with the current status of research? [in Norwegian]. *Tidsskrift for Den Norske Laegeforening.* 2008;128(6):694-697.

Karas M, Amir H, Fishman D, Danilenko M, Segal S, Nahum A, Koifmann A, Giat Y, Levy J, Sharoni Y. Lycopene interferes with cell cycle progression and insulin-like growth factor I signaling in mammary cancer cells. *Nutr Cancer.* 2000;36(1):101-111.

Kawaoka T, Yoshino S, Kondo H, Yamamoto K, Hazama S, Oka M. Clinical evaluation of intrapleural or peritoneal repetitive administration of Lentinan and OK-432 for malignant effusion [in Japanese]. *Gan to Kagaku Ryoho [Japanese Journal of Cancer & Chemotherapy].* 2005;32(11):1565-1567.

Kirsh VA, Mayne ST, Peters U, Chatterjee N, Leitzmann MF, Dixon LB, Urban DA, Crawford ED, Hayes RB. A prospective study of lycopene and tomato product intake and risk of prostate cancer. *Cancer Epidemiol Biomarkers Prev.* 2006;15(1):92-98.

Kodoma N, Komuta K, Nanba H. Can maitake MD-fraction aid cancer patients? *Altern Med Rev.* 2002;7(3):236-239.
    Comment in:
    Altern Med Rev. 2002;7(6):236-451; author reply 452-454.

Konno S. Potential growth inhibitory effect of maitake D-fraction on canine cancer cells. *Vet Ther.* 2004;5(4):263-271.

Ko YT, Lin YL. 1,3-beta-glucan quantification by a fluorescence microassay and analysis of its distribution in foods. *J Agric Food Chem.* 2004;52(11):3313-3318.

Kresty LA, Morse MA, Morgan C, Carlton PS, Lu J, Gupta A, Blackwood M, Stoner GD. Chemoprevention of esophageal tumorigenesis by dietary administration of lyophilized black raspberries. *Cancer Res.* 2001;61(16):6112-6119.

Kurahashi N, Sasazuki S, Iwasaki M, Inoue M, Tsugane S; JPHC Study Group. Green tea consumption and prostate cancer risk in Japanese men: a prospective study. *Am J Epidemiol.* 2008;167(1):71-77.

Kuriyama S, Shimazu T, Ohmori K, Kikuchi N, Nakaya N, Nishino Y, Tsubono Y, Tsuji I. Green tea consumption and mortality due to cardiovascular disease, cancer, and all causes in Japan: the Ohsaki study. *JAMA.* 2006;296(10):1255-1265.

Kushi LH, Byers T, Doyle C, Bandera EV, McCullough M, McTiernan A, Gansler T, Andrews KS, Thun MJ; American Cancer Society 2006 Nutrition and Physical Activity Guidelines Advisory Committee. American Cancer Society guidelines on Nutrition and Physical Activity for cancer prevention: reducing the risk of cancer with healthy food choices and physical activity. *CA Cancer J Clin.* 2006;56(5):254-281.

La Vecchia C, Tavani A. Coffee and cancer risk: an update. *Eur J Cancer Prev.* 2007;16(5):385-389.

Labrecque L, Lamy S, Chapus A, Mihoubi S, Durocher Y, Cass B, Bojanowski MW, Gingras D, Béliveau R. Combined inhibition of PDGF and VEGF receptors by ellagic acid, a dietary-derived phenolic compound. *Carcinogenesis.* 2005;26(4):821-826.

Larsson SC, Bergkvist L, Wolk A. Consumption of sugar and sugar-sweetened foods and the risk of pancreatic cancer in a prospective study. *Am J Clin Nutr.* 2006;84(5):1171-1176.

Lawenda BD, Kelly KM, Ladas EJ, Sagar SM, Vickers A, Blumberg JB. Should supplemental antioxidant administration be avoided during chemotherapy and radiation therapy? *J Natl Cancer Inst.* 2008;100(11):773-783.

Lin X, Gingrich JR, Bao W, Li J, Haroon ZA, Demark-Wahnefried W. Effect of flaxseed supplementation on prostatic carcinoma in transgenic mice. *Urology.* 2002;60(5):919-924.

Liu Z, Hornick C, Woltering E. Noni tree: potential cancer preventative, therapy. LSU Agricultural Center Web site. http://www.lsuagcenter.com/en/communications/publications/agmag/Archive/2005/Winter/Noni+Tree+Potential+Cancer+Preventative+Therapy.htm. Updated April 04, 2006. Accessed December 5, 2009.

Lumb AB. Effect of dried ginger on human platelet function. *Thromb Haemost.* 1994;71(1):110-111.

Lycopene: an antioxidant for good health. American Dietetic Association Web site. http://www.eatright.org/cps/rde/xchg/ada/hs.xsl/nutrition_5328_ENU_HTML.htm. Posted 2002. Accessed December 5, 2009.

MacGregor CA, Canney PA, Patterson G, McDonald R, Paul J. A randomised double-blind controlled trial of oral soy supplements versus placebo for treatment of menopausal symptoms in patients with early breast cancer. *Eur J Cancer.* 2005;41(5):708-714.

MacLean CH, Newberry SJ, Mojica WA, Khanna P, Issa AM, Suttorp MJ, Lim YW, Traina SB, Hilton L, Garland R, Morton SC. Effects of Omega-3 fatty acids on cancer risk: a systematic review. *JAMA*. 2006;295(4):403-415.
Erratum in:
JAMA. 2006;295(16):1900.

Mandal S, Stoner GD. Inhibition of N-nitrosobenzylmethylamine-induced esophageal tumorigenesis in rats by ellagic acid. *Carcinogenesis*. 1990;11(1):55-61.

Manusirivithaya S, Sripramote M, Tangjitgamol S, Sheanakul C, Leelahakorn S, Thavaramara T, Tangcharoenpanich K. Antiemetic effect of ginger in gynecologic oncology patients receiving cisplatin. *Int J Gynecol Cancer*. 2004;14(6):1063-1069.

Matsushita K, Kuramitsu Y, Ohiro Y, Obara M, Kobayashi M, Li YQ, Hosokawa M. Combination therapy of active hexose correlated compound plus UFT significantly reduces the metastasis of rat mammary adenocarcinoma. *Anticancer Drugs*. 1998;9(4):343-350.

Meijerman I, Beijen JH, Schellens JH. Herb-drug interactions in oncology: focus on mechanisms of induction. *Oncologist*. 2006;11(7):742-752.

Mertens-Talcott SU, Lee JH, Percival SS, Talcott ST. Induction of cell death in Caco-2 human colon carcinoma cells by ellagic acid rich fractions from muscadine grapes (Vitis rotundifolia). *J Agric Food Chem*. 2006;54(15):5336-5343.

Messina M, Bennink M. Soyfoods, isoflavones and risk of colonic cancer: a review of the in vitro and in vivo data. *Baillieres Clin Endocrinol Metab*. 1998;12(4):707-728.

Messina M. Soy, soy phytoestrogens (isoflavones), and breast cancer. *Am J Clin Nutr*. 1999;70(4):574-575.

Michaud DS, Pietinen P, Taylor PR, Virtanen M, Virtamo J, Albanes D. Intakes of fruits and vegetables, carotenoids and vitamins A, E, C in relation to the risk of bladder cancer in the ATBC cohort study. *Br J Cancer*. 2002;87(9):960-965.

Michaud DS, Spiegelman D, Clinton SK, Rimm EB, Willett WC, Giovannucci EL. Fruit and vegetable intake and incidence of bladder cancer in a male prospective cohort. *J Natl Cancer Inst*. 1999;9(7):605-613.

Miller LG. Herbal medicinals: selected clinical considerations focusing on known or potential drug-herb interactions. *Arch Intern Med*. 1998;158(20):2200-2211.

Millonig G, Stadlmann S, Vogel W. Herbal hepatotoxicity: acute hepatitis caused by a Noni preparation (Morinda citrifolia). *Eur J Gastroenterol Hepatol*. 2005;17(4):445-447.

Moses AW, Slater C, Preston T, Barber MD, Fearon KC. Reduced total energy expenditure and physical activity in cachectic patients with pancreatic cancer can be modulated by an energy and protein dense oral supplement enriched with n-3 fatty acids. *Br J Cancer*. 2004;90(5):996-1002.

Moyad MA. Soy, disease prevention, and prostate cancer. *Semin Urol Oncol*. 1999;17(2):97-102.

Mueller BA, Scott MK, Sowinski KM, Prag KA. Noni juice (Morinda citrifolia): hidden potential for hyperkalemia? *Am J Kidney Dis.* 2000;35(2):310-312.

Comment in:
Am J Kidney Dis. 2000;35(2):330-332.

Mukhtar H, Del Tito BJ Jr, Marcelo CL, Das M, Bickers DR. Ellagic acid: a potent naturally occurring inhibitor of benzo[a]pyrene metabolism and its subsequent glucuronidation, sulfation and covalent binding to DNA in cultured BALB/C mouse keratinocytes. *Carcinogenesis.* 1984;5(12):1565-1571.

Murakami A, Ohigashi H. Targeting NOX, INOS and COX-2 in inflammatory cells: chemoprevention using food phytochemicals. *Int J Cancer.* 2007;121(11):2357-2363.

Nagahashi S, Suzuki H, Nishiwaki M, Okuda K, Kurosawa Y, Terada S, Sugihara T, Andou K, Hibi T. TS-1/CDDP/Lentinan combination chemotherapy for inoperable advanced gastric cancer [in Japanese]. *Gan to Kagaku Ryoho [Japanese Journal of Cancer & Chemotherapy].* 2004;31(12):1999-2003.

Nagano J, Kono S, Preston DL, Mabuchi K. A prospective study of green tea consumption and cancer incidence, Hiroshima and Nagasaki (Japan). *Cancer Causes Control.* 2001;12(6):501-508.

National Cancer Institute. Fact sheet: red wine and cancer prevention. National Cancer Institute Web site. http://www.cancer.gov/cancertopics/factsheet/red-wine-and-cancer-prevention. Posted November 27, 2002. Accessed December 5, 2009.

National Cancer Institute. Fact sheet: tea and cancer prevention. National Cancer Institute Web site. http://www.cancer.gov/cancertopics/factsheet/tea-and-cancer-prevention. Posted December 6, 2002. Accessed December 5, 2009.

Ngo SN, Williams DB, Cobiac L, Head RJ. Does garlic reduce risk of colorectal cancer? A systematic review. *J Nutr.* 2007;137(10):2264-2269.

Nihal M, Ahmad N, Mukhtar H, Wood GS. Anti-proliferative and proapoptotic effects of (-)-epigallocatechin-3-gallate on human melanoma: possible implications for the chemoprevention of melanoma. *Int J Cancer.* 2005;114(4):513-521.

Narayanan BA, Re GG. IGF-II down regulation associated cell cycle arrest in colon cancer cells exposed to phenolic antioxidant ellagic acid. *Anticancer Res.* 2001;21(1A):359-364.

Natural Standard. Foods, herbs, and supplements: flaxseed and flaxseed oil. Natural Standard Web site. http://3rdparty.naturalstandard.com/frameset.asp. Accessed January 4, 2010.

Natural Standard. Foods, herbs, and supplements: ginger. Natural Standard Web site. http://3rdparty.naturalstandard.com/frameset.asp. Accessed January 4, 2010.

Natural Standard. Foods, herbs, and supplements: green tea. Natural Standard Web site. http://3rdparty.naturalstandard.com/frameset.asp. Accessed January 4, 2010.

Natural Standard. Foods, herbs, and supplements: soy (glycine max). Natural Standard Web site. http://3rdparty.naturalstandard.com/frameset.asp. Accessed January 4, 2010.

Nelson S. Chemical constituents of noni (morinda citrifolia). College of Tropical Agriculture and Human Resources, University of Hawai at Mānoa Web site. http://www.ctahr.hawaii.edu/noni/. Updated December 7, 2006. Accessed December 5, 2009.

Nestle M. Broccoli sprouts in cancer prevention. *Nutr Rev.* 1998;56(4 Pt 1):127-130.

Nikander E, Kilkkinen A, Metsä-Heikkilä M, Adlercreutz H, Pietinen P, Tiitinen A, Ylikorkala O. A randomized placebo-controlled crossover trial with phytoestrogens in treatment of menopause in breast cancer patients. *Obstet Gynecol.* 2003;101(6):1213-1220.

Noni. Memorial Sloan-Kettering Cancer Center Web site. http://www.mskcc.org/mskcc/html/69312.cfm. Updated March 24, 2009. Accessed December 5, 2009.

Noni. WholeHealthMD Web site. http://www.wholehealthmd.com/ME2/dirmod.asp?sid=17E09E7CFFF640448 FFB0B4FC1B7FEF0&nm=Reference+Library&type=AWHN_Supplements&mod=Supplements&mid=&id=5B78 D2210C824CBF90BA823C8D2D7086&tier=2. Updated September 14, 2005. Accessed December 5, 2009.

Norman PE, Powell JT. Vitamin D, shedding light on the development of disease in peripheral arteries. *Arterioscler Thromb Vasc Biol.* 2005;25(1):39-46.
> Erratum in:
> *Arterioscler Thromb Vasc Biol.* 2005;25(4):875.

Norrish AE, Jackson RT, Sharpe SJ, Skeaff CM. Prostate cancer and dietary carotenoids. *Am J Epidemiol.* 2000;151(2):119-123.

Ngo SN, Williams DB, Cobiac L, Head RJ. Does garlic reduce risk of colorectal cancer? A systematic review. *J Nutr.* 2007;137(10):2264-2269.

Oh K, Willett WC, Fuchs CS, Giovannucci E. Dietary marine n-3 fatty acids in relation to risk of distal colorectal adenoma in women. *Cancer Epidemiol Biomarkers Prev.* 2005;14(4):835-841.

O'Hara MA, Kiefer D, Farrell K, Kemper K. A review of 12 commonly used medicinal herbs. *Arch Fam Med.* 1998;7(6):523-536.

Omega-3. Memorial Sloan Kettering Cancer Center Web site. http://www.mskcc.org/mskcc/html/69316.cfm. Updated August 19, 2009. Accessed December 5, 2009.

Paiva SA, Russell RM. Beta-carotene and other carotenoids as antioxidants. *J Am Coll Nutr.* 1999;18(5):426-433.

Pantuck AJ, Leppert JT, Zomorodian N, Aronson W, Hong J, Barnard RJ, Seeram N, Liker H, Wang H, Elashoff R, Heber D, Aviram M, Ignarro L, Belldegrun A. Phase II study of pomegranate juice for men with rising prostate-specific antigen following surgery or radiation for prostate cancer. *Clin Cancer Res.* 2006;12(13):4018-4026.

Papoutsi Z, Kassi E, Tsiapara A, Fokialakis N, Chrousos GP, Moutsatsou P. Evaluation of estrogenic/antiestrogenic activity of ellagic acid via the estrogen receptor subtypes ERalpha and ERbeta. *J Agric Food Chem.* 2005;53(20):7715-7720.

Parnaud G, Li P, Cassar G, Rouimi P, Tulliez J, Combaret L, Gamet-Payrastre L. Mechanism of sulforaphane-induced cell cycle arrest and apoptosis in human colon cancer cells. *Nutr Cancer.* 2004;48(2):198-206.

Pendleton JM, Tan WW, Anai S, Chang M, Hou W, Shiverick KT, Rosser CJ. Phase II trial of isoflavone in prostate-specific antigen recurrent prostate cancer after previous local therapy. *BMC Cancer.* 2008;8:132.

Peters U, Leitzmann MF, Chatterjee N, Wang Y, Albanes D, Gelmann EP, Friesen MD, Riboli E, Hayes RB. Serum lycopene, other carotenoids, and prostate cancer risk: a nested case-control study in the prostate, lung, colorectal, and ovarian cancer screening trial. *Cancer Epidemiol Biomarkers Prev.* 2007;16(5):962-968.

Phytochemicals and cardiovascular disease. American Heart Association Web site. http://www.americanheart.org/ presenter.jhtml?identifier=4722. Accessed December 5, 2009.

Pisters KM, Newman RA, Coldman B, Shin DM, Khuri FR, Hong WK, Glisson BS, Lee JS. Phase I trial of oral green tea extract in adult patients with solid tumors. *J Clin Oncol.* 2001;19(6):1830-1838.

Quella SK, Loprinzi CL, Barton DL, Knost JA, Sloan JA, LaVasseur BI, Swan D, Krupp KR, Miller KD, Novotny PJ. Evaluation of soy phytoestrogens for the treatment of hot flashes in breast cancer survivors: A North Central Cancer Treatment Group Trial. *J Clin Oncol.* 2000;18(14):1068-1074.

Rajakumar K. Vitamin D, cod-liver oil, sunlight, and rickets: a historical perspective. *Pediatrics.* 2003;112(2):e132-e135.

Riggs DR, DeHaven JI, Lamm DL. Allium sativum (garlic) treatment for murine transitional cell carcinoma. *Cancer.* 1997;79(10):1987-1994.

Schernhammer ES, Hu FB, Giovannucci E, Michaud DS, Colditz GA, Stampfer MJ, Fuchs CS. Sugar-sweetened soft drink consumption and risk of pancreatic cancer in two prospective cohorts. *Cancer Epidemiol Biomarkers Prev.* 2005;14(9):2098-2105.

Schröder FH, Roobol MJ, Boevé ER, de Mutsert R, Zuijdgeest-van Leeuwen SD, Kersten I, Wildhagen MF, van Helvoort A. Randomized, double-blind, placebo-controlled crossover study in men with prostate cancer and rising PSA: effectiveness of a dietary supplement. *Eur Urol.* 2005;48(6):922-930; discussion 930-931.

Schulz M, Lahmann PH, Boeing H, Hoffmann K, Allen N, Key TJ, Bingham S, Wirfält E, Berglund G, Lundin E, Hallmans G, Lukanova A, Martínez Garcia C, González CA, Tormo MJ, Quirós JR, Ardanaz E, Larrañaga N, Lund E, Gram IT, Skeie G, Peeters PH, van Gils CH, Bueno-de-Mesquita HB, Büchner FL, Pasanisi P, Galasso R, Palli D, Tumino R, Vineis P, Trichopoulou A, Kalapothaki V, Trichopoulos D, Chang-Claude J, Linseisen J, Boutron-Ruault MC, Touillaud M, Clavel-Chapelon F, Olsen A, Tjønneland A, Overvad K, Tetsche M, Jenab M, Norat T, Kaaks R, Riboli E. Fruit and vegetable consumption and risk of epithelial ovarian cancer: the European Prospective Investigation into Cancer and Nutrition. *Cancer Epidemiol Biomarkers Prev.* 2005;14(11 Pt 1):2531-2535.

Shalansky S, Lynd L, Richardson K, Ingaszewski A, Kerr C. Risk of warfarin-related bleeding events and supratherapeutic international normalized ratios associated with complementary and alternative medicine: a longitudinal analysis. *Pharmacotherapy.* 2007;27(9):1237-1247.

Shapiro TA, Fahey JW, Dinkova-Kostova AT, Holtzclaw WD, Stephenson KK, Wade KL, Ye L, Talalay P. Safety, tolerance, and metabolism of broccoli sprout glucosinolates and isothiocyanates: a clinical phase I study. *Nutr Cancer.* 2006;55(1):53-62.

Shapiro TA, Fahey JW, Wade KL, Stephenson KK, Talalay P. Human metabolism and excretion of cancer chemoprotective glucosinolates and isothiocyanates of cruciferous vegetables. *Cancer Epidemiol Biomarkers Prev.* 1998;7(12):1091-1100.

Sharma SS, Gupta YK. Reversal of cisplatin-induced delay in gastric emptying in rats by ginger (*Zingiber officinale*). *J Ethnopharmacol*. 1998;62(1):49-55.

Shiitake mushroom. Memorial Sloan-Kettering Cancer Center Web site. http://www.mskcc.org/mskcc/html/69377.cfm. Updated July 14, 2008. Accessed December 5, 2009.

Shukla Y, Singh M. Cancer preventive properties of ginger: a brief review. *Food Chem Toxicol*. 2007;45(5):683-690.

Singh SV, Srivastava SK, Choi S, Lew KL, Antosiewicz J, Xiao D, Zeng Y, Watkins SC, Johnson CS, Trump DL, Lee YJ, Xiao H, Herman-Antosiewicz A. Sulforaphane-induced cell death in human prostate cancer cells is initiated by reactive oxygen species. *J Biol Chem*. 2005;280(20):19911-19924.

Slattery ML, Benson J, Curtin K, Ma KN, Schaeffer D, Potter JD. Carotenoids and colon cancer. *Am J Clin Nutr*. 2000;71(2):575-582.

Smith C, Crowther C, Willson K, Hotham N, McMillian V. A randomized controlled trial of ginger to treat nausea and vomiting in pregnancy. *Obstet Gynecol*. 2004;103(4):639-645.

Soy. Memorial Sloan-Kettering Cancer Center Web site. http://www.mskcc.org/mskcc/html/69383.cfm. Updated December 2, 2009. Accessed December 5, 2009.

Soy. PDRhealth Web site. http://www.pdrhealth.com/drugs/altmed/altmed-mono.aspx?contentFileName=ame0457.xml&contentName=Soy. Accessed December 5, 2009.

Stadlbauer V, Fickert P, Lackner C, Schmerlaib J, Krisper P, Trauner M, Stauber RE. Hepatotoxicity of NONI juice: report of two cases. *World J Gastroenterol*. 2005;11(30):4758-4760.

Steele VE, Kelloff GJ, Balentine D, Boone CW, Mehta R, Bagheri D, Sigman CC, Zhu S, Sharma S. Comparative chemopreventive mechanisms of green tea, black tea and selected polyphenol extracts measured by in vitro bioassays. *Carcinogenesis*. 2000;21(1):63-67.

Steinmetz KA, Kushi LH, Bostick RM, Folsom AR, Potter JD. Vegetables, fruit, and colon cancer in the Iowa Women's Health Study. *Am J Epidemiol*. 1994;139(1):1-15.

Su BN, Pawlus AD, Jung HA, Keller WJ, McLaughlin JL, Kinghorn AD. Chemical constituents of the fruits of Morinda citrifolia (Noni) and their antioxidant activity. *J Nat Prod*. 2005;68(4):592-595.

Sulforaphane. PDRhealth Web site. http://www.pdrhealth.com/drug_info/nmdrugprofiles/nutsupdrugs/sul_0243.shtml. Accessed June 12, 2007. Content no longer available.

Sulforaphane. Wikipedia Web site. http://en.wikipedia.org/wiki/Sulforaphane. Accessed December 5, 2009.

Sun CL, Yuan JM, Koh WP, Yu MC. Green tea, black tea and breast cancer risk: a meta-analysis of epidemiological studies. *Carcinogenesis*. 2006;27(7):1310-1315. Epub 2005 Nov 25.

Sundaram SG, Milner JA. Diallyl disulfide induces apoptosis of human colon tumor cells. *Carcinogenesis*. 1996;17(4):669-673.

Suzuki Y, Tsubono Y, Nakaya N, Koizumi Y, Suzuki Y, Shibuya D, Tsuji I. Green tea and the risk of colorectal cancer: pooled analysis of two prospective studies in Japan. *J Epidemiol*. 2005;15(4):118-124.

Suzuki Y, Tsubono Y, Nakaya N, Suzuki Y, Koizumi Y, Tsuji I. Green tea and the risk of breast cancer: pooled analysis of two prospective studies in Japan. *Br J Cancer.* 2004;90(7):1361-1363.

Taguchi T. Clinical efficacy of lentinan on patients with stomach cancer: end-point results of a four-year follow-up survey. *Cancer Detect Prev Suppl.* 1987;1:333-349.

Takeuchi A, Tsuchiya H, Yamamoto N, Hayashi K, Yamauchi K, Kawahara M, Miyamoto K, Tomita K. Caffeine-potentiated chemotherapy for patients with high-grade soft tissue sarcoma: long-term clinical outcome. *Anticancer Res.* 2007;27(5B):3489-3495.

Tanaka S, Haruma K, Yoshihara M, Kajiyama G, Kira K, Amagase H, Chayama K. Aged garlic extract has potential suppressive effect on colorectal adenomas in humans. *J Nut.* 2006;136(3 Suppl):821S-826S.

Tang L, Zhang Y, Jobson HE, Li J, Stephenson KK, Wade KL, Fahey JW. Potent activation of mitochondria-mediated apoptosis and arrest in S and M phases of cancer cells by a broccoli sprout extract. *Mol Cancer Ther.* 2006;5(4):935-944.

Tapsell LC, Hemphill I, Cobiac L, Patch CS, Sullivan DR, Fenech M, Roodenrys S, Keogh JB, Clifton PM, Williams PG, Fazio VA, Inge KE. Health benefits of herbs and spices: the past, the present, the future. *Med J Aust.* 2006;185(4 Suppl):S4-S24.

Tavani A, La Vecchia C. Coffee and cancer: a review of epidemiological studies, 1990–1999. *Eur J Cancer Prev.* 2000;9(4):241-256.

Tavlan A, Tuncer S, Erol A, Reisli R, Aysolmaz G, Otelcioglu S. Prevention of postoperative nausea and vomiting after thyroidectomy: combined antiemetic treatment with dexamethasone and ginger versus dexamethasone alone. *Clinical Drug Investig.* 2006;26(4):209-214.

Thanos J, Cotterchio M, Boucher BA, Kreiger N, Thompson LU. Adolescent dietary phytoestrogen intake and breast cancer risk (Canada). *Cancer Causes Control.* 2006;17(10):1253-1261.

Thompson LU, Chen JM, Li T, Strasser-Weippl K, Goss PE. Dietary flaxseed alters tumor biological markers in postmenopausal breast cancer. *Clin Cancer Res.* 2005;11(10):3828-3835.

Thresiamma KC, George J, Kuttan R. Protective effect of curcumin, ellagic acid and bixin on radiation induced genotoxicity. *J Exp Clin Cancer Res.* 1998;17(4):431-434.

Tsubono Y, Nishino Y, Komatsu S, Hsieh CC, Kanemura S, Tsuji I, Nakatsuka H, Fukao A, Satoh H, Hisamichi S. Green tea and the risk of gastric cancer in Japan. *N Engl J Med.* 2001;344(9):632-636.

United States Department of Agriculture. Get on the grain train: dietary guidelines for Americans. Home and Garden Bulletin No. 267-2. May 2002. Center for Nutrition Policy and Promotion Web site. http://www.cnpp.usda.gov/Publications/DietaryGuidelines/2000/2000DGBrochureGrainTrain.pdf. Accessed December 5, 2009.

US Department of Health and Human Services and United States Department of Agriculture. Dietary Guidelines for Americans, 2005. US Department of Health and Human Services Web site. http://www.health.gov/dietaryguidelines/dga2005/document/default.htm. Published January 2005. Accessed December 5, 2009.

US Food and Drug Administration. FDA Talk Paper: FDA approves new health claim for soy protein and coronary heart disease. Rockville, MD: National Press Office; October 20, 1999. Talk Paper T99-48.

Vaishampayan U, Hussain M, Banerjee M, Seren S, Sarkar FH, Fontana J, Forman JD, Cher ML, Powell I, Pontes JE, Kucuk O. Lycopene and soy isoflavones in the treatment of prostate cancer. *Nutr Cancer.* 2007;59(1):1-7.

Van Patten CL, Olivotto IA, Chambers GK, Gelmon KA, Hislop TG, Templeton E, Wattie A, Prior JC. Effect of soy phytoestrogens on hot flashes in postmenopausal women with breast cancer: a randomized, controlled clinical trial. *J Clin Oncol.* 2002;20(6):1449-1455.

West BJ, Jensen CJ, Westendorf J. Noni juice is not hepatotoxic. *World J Gastroenterol.* 2006;12(22):3616-3619.

Wu AH, Pike MC, Williams LD, Spicer D, Tseng CC, Churchwell MI, Doerge DR. Tamoxifen, soy, and lifestyle factors in Asian American women with breast cancer. *J Clin Oncol.* 2007;25(21):3024-3030.
     Erratum in:
     J Clin Oncol. 2007;25(30):4862.

Wu AH, Wan P, Hankin J, Tseng CC, Yu MC, Pike MC. Adolescent and adult soy intake and risk of breast cancer in Asian-Americans. *Carcinogenesis.* 2002;23(9):1491-1496.

Wu AH, Yu MC, Tseng CC, Hankin J, Pike MC. Green tea and risk of breast cancer in Asian Americans. *Int J Cancer.* 2003;106(4):574-579.

Wu AH, Yu MC, Tseng CC, Pike MC. Epidemiology of soy exposures and breast cancer risk. *Br J Cancer.* 2008;98(1):9-14.

Yan L, Yee JA, Li D, McGuire MH, Thompson LU. Dietary flaxseed supplementation and experimental metastasis of melanoma cells in mice. *Cancer Lett.* 1998;124(2):181-186.

Yang CS, Ju J, Lu G, Xiao H, Hao X, Sang S, Lambert JD. Cancer prevention by tea and tea polyphenols. *Asia Pac J Clin Nutr.* 2008;17 Suppl 1:245-248.

Yetiv JZ. Clinical applications of fish oils. *JAMA.* 1988;260(5):665-670.

You WC, Brown LM, Zhang L, Li JY, Jin ML, Chang YS, Ma JL, Pan KF, Liu WD, Hu Y, Crystal-Mansour S, Pee D, Blot WJ, Fraumeni JF Jr, Xu GW, Gail MH. Randomized double-blind factorial trial of three treatments to reduce the prevalence of precancerous gastric lesions. *J Natl Cancer Inst.* 2006;98(14):974-983.

Younos C, Rolland A, Fleurentin J, Lanhers MC, Misslin R, Mortier F. Analgesic and behavioral effects of Morinda citrifolia. *Planta Med.* 1990;56(5):430-434.

Yüce B, Gülberg V, Diebold J, Gerbes AL. Hepatitis induced by Noni juice from Morinda citrifolia: a rare cause of hepatotoxicity or the tip of the iceberg? *Digestion.* 2006;73(2-3):167-170.

Zhou Y, Li N, Zhuang W, Liu G, Wu T, Yao X, Du L, Wei M, Wu X. Green tea and gastric cancer risk: meta-analysis of epidemiologic studies. *Asia Pac J Clin Nutr.* 2008;17(1):159-165.

Chapter Four

How Food Is Grown and Treated

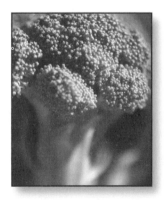

AS YOU CONSIDER NUTRITION and its important effects on cancer and its treatment, you may also be thinking about the quality and safety of the food you eat. You may wonder if the way food is raised, grown, or treated might affect your health or treatment. This chapter will focus on factors related to food quality and its safety and why they are important for people dealing with a cancer diagnosis. Food safety guidelines for people undergoing cancer treatment are discussed in chapter 10.

Pesticides

The Environmental Protection Agency (EPA) defines a pesticide as any substance or mixture of substances intended to prevent, destroy, repel, or reduce any pest. Pests can be animals (such as insects and mice), unwanted plants (weeds), fungi, or microorganisms like bacteria and viruses. Though often misunderstood as referring only to insecticides, the term pesticide also applies to herbicides (chemicals that kill weeds) and fungicides (chemicals that kill fungi).

Pesticides are applied to many commercially grown vegetable and fruit crops to help protect them from insects, diseases, weeds, and mold. Pesticides are closely regulated by the EPA, the U.S. Food and Drug Administration (FDA), and the United States Department of Agriculture (USDA).

Are Pesticides Safe?

Pesticides play a valuable role in sustaining the food supply. Pesticide residues in the vegetables and fruits you buy or grow pose very little risk to human health. Although vegetables and fruits sometimes contain low levels of pesticides, no evidence has shown that the low doses of pesticides and herbicides found in foods increase the risk for cancer or recurrence. The health benefits of a balanced diet rich in vegetables and fruits, both for overall health and for cancer protection, far outweigh the largely theoretical risks posed by occasional, very low pesticide residues in foods.

If you are concerned about pesticides, using organically grown foods will reduce your exposure to them. If you are concerned about pesticide residues on nonorganic foods, here are some steps you can take to reduce your exposure:

- Wash vegetables and fruits with large amounts of cold or lukewarm running tap water or place them in a large container of water to which you have added a product for washing fresh produce. Scrub with a dish brush or vegetable brush if the outer skin or peel of the food will be consumed, such as with apples, cucumbers, or potatoes. To avoid the expense of produce-washing products, dish soap also can be used in very small amounts (one drop in two to three gallons of water). If the amount used is very small, it can safely help to remove dirt, pesticides, and insects. Just be very sure to rinse well. Discard the outermost leaves of leafy vegetables, such as lettuce and cabbage.

- Even if produce is labeled as prewashed, reduce your risk of food-borne illness by washing all produce thoroughly again before serving.
- Place washed fruit and vegetables in containers or bags for storage—putting a paper towel inside the bag with the produce helps to ensure complete drying and increases shelf life.

SHOPPER'S GUIDE TO PESTICIDES

According to the Environmental Working Group, the following "dirty dozen" non-organic fruits and vegetables contain the *highest* amount of pesticides. The "clean fifteen" non-organic fruits and vegetables contain the *smallest* amount of pesticide residue.

DIRTY DOZEN
1. Peach
2. Apple
3. Bell Pepper
4. Celery
5. Nectarine
6. Strawberries
7. Cherries
8. Kale
9. Lettuce
10. Grapes (imported)
11. Carrot
12. Pear

CLEAN FIFTEEN
1. Onion
2. Avocado
3. Sweet Corn
4. Pineapple
5. Mango
6. Asparagus
7. Sweet Peas
8. Kiwi
9. Cabbage
10. Eggplant
11. Papaya
12. Watermelon
13. Broccoli
14. Tomato
15. Sweet Potato

Reprinted, with permission, from Environmental Working Group. *Shopper's Guide to Pesticides.* http://www.foodnews.org/.

Fruit and Vegetable Washes

Because of recent concerns regarding outbreaks of E. coli and salmonella in fresh produce, some people undergoing cancer treatment may be instructed by their health care team to take special precautions when preparing fresh vegetables and fruit, even if they are going to be cooked before they are eaten. People with treatment-related low white blood cell counts are at higher risk for food-borne illness. While this extra effort may not always be necessary, it can help ensure that your fresh produce is clean. Your health care provider may advise you to use a drop of dish soap and thoroughly rinse the produce before using it, especially if it is to be eaten raw. This extra effort helps loosen and remove pesticides and even pathogens ("bad bugs"). Other people may be asked to use a "vegetable and fruit wash" product. These products can often be found in the produce section of the grocery store, or you can make a homemade wash to clean fresh produce (see below). Please follow your health care team's specific instructions. See chapter 10 for more information on food safety at home.

Produce Spray Recipe

In a spray bottle, gently mix together one tablespoon of lemon juice, two tablespoons of baking soda, and one cup of water. Spray the mixture on the produce and allow to sit for two to five minutes. Lightly scrub the produce with a clean sponge or vegetable brush. Rinse produce thoroughly under cool water. Pat dry.

Produce Wash Recipe

Mix together one-half cup of white vinegar and three tablespoons of salt; stir until salt has dissolved. Add vinegar and salt mixture to a sink full of cool water. Stir to mix. Soak produce for fifteen to twenty minutes. Rinse in cool water. Pat dry.

Genetically Modified Foods

Foods that are genetically modified are those that are changed in the laboratory to resist pests or disease, increase nutrients, or improve quality or shelf life. They are made by adding genes from other plants or organisms. Forty genetically modified foods, including varieties of tomatoes, soy, and corn, have been approved for sale in the United States.

Are Genetically Modified Foods Safe?

Genetically modified foods pose the same risks or benefits to human health as do other foods. The presence of allergens, natural toxins, or even antinutrients (which inhibit the absorption of nutrients) is common in our food supply.

A LOCAL RESOURCE

Consider calling or contacting your local health department or Cooperative Extension office if you have concerns about food safety. These services are available throughout the United States and are a wonderful resource for answers to questions about food quality, safety, and preparation. They can even guide you in growing your own produce! You may also contact your health care team with specific questions or concerns. To locate your local Cooperative Extension office, visit the USDA's Cooperative State Research, Education, and Extension Service Web site at www.csrees.usda.gov/Extension/ or call 800-FED-INFO (800-333-4636).

Scientists expect that genetic modifications will increasingly be used to enhance the nutritional value of foods. For example, a genetically modified potato that contains a lot of protein is being developed. Golden rice that contains DNA from daffodils (which are rich in beta carotene) could be used to help combat a vitamin A deficiency that causes up to five hundred thousand new cases of blindness each year, mostly among children living in Africa and Asia.

Before a genetically modified food is marketed to consumers, a company's scientists must seek to determine whether the food poses any heightened safety risks. The FDA published guidelines in 1992 to ensure that companies who develop genetically modified foods work with the agency to assess their safety.

The FDA, EPA, and USDA share oversight of genetically modified foods. Although current tests have been adequate for evaluating genetically modified foods that have undergone relatively simple compositional changes, new technologies are being developed to evaluate the increasingly complex compositional changes expected. There is neither scientific evidence nor is there a suggestion that long-term harm, such as higher cancer rates or recurrence, results from eating genetically modified foods.

Increasingly, the produce industry and other food commodity groups are working to select or breed more nutrient-packed produce. For example, one can find tomatoes that are higher in lycopene, purple carrots that are rich in anthocyanins, or broccoflower—a cross between broccoli and cauliflower—on supermarket shelves.

FACTS ABOUT FUNCTIONAL FOODS AND PHYTOCHEMICALS

Functional foods are foods that have been modified (for example, fortified, bred, or bioengineered) to offer health benefits. The idea of vitamin-fortified foods is not new, but scientists have taken the concept many steps further. Some examples of functional foods are already in supermarkets—for example, calcium-fortified orange juice, herbal tea with antioxidants, and eggs with omega-3 fatty acids. Functional foods are created with the hope of improving upon the benefits nature has already provided.

There are approximately forty-four nutrients that are essential for health, but thousands of phytochemicals may also provide health benefits. For example, plant scientists and growers are developing a type of broccoli that will have a higher-than-normal level of phytochemicals called glucosinolates, which may help prevent cancer. More research is needed to determine whether this "functional food" can truly affect cancer development in humans.

Some scientists believe that phytochemicals known as isoflavones have the potential to reduce cancer risk. Found mainly in soybeans, isoflavones are credited with possessing an array of health benefits, including lowering the risk of prostate, breast, and other major cancers. Bioengineers are working to isolate soy genes that create possible tumor-blocking chemicals. The goal is to insert the protective soy genes into wheat, corn, and other grains to create anticancer foods.

There are thousands of phytochemicals in the food supply, and scientists are just beginning to understand which are the most effective in preventing disease. Further work is still needed to determine whether regular consumption of phytochemical-enriched foods will improve health in humans. For example, one study showed that eating lycopene-enhanced tomatoes increased lycopene levels in the blood, but it did not show a reduction in the stress caused by oxidation (as measured by blood samples). It is still unknown whether eating lycopene-enhanced tomatoes reduces the risk for prostate cancer. Generally, these enriched foods provide a higher concentration of the select compounds than non-enriched products, but they are unlikely to provide anywhere near the amount as a dietary supplement of the same compound. The risks associated with enriched foods are likely small but need further investigation.

While scientists wait for the results of research regarding functional foods, the best way to provide your body with a wide variety of phytochemicals is to eat a balanced diet that includes whole grains, nuts, legumes, and at least five servings of vegetables and fruits a day, as well as lean protein sources.

Food Additives

In the broadest sense, a food additive is any substance added to food. Legally, the term refers to "any substance the intended use of which results or may reasonably be expected to result—directly or indirectly—in its becoming a component or otherwise affecting the characteristics of any food." This definition includes any substance used in the production, processing, treatment, packaging, transportation, or storage of food.

Additives are used in foods for five main reasons:

1. to improve consistency and texture (emulsifiers, stabilizers, and texturizers that keep foods creamy and mixed; thickeners; humectants that keep foods moist; leavening agents; and anti-caking agents)
2. to replace nutrients lost during refining or milling
3. to preserve food and keep it from spoiling
4. to provide leavening or control acidity or alkalinity
5. to enhance color (colorings or bleaches) or flavor (flavorings, flavor enhancers, or sweeteners)

Some additives have been used for many years in the United States and have played an important role in fortifying certain foods in order to reduce nutritional deficiencies. For example, folic acid and iron are added to some breakfast cereals. Other times, nutrients are added to provide an extra source of a key nutrient in the diet. An example is the addition of calcium to orange juice. All additives are subject to ongoing safety review as scientific understanding and methods of testing continue to improve. In fact, the federal regulations that ensure the safety of food additives are stricter than those that apply to dietary supplements.

Many additives listed on ingredient labels may seem foreign but are actually quite familiar. For example, ascorbic acid is another name for vitamin C, alpha tocopherol is another name for vitamin E, and beta carotene is a source of vitamin A. Technically, all food is made up of chemicals. Carbon, hydrogen, and other chemical elements provide the basic building blocks for everything in life.

Indirect food additives are those that become part of food in trace amounts because of packaging, storage, or other handling. Food packaging manufacturers must prove to the FDA that all materials that come into contact with food are safe. Little is known about these indirect food additives and health.

Examples of Food Additives and Common Uses

ADDITIVE USES	ADDITIVE EXAMPLES	FOODS WHERE THEY MIGHT BE FOUND
To improve food consistency and texture	Alginates, lecithin, mono- and diglycerides, methyl cellulose, carrageenan, glyceride, pectin, guar gum, sodium aluminosilicate	Baked goods, cake mixes, salad dressings, ice cream, processed cheese, coconut, table salt
To replace nutrients lost during refining or milling	Vitamins A and D, thiamine, niacin, riboflavin, pyridoxine, folic acid, ascorbic acid, calcium carbonate, zinc oxide, iron	Flour, bread, biscuits, breakfast cereals, pasta, margarine, milk, iodized salt, gelatin desserts
To preserve food and keep it from spoiling	Propionic acid and its salts, ascorbic acid, butylated hydroxy anisole (BHA), butylated hydroxytoluene (BHT), benzoates, sodium nitrates, citric acid	Bread, cheese, crackers, frozen and dried fruit, margarine, lard, potato chips, cake mixes, meat
To provide leavening or control acidity or alkalinity	Yeast, sodium bicarbonate, citric acid, fumaric acid, phosphoric acid, lactic acid, tartrates	Cakes, cookies, quick breads, crackers, butter, chocolates, soft drinks
To enhance color or flavor	Cloves, ginger, fructose, aspartame, saccharin, FD&C red no. 40, monosodium glutamate, caramel, annatto, limonene, turmeric	Spice cake, gingerbread, soft drinks, yogurt, soup, confections, baked goods, cheeses, jams, gum

Are Food Additives Safe?

To market a new food or color additive, a manufacturer must first petition the FDA for approval. Animal studies in which large doses of the additive are given for long periods are often necessary to show that a substance would not cause harmful effects at expected levels of human consumption. Studies of human consumption of the additive may also be submitted to the FDA.

After an additive is approved, the FDA may issue specific regulations on the types of foods in which it can be used, the maximum amounts to be used, and how it should be identified on food labels. Additives to be used in meat and poultry products also must receive specific authorization by the USDA. Once an additive is on the market, federal officials carefully monitor the extent of Americans' consumption of it and the results of any new research on its safety to ensure its use continues to be within safe limits.

Additives are usually present in very small quantities in food, and no convincing evidence has shown that any additive causes human cancers or recurrence at these levels. Some individuals may, however, have adverse reactions (such as headache or nausea) to some additives.

Irradiated Foods

Radiation is increasingly used to kill harmful organisms on foods. Irradiation is used to extend the shelf life of foods such as produce. Radiation does not remain in the food after it is treated. Consuming irradiated foods does not expose you to radiation. No research has been conducted in people to determine whether eating irradiated foods alters your cancer risk.

Many health experts agree that irradiation can be an effective way to help reduce foodborne hazards and ensure that harmful organisms are not in the foods we buy. During irradiation, foods are exposed briefly to a radiant energy source, such as gamma rays or electron beams, within a shielded facility. Irradiation is not a substitute for proper food manufacturing and handling. But the process, especially when used to treat meat and poultry products, can kill harmful bacteria, greatly reducing potential hazards.

Irradiation does not make foods radioactive, just as an airport luggage scanner does not make luggage radioactive, and it does not cause harmful chemical changes. The process may cause a small loss of nutrients, but no more so than other processing methods, such as cooking, canning, or heat pasteurization. Federal rules require irradiated foods to be labeled as such.

Are Irradiated Foods Safe?

Irradiation of fresh meat and poultry has been approved by the FDA. It is also allowed for a variety of other foods, including fresh vegetables and fruits and spices. Irradiation is safe and effective in decreasing or eliminating harmful bacteria, and it also reduces spoilage and decreases insects and parasites. In certain vegetables and fruits, it inhibits sprouting and delays ripening. For example, irradiated strawberries stay unspoiled for up to three weeks, versus three to five days for untreated berries. Food irradiation is allowed in nearly forty countries and is endorsed by the World Health Organization, the American Medical Association, and many other organizations.

Organic Foods

Organic food differs from conventionally produced food in the way it is grown, handled, and processed. The term organic is often used to refer to plant foods grown without pesticides and genetic modifications. It is also used to refer to meat, poultry, eggs, and dairy products produced without the use of antibiotics or growth hormones. Organic farming does not use bioengineering, ionizing radiation, conventional pesticides, or fertilizers made with synthetic ingredients or sewage sludge.

The term "natural" does not mean "organic." Food labeled as organic has been certified as meeting USDA organic standards. The term natural is not defined by law or in FDA regulations, so there are no restrictions or guidelines governing its use.

The USDA standards for the organic label apply to foods grown in the United States or imported from other countries. Before a product can be labeled organic, a government-approved certifier inspects the farm where the food is grown to make sure the farmer is following all USDA organic standards. Companies that handle or process organic food before it gets to your local supermarket or restaurant must be certified, too.

Are Organic Foods Safe?

Organic foods contain fewer contaminants than conventionally produced foods. However, the USDA makes no claims that organically produced food is safer or more nutritious than conventionally produced food. Organic produce, like any produce, should be washed before eating. It may be organic, but it still could be contaminated by dirt, insects, or even stray pesticide residues.

A recent report indicates that organic produce may contain higher levels of antioxidants than traditionally grown foods. However, these differences were small, and more research is needed to confirm these findings. Most likely, the higher nutrient content relates to the fact that organic foods are consumed earlier after harvest than are nonorganic foods, simply because the quality of organics can reduce rapidly. Generally, the closer produce is to the time of harvest, the higher the nutrient content, regardless of whether it is organic.

During cancer treatment, some people choose to eat organic foods to reduce exposure to pesticides. This is certainly an acceptable approach, but it may or may not change health, and it will likely increase food costs. The bottom line is this: if consuming mostly organic foods provides you with greater peace of mind, do it.

Labeling Organic Foods

What's in a label? A lot, according to the USDA. Here are the differences among organically labeled foods, as dictated by the USDA National Organic Program.

IF THE LABEL READS "100 PERCENT ORGANIC"	IF THE LABEL READS "ORGANIC"	IF THE LABEL READS "MADE WITH ORGANIC INGREDIENTS"
Must contain only organically produced ingredients and processing aids, excluding water and salt	Must contain at least 95 percent organically produced ingredients, excluding water and salt	Must contain at least 70 percent organic ingredients, excluding water and salt
Cannot be produced using specifically excluded methods, sewage sludge, or ionizing radiation	Cannot be produced using specifically excluded methods, sewage sludge, or ionizing radiation	Cannot be produced using specifically excluded methods, sewage sludge, or ionizing radiation
Label can display the USDA seal or the seal of the certifying agent	Label can display the USDA seal or the seal of the certifying agent	The percentage of organic content and certifying agent seal may be used on the package but the USDA seal cannot be used

- Products that contain less than 70 percent organic ingredients cannot use the term "organic" on the label, but they can list specific ingredients (on the ingredient label) that are organically produced.
- There are no restrictions on the use of other truthful labeling claims such as "no drugs or hormones used" or "free-range."

Adapted from the United States Department of Agriculture National Organic Program. "Organic Labeling and Marketing Information." 2008. www.ams.usda.gov/nop.

References

American Cancer Society. *Good for You! Reducing Your Risk of Developing Cancer*. Atlanta, GA: American Cancer Society; 2002.

American Dietetic Association. Position of the American Dietetic Association: agriculture and food biotechnology. *J Am Diet Assoc*. 2006;106(2):285-293.

Anderson J, Deskins B. *The Nutrition Bible: A Comprehensive, No-Nonsense Guide to Foods, Nutrients, Additives, Preservatives, Pollutants, and Everything Else We Eat and Drink*. New York: William Morrow and Company, Inc; 1995.

Brody JE. For unrefined healthfulness: refined grains. *The New York Times*. March 4. 2003: F5.

Fruit and vegetable benefits. Fruits and Veggies Matter Web site. http://www.fruitsandveggiesmatter.gov/benefits/index.html. Accessed December 4, 2009.

Home food safety 101. American Dietetic Association Web site. http://www.eatright.org/Public/content.aspx?id=10948. Accessed December 7, 2009.

International Food Information Council Foundation. Consumer's guide to food safety risks. Food Insight Web site. http://www.foodinsight.org/Resources/Detail.aspx?topic=A_Consumer_s_Guide_to_Food_Safety_Risks. Posted October 1, 2007. Accessed December 6, 2009.

Pesticides on fruits and vegetables. *Nutrition News Focus*. November 1998.

Souping up your immune system. American Cancer Society Web site. http://www.cancer.org/docroot/NWS/content/NWS_1_1x_Souping_Up_Your_Immune_System.asp. Published November 24, 1998. Content no longer available.

United States Department of Agriculture, National Organic Program. Organic labeling and marketing information. US Department of Agriculture Web site. http://www.ams.usda.gov/AMSv1.0/getfile?dDocName=STELDEV3004446&acct=nopgeninfo. Published October 2002. Updated April 2008. Accessed December 7, 2009.

US Environmental Protection Agency. Pesticides and food: what your family needs to know. http://www.epa.gov/pesticides/food/. Accessed December 7, 2009.

US Environmental Protection Agency. Pesticides on food: consumer information. January 1998. US Environmental Protection Agency Web site. http://www.epa.gov/fedrgstr/EPA-PEST/1998/January/ Day-14/6020.pdf. Content no longer available.

US Food and Drug Administration and International Food Information Council. Food ingredients and colors. US Food and Drug Administration Web site. http://www.fda.gov/Food/FoodIngredientsPackaging/ucm094211.htm. Updated October 7, 2009. Accessed December 7, 2009.

US Food and Drug Administration. Irradiation and food safety: answers to frequently asked questions. US Food and Drug Administration Web site. http://www.fsis.usda.gov/Fact_Sheets/Irradiation_and_Food_Safety/index.asp. Updated September 2005. Accessed December 7, 2009.

US General Accounting Office. Genetically modified foods: experts view regimen of safety tests as adequate, but FDA's evaluation process could be enhanced. Report no. GAO-02-566. US General Accounting Office Web site. http://www.gao.gov/docdblite/summary.php?recflag=&accno=A03410&rptno=GAO-02-566. Published May 23, 2002. Accessed December 7, 2009.

Washing produce, cutting boards, storage containers. American Dietetic Association Web site. http://www.eatright.org/Public/content.aspx?id=10957. Accessed December 7, 2009.

Chapter Five

Dietary Supplements: Vitamins, Minerals, and Herbs

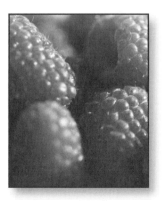

MANY PEOPLE WITH A CANCER DIAGNOSIS TAKE DIETARY SUPPLEMENTS such as vitamins, minerals, and herbs with the hope of halting or even reversing the course of their disease and to replace nutrients. Others take dietary supplements because they want to actively participate in treatment, improve their overall nutrition, or to reduce fatigue and increase energy. In many instances, friends or family members encourage people with cancer to try various supplements. In one recent study, up to 77 percent of people with a cancer diagnosis reported taking a multivitamin/mineral supplement daily. Many people with cancer take dietary supplements despite a lack of evidence that they are needed. For example, a recent study showed no improvement in radiation therapy–related fatigue with multivitamin use. Some dietary supplements, such as multivitamin/mineral supplements that meet United States Department of Agriculture (USDA) requirements, are useful and important. Other supplements are touted as cancer treatments or cures. At this time, there is no proof that a dietary supplement will cure cancer.

Because of all the possible pros and cons, the use of dietary supplements during and after cancer should be determined on a case-by-case basis, with input from the doctor or health care team and the person with cancer.

Dietary Supplements

Dietary supplements are a diverse group of substances and products, including vitamins, minerals, and herbs. They are not grouped together for any medical or scientific reason. Rather, Congress has lumped this diverse group of substances together based on the way it regulates these products.

According to the definition Congress established in 1994 in the Dietary Supplement Health and Education Act (DSHEA), a dietary supplement is—

a product taken by mouth that contains a 'dietary ingredient' intended to supplement the diet. The 'dietary ingredients' in these products may include vitamins, minerals, herbs or other botanicals, amino acids, and substances such as enzymes, organ tissues, glandulars, and metabolites. Dietary supplements can also be extracts or concentrates, and may be found in many forms such as tablets, capsules, softgels, gelcaps, liquids, or powders. They can also be in other forms, such as a bar, but if they are, information on their label must not represent the product as a conventional food or a sole item of a meal or diet. Whatever their form may be, DSHEA places dietary supplements in a special category under the general umbrella of 'foods,' not drugs, and requires that every supplement be labeled a dietary supplement.

In this chapter, the risks and purported benefits of dietary supplements will be outlined—especially select vitamins, minerals, and herbs that people with cancer often read about or hear about. As you read the rest of this chapter, there are two important things for you to remember:

1. **Whereas many dietary supplements may be touted as cancer cures, there is no evidence that any dietary supplement can cure cancer.**

2. **Self-medication with dietary supplements can be potentially risky and harmful, especially for people undergoing cancer treatment.**

Some Common Questions: Nutritional and Herbal Supplements

Q: Can I take a multivitamin/mineral supplement while I am going through cancer treatment, even if my blood counts (white blood cells, hemoglobin, or platelets) are low?

A: Yes. It may be difficult during and after cancer treatment to consume a diet with adequate amounts of micronutrients. Therefore, health experts, including the American Cancer Society, conclude that there most likely is a benefit from taking a standard multivitamin/mineral supplement that contains no more than 100 percent of the Recommended Daily Values.

Q: Is it okay to take herbals and dietary supplements (for example, amino acids or high-dose vitamins and minerals) when my blood counts are low because of cancer treatment?

A: Always talk to your doctor before taking any dietary supplements, especially while you are undergoing treatment. Your health care team would most likely recommend stopping all herbals and dietary supplements during your cancer treatment. Interaction between these products and medications that your doctor has prescribed may interfere with or reduce the effectiveness of your cancer treatment. Some products have been shown to have adverse side effects in some people, including bleeding, liver or kidney dysfunction, or fluid retention. Finally, herbal and dietary supplements are not regulated by the FDA, and they may contain ingredients or additives that are not listed on the label and may be harmful.

Vitamin and Mineral Supplements

Vitamins and minerals are essential to health and are crucial in the normal functioning of our bodies. When you eat a balanced diet of vegetables, fruits, grains, dairy, and animal products, you get most of the vitamins and minerals you need in their most effective forms. Vitamins and minerals work together in the body in complex ways, affecting the absorption and processing of each other and, in turn, affecting the way the body runs. When you get vitamins and minerals through foods, the body is better able to maintain a balance of these nutrients.

Your doctor, registered dietitian, or pharmacist may advise you to supplement your diet with certain vitamins and minerals during treatment. This is especially likely if you are unable to eat a diet that is adequate in nutrients. In most cases, a multivitamin/mineral supplement that contains 100 percent of the Recommended Daily Value requirements for vitamins, as well as smaller amounts of calcium and other minerals and trace elements is sufficient to meet daily needs for health. Remember this is *in addition to* or *to supplement* a healthy diet.

Keep in mind the following tips when considering taking a multivitamin/mineral supplement:

- Tell your health care team if you are taking a multivitamin/mineral or any other supplement. If you are already taking supplements, bring the products with you to your doctor or clinic visit for approval of the dose and to ensure that the ingredients do not interfere with your health or cancer treatment.
- Expensive multivitamin/mineral supplements are not necessarily a better quality product than generic or store brands.
- Make sure the label specifies that the multivitamin/mineral contains approximately 100 percent of the Recommended Daily Value of essential vitamins and minerals.
- Beware of ambitious claims for a multivitamin/mineral supplement or any unusual ingredients.
- Talk to your health care team to find out whether you need any nutrients beyond a multivitamin/mineral.

Vitamins

Vitamins help the body use energy (calories) from carbohydrates, fats, and proteins. Vitamins are needed for a wide range of body functions. Thirteen vitamins and minerals exist, and each plays a different role in helping the body function. (See the vitamin and mineral charts on pages 106–109 for more information on specific nutrients.)

Vitamins are either fat soluble or water soluble. Because vitamins B and C are water soluble, the body can store only minimal amounts of these nutrients, and it is best if these vitamins are consumed in our diets every day. Vitamins A, D, E, and K are fat soluble, meaning the body can store them in its fat stores for a longer period.

Nutritional information can be found on all multivitamin/mineral supplement labels. Remember to look at the "serving size." Some supplements require that you take multiple pills to get the amount listed for each vitamin and mineral. The labels list the amount of each nutrient the supplement contains, along with an estimated percentage of the daily requirement (Recommended Daily Value) for each nutrient. The Daily Values are the amounts of nutrients most people need to consume to be adequately nourished.

Taking additional water-soluble nutrients (beyond the Recommended Daily Value) is generally okay, but there have been some instances of adverse health effects. For example, excess vitamin B6 has been associated with reversible peripheral neuropathy, and excess vitamin C has been linked to kidney stone formation. The risk of adverse effects is slightly higher if you take additional fat-soluble vitamins; because they can be stored in the body, levels of exposure have the potential to be higher. For example, excess vitamin A in pregnant women is associated with birth defects, excess vitamin E has been associated with increased risk for hemorrhagic stroke, and too much vitamin D has been associated with kidney stone formation in some individuals. Moderation is the best advice.

People with cancer may have increased vitamin needs; your health care team can help you determine whether you need more than a single daily multivitamin/mineral to meet your individual requirements.

VITAMIN D

Vitamin D has received increasing attention as a potential cancer-preventing nutrient. While called a fat-soluble vitamin, vitamin D actually works more like a hormone in the body. Most people get vitamin D from fortified dairy products. Other sources include fatty fish oils, including cod liver oil. It can be difficult for our bodies to get enough vitamin D because of the limited dietary sources and because our bodies can only "activate" vitamin D by absorbing sunlight through our skin. Older people, people who live in areas of the country with low levels of sun exposure, those who use sunscreen on a regular basis, and even overweight people or those with dark-pigmented skin are at risk for having inadequate vitamin D levels. Many doctors are now measuring vitamin D levels in their patients to evaluate whether dietary supplements or moderate sun exposure is needed. Refer to page 279 in chapter 12 for more information on vitamin D for cancer survivors.

Minerals

Minerals play a role in several of the body's metabolic processes. The body needs only small amounts of most minerals, and eating a varied diet typically provides them. The one exception might be calcium. Calcium requirements range from eight hundred to fifteen hundred milligrams daily. Many people have difficulty meeting this requirement through diet alone, so supplementation is often necessary. The body can store minerals for use when your body needs them.

Cancer treatments such as surgery and chemotherapy can diminish the body's stores of vitamins and minerals. If your diet is insufficient in vitamins and/or minerals, your doctor or registered dietitian may recommend a dietary supplement. Many people take a combined vitamin and mineral supplement to ensure they are getting all the nutrients they need, especially when they feel they are not eating a balanced diet during treatment.

Even some people not in cancer treatment wonder whether they should take a multivitamin/mineral supplement, especially if they do not eat the healthiest diet. One study suggested that taking a multivitamin/mineral supplement for more than ten years protected against colorectal cancer. A more recent analysis from the Women's Health Initiative, which included more than one hundred thousand postmenopausal women who were generally well-nourished, did not find evidence that short- or longer-term use of multivitamin/mineral supplements reduces risk for any cancer.

Antioxidant Supplements

Antioxidants are nutrients in vegetables and fruits that appear to protect cells in the body from free radicals. Antioxidants include vitamin C, vitamin E, selenium, vitamin A and carotenoids, and many other phytochemicals (chemicals from plants). Five or more servings of vegetables and fruits a day and a standard multivitamin/mineral supplement with 100 percent of the Recommended Daily Value will give your body the nutrients it needs to stay strong and healthy. (See page 69 for more information about antioxidants.)

Taking large doses of antioxidant supplements may be dangerous and is not recommended for people undergoing chemotherapy, biotherapy, or radiation therapy. For example, several studies have shown evidence of potential interactions between antioxidant supplements, such as vitamins C, E, and A, and radiation therapy and chemotherapy. Since antioxidants protect cells from damage, or oxidation, they could also protect cancer cells from the damaging effects of cancer treatments.

Your health care team will develop a nutrition plan that meshes with your particular cancer treatment and is based on sound science. Talk with your health care team to determine the best time to take antioxidant supplements, and remember that large doses of any nutrient are not helpful and may be dangerous. Before and after treatment, antioxidants may be of benefit, but they should be limited or avoided during treatment.

Vitamins, Their Sources, and Their Functions

VITAMIN	FUNCTION
Vitamin C (water soluble)	• Provides antioxidant action • Helps synthesize tissue and neurotransmitters • Increases iron absorption
Vitamin A (fat soluble)	• Aids in cell differentiation affecting growth, reproduction, bone health, skin, and immunity • Plays a major role in eye health • Provides antioxidant action
Thiamin (Vitamin B1) (water soluble)	• Provides coenzyme activity in the metabolism of carbohydrates and proteins • Aids in energy production
Riboflavin (Vitamin B2) (water soluble)	• Used to convert glucose and fatty acids to energy
Niacin (Vitamin B3) (water soluble)	• Used in the synthesis and/or degradation of carbohydrates, fat and protein • Used to help lower blood lipids
Cobalamin (Vitamin B12) (water soluble)	• Functions in the synthesis process of some critical enzymes • Works with folate to help form DNA • Assists in the catabolism of some fats and proteins
Folate/Folic acid (water soluble)	• Helps prevent neural tube defects • May help protect the heart by reducing levels of homoysteine • Helps to metabolize protein and purines • Aids in DNA syntheses and cell division

* IU indicates International Units of Measure.

FOOD SOURCES	DIETARY REFERENCE INTAKE (DRI) (PER DAY)
Papayas, strawberries, oranges, broccoli, mangoes, Brussels sprouts	• 90 mg for men • 75 mg for women
Liver, sweet potatoes, carrots, spinach, mangoes	• 900 mcg (3000 IU*) for men • 700 mcg (2333 IU) for women
Pork loin, green peas, brown rice, pinto beans, baked potatoes	• 1.2 mg for men • 1.1 mg for women
Milk, eggs, spinach, spaghetti, salmon, chicken	• 1.3 mg for men • 1.1 mg for women
Chicken, tuna, beef, peanuts, avocado, bagels	• 16 mg of niacin equivalents for men • 14 mg of niacin equivalents for women
Oysters, Alaskan crab, beef, salmon, eggs	• 2.4 mcg for men and women
Spinach, oranges, romaine lettuce, peanut butter	• 400 mcg for men and women

Vitamins, Their Sources, and Their Functions (continued)

VITAMIN	FUNCTION
Vitamin D (fat soluble)	• Helps to maintain calcium balances in the body
Vitamin E (fat soluble)	• Provides antioxidant action • Aids in immune function • May help protect against heart disease

* IU indicates International Units of Measure.

Minerals, Their Sources, and Their Functions

MINERAL	PURPOSE
Iron	• Helps red blood cell formation • Critical part of many proteins and enzymes needed to maintain health
Selenium	• Provides antioxidant action • Helps thyroid function • Assists in immune function
Zinc	• Helps with enzyme activity • Assists in protein and DNA synthesis • Aids in wound healing • Helps in cell division
Calcium	• Aids in muscle contraction • Aids in blood vessel expansion and contraction • Helps with secretion of hormones and enzymes • Storage in the bones and teeth helps maintain strong bones and teeth

FOOD SOURCES	DIETARY REFERENCE INTAKE (DRI) (PER DAY)
Egg yolks, liver, fatty fishes, fortified milk	• 200 IU* for adults under fifty years of age • 400 IU for adults aged fifty-one to seventy • 600 IU for adults over the age of seventy
Wheat germ and oil, sunflower seeds and oil, hazelnuts, papayas	• 15 mg (22 IU) for men and women

FOOD SOURCES	DIETARY REFERENCE INTAKE (DRI) (PER DAY)
Chicken livers, oysters, beef, turkey (dark meat), ready-to-eat iron-fortified cereals, assorted legumes (beans) and lentils	• 8 mg for men • 18 mg for women between the ages of eighteen and fifty • 8 mg for women aged fifty-one and older
Brazil nuts, tuna, beef, spaghetti with meat sauce, cod, turkey	• 55 mcg for men and women
Oysters, beef, Alaskan crab, pork, fortified breakfast cereals	• 11 mg for men • 8 mg for women
Yogurt, sardines, cheese, milk, calcium-fortified orange juice and tofu	• 1000 mg for men and women between the ages of nineteen and fifty • 1200 mg for men and women aged fifty-one and older

Herbal Supplements

Botanical medicine is the use of plants or plant parts to treat illness and related symptoms. Research on whether these supplements are helpful or potentially harmful is limited, even though they may have been in use for some time.

There are two general groups of herbs: culinary herbs, which are used to season food, and medicinal herbs, which are used to treat illness. Culinary herbs are harmless when eaten in amounts typically used in cooking and can help to promote good health. Herbal supplements contain higher concentrations of a given herb or even a specific phytochemical within the herb than would generally be consumed through diet. Some herbal supplements fall into both categories. For example, turmeric is used in cooking and is under active study as a medicinal supplement, both to reduce inflammation and as a potential agent to decrease cancer risk—called a "chemopreventive" agent in cancer prevention research. The phytochemical D-limonone, which is found in citrus fruits, is similar; the orange zest used in cooking is also under study in cancer prevention in a more concentrated form.

Herbs have been used to treat disease in every culture throughout the history of civilization. Today, herbs are found in a variety of products, such as pills, liquid extracts, teas, and ointments. Herbs are sold dried, finely chopped, powdered, and in capsule or liquid form. Products may include only a specific plant part, such as the leaf or root, the entire plant, or a combination of different plants. They may be marketed as single substances or in combination with other materials, such as vitamins, minerals, amino acids, and non-nutrient ingredients. While many herbal products are harmless and safe, others are associated with harmful side effects and can interfere with cancer therapies such as chemotherapy and radiation therapy, as well as with recovery from surgery. Herbal supplements may be sold with claims of alleviating side effects of cancer treatment or as treatments for cancer itself. However, it is important to remember two points:

- Herbal supplements do not slow or reverse the spread of cancer.
- Herbs' effects on the growth of cancer or cancer cells is under study, and their use should be discussed with your health care team.

The basic difference between herbal supplements and medicines prescribed by a doctor or naturopathic doctor is that herbals contain the entire plant or plant part, while prescription and over-the-counter medicines made by pharmaceutical companies contain only a purified active ingredient that has been studied and proven safe and effective. Many important prescription pharmaceuticals come from natural plants or herbs. For example, the following chemotherapy drugs are derived from plants: vincristine (Oncovin) and vinblastine (Velban) from periwinkle; paclitaxel (Taxol) and docetaxel (Taxotere) from yew trees; irinotecan (Camptosar) and topotecan (Hycamtin) from *Camptotheca acuminate* (a tree native to China and Tibet); and etoposide (VePesid) from May apple.

Herbal supplements should be avoided entirely during cancer treatment, with the exception of culinary herbs consumed as a flavoring in food. Some herbs can interfere with chemotherapy or with the blood's ability to coagulate during surgery. Because not enough is known about these effects, health care providers recommend caution. People with cancer who are in active treatment or who have completed therapy but are considering herbal remedies, even for relief of symptoms or short-term problems, should first talk with their health care team.

HERBS TO BE AVOIDED DURING TREATMENT

The Seattle Cancer Care Alliance advises that the following herbal and botanical products should not be used under any circumstance by individuals undergoing high-dose chemotherapy or stem cell (bone marrow) transplantation because of known dangerous side effects:

alfalfa	kava kava
borage	laetrile (apricot pits)
chaparral	licorice root
Chinese herbs	L-tryptophan
coltsfoot	lobelia
comfrey	maté tea
DHEA (dehydroepiandrosterone)	pau d'arco
dieter's tea (contains senna,aloa, buckthorn, cascara, castor oil, rhubarb root)	pennyroyal
	sassafras
ephedra or MaHuange	St. John's wort
groundsel or life root	yohimbe and yohimbine
	valerian or heliotrope

Reprinted from Seattle Cancer Care Alliance. "Adult and Pediatric Guidelines for the Use of Herbal and Nutrient Supplements During Hematopoietic Stem Cell Transplantation (HSCT) and High-Dose Chemotherapy." www.seattlecca.org.

Risks of Dietary Supplements

Regardless of your cancer treatment regimen, consult with your doctor or registered dietitian regarding the potential benefits and risks of each dietary supplement you are considering or currently using. Review all dietary supplements with your health care team before beginning your treatment.

Some doctors may not be familiar with the uses, risks, and potential benefits of all dietary supplements. Bridge this gap by gathering as much information as possible from reliable sources on the dietary supplement therapy you are considering. (See the rest of this chapter and chapter 14 for reliable information sources.) Then ask for your doctor's professional opinion as to whether the dietary supplements are safe and medically sound, and how or if it might be safely integrated into your current treatment regimen. Take time to talk to other members of your health care team, such as a registered dietitian or your pharmacist, who will likely be knowledgeable about dietary supplements. Taking dietary supplements without consulting your health care team can be harmful. Bring your dietary supplements with you to your health care appointment so you can review each supplement to determine its potential efficacy, any safety issues of concern, and its appropriateness as part of your individual treatment plan.

Dietary Supplements Can Interfere with Medications

Many people assume that dietary supplements can safely be taken along with prescription medication. Unfortunately, this is not always true. Some supplements can change the way chemotherapy drugs or radiation therapy affects your body and can possibly cause your treatment to be less effective. For example, certain herbal supplements can block or speed up the body's absorption of some medications, causing a person to have too much or too little of the drug in their bloodstream. Certain dietary supplements can cause skin sensitivity and severe reactions to radiation exposure. Patients undergoing chemotherapy are at significant risk for drug interaction if they take dietary supplements, especially those containing high levels of antioxidants or folic acid.

There are specific instances where dietary supplements or food choices may reduce side effects or improve the way a drug works. For example, people on steroid therapy are encouraged to get adequate calcium, those on diuretics may need supplemental potassium, and individuals with anemia (iron deficiency) may be prescribed iron supplements. It can be complicated. Talk with your doctor, registered dietitian, or pharmacist about any dietary supplements you wish to take or any changes in the supplements you are taking.

Unlike prescription medications, most companies that produce dietary supplements do not conduct research to determine whether the supplements interact with pharmaceutical drugs. For many herbal supplements, the risks of taking them with prescribed medications are largely unknown. More information is slowly emerging as the use of herbs continues to rise and regulatory agencies such as the Food and Drug Administration (FDA) compile reports of interactions, or adverse events.

Like pharmaceutical drugs, dietary supplements have pros, cons, and side effects. They should only be used when the correct dose and frequency of administration has been safely determined. However, unlike drugs, dietary supplements are usually self-prescribed and administered with little or no input from informed medical sources. There is a lot of misinformation about the safe usage and potential risks of dietary supplements. Unfortunately, the misuse of dietary supplements or the use of dangerous supplements can lead to serious adverse reactions and even death.

The "Natural Is Safe" or "Natural Is Better" Myth

Many people believe that a substance sold in its unrefined, naturally occurring state is better or safer than a manufactured or refined substance. However, supplements that claim to be "all-natural" are not necessarily better or safer for human consumption than refined or manufactured substances. Some of the most toxic substances in the world occur naturally. Poisonous mushrooms, for example, are completely natural but are not safe or beneficial to humans.

Traditional or historical use is, likewise, not a reliable gauge of safety. Tobacco was used for many years in Native American traditional medicine, but now we know it causes one third of cancer deaths in the United States.

Most plants contain hundreds or thousands of chemical compounds, many of which influence functioning of the human body. Some of these compounds provide beneficial effects, whereas others can be toxic. Many drugs currently used in oncology and other fields of medicine come from plant sources. To develop these drugs, it takes decades of research to learn which plant components are beneficial and to separate the beneficial compounds from the harmful ones.

Some vitamin and mineral supplements may be described as "natural" or as "not synthetic." Scientists learned the chemical structure of vitamins decades ago. Most of these vitamins can be made synthetically, meaning by chemical reactions of other substances. Whether a vitamin or mineral molecule is purified from a plant source or made in the laboratory, it has the same chemical properties and the same effects on your body. What is more important is that the product has consistent and accurate dosages and is free of contaminants.

Check the product labels for both the quantity and concentration of active ingredients contained in each product. There are many sources of quality information about dietary supplements, including the American Cancer Society. Memorial Sloan-Kettering Cancer Center also has a great deal of information in the Herbs and Botanical Information section of its Web site (www.mskcc.org/mskcc/html/11570.cfm).

Dietary Supplements That May Be of Use for People with Cancer

NUTRIENT OR BOTANICAL	BENEFITS
Calcium	Promotes healthy bone structure during and after cancer treatment
Vitamin D	Promotes bone health and may boost immune function during and after treatment
Ginger	Shown to help reduce nausea associated with treatment
Melatonin	May promote better sleep patterns after treatment

Regulation of Dietary Supplements

In the United States, all over-the-counter and prescription drugs are regulated by the FDA. The safety or efficacy of new drugs must be proved *before* they are available to consumers. Dietary supplements (including vitamins, minerals, and herbs) are not categorized as drugs, however, and so they are not subject to the same stringent safety and effectiveness requirements as pharmaceuticals.

Manufacturers are not required to test new ingredients of supplements in clinical trials. Because Congress has decided to recognize all dietary supplements as "generally safe," they do not need to be tested under conditions that would put their possible risks and contraindications under rigorous examination. Dietary supplement manufacturers are not required to include information on a product's packaging about its contents or possible dangers. Unlike approved medicines, supplements may contain harmful ingredients or contaminants along with ingredients thought to be helpful.

The Dietary Supplement Health and Education Act (DSHEA) gives the FDA permission to stop production of a dietary supplement, but *only* when the FDA proves that the product poses a significant risk to the health of Americans. The result is a system in which dietary supplements are assumed to be safe until they are proven unsafe. Therefore, it falls to the consumer to gather accurate information about the safe usage of dietary supplements, as well as about which manufacturers can be trusted to produce high-quality supplements.

Good Manufacturing Practices

In 2007, the Department of Health and Human Services established a set of standards (called Good Manufacturing Practices or GMPs) by which dietary supplements must be manufactured, packaged, and labeled. Large and medium companies have been required to follow the guidelines since 2008 (for large companies) and 2009 (for medium companies), and smaller companies (with fewer than twenty full-time employees) were given until June 2010 to comply with the new standards.

The goal of the GMPs is to guarantee the identity, purity, strength, and composition of manufactured dietary supplements. The GMPs for dietary supplements fall somewhere between the tolerance standards for food production and the stringent consistency standards applied to pharmaceuticals.

The U.S. Pharmacopeia (USP) is a nonprofit organization that establishes standards for medicines and dietary supplements that are recognized in U.S. federal law. Updated continuously to reflect industry and public health needs, USP standards provide specifications for strength, quality, purity, packaging, and labeling. USP also offers a Dietary Supplement Verification program through which dietary supplement manufacturers can voluntarily submit their products for laboratory testing, documentation review, and a GMP audit.

Products that meet USP's criteria are awarded the USP Verified Dietary Supplement mark to use on packaging and marketing (see image). This mark lets consumers know the product contains the ingredients listed on the label, in the declared potency and amounts; does not contain harmful levels of specified contaminants, such as, but not limited to, heavy metals, microbes, and pesticides; will break down and release into the body within a specified amount of time; and has been made according to the FDA's current GMPs, using sanitary and well-controlled procedures. A list of USP Verified products can be found at www.uspverified.org.

The National Sanitation Foundation (NSF) also tests supplements to verify the authenticity and quantity of ingredients listed on product labels and to ensure the products do not contain undeclared ingredients or unacceptable levels of contaminants. In addition, NSF inspects manufacturing facilities for conformance with GMP. Supplements that have received the NSF mark may be found at www.nsf.org/Certified/Dietary/.

Claims: What They Mean and Don't Mean

Before you buy a dietary supplement, read the label carefully. It is easy to misunderstand or misinterpret the claims made about a product. The manufacturers of dietary supplements are allowed to make four kinds of claims on the labels of their products: nutritional claims, claims of well-being, health claims, and structure or function claims.

Nutritional claims are statements about the effects dietary supplements, vitamins, and minerals have on known nutrient-deficiency diseases. For example, "vitamin C prevents scurvy." These claims do not need to be preapproved by the FDA. However, the label must also make clear how prevalent the disease is in the United States to help consumers weigh the risk of contracting the disease against the potential risks of the supplement itself.

Claims of well-being are just that: claims that relate to overall well-being. Unevaluated statements such as "makes you feel better" may or may not be factually accurate. Claims of well-being do not require preapproval by the FDA or any other government agency.

Health claims are allowed to state the specific effects of a dietary factor on the body. Some examples are "a diet low in sodium may reduce the risk of high blood pressure," that "oat bran and whole oat products reduce cholesterol," that "food containing sugar alcohol in place of sugar reduces the risk of tooth decay," or that "eating vegetables and fruits reduces a person's risk of cancer and heart disease." The FDA must preapprove all health claims and requires that they be supported by evidence from scientific studies.

Structure or function claims are claims about the effect of the dietary supplement on the structure or function of the body. Such claims can imply but cannot specifically state their effects. Examples are, "beverages with antioxidants improve overall health," "grapes and grape juice support normal, healthy cardiovascular function," or "calcium builds strong bones." The FDA published a ruling in January 2000 that clarified exactly what kinds of structure or function claims are acceptable for dietary supplements. Dietary supplements may not make any claims regarding the treatment of disease. However, the following product descriptions are acceptable as structure or function claims for dietary supplements:

- the product's mechanism of action ("works as an antioxidant")
- the product's effects on cellular structure ("helps membrane stability")
- the product's effects on the body's physiology ("promotes normal urinary flow")
- the product's effects on chemical or laboratory parameters ("supports normal blood glucose")
- claims of maintenance ("helps maintain a healthy circulatory system") or other nondisease claims ("helps you relax")
- claims for common conditions and symptoms related to life stages ("reduces irritability, bloating, and cramping associated with premenstrual syndrome")

Structure or function claims are controversial and also confusing to consumers. They are not reviewed by the FDA and must be accompanied by the disclaimer, "This statement has not been evaluated by the Food and Drug Administration. This product is not intended to diagnose, treat, cure, or prevent any disease."

The FDA requires that this disclaimer be printed on supplement labels because it is easy for consumers to misunderstand structure or function claims. For example, many consumers believe that a statement such as "helps maintain vision acuity" means the product has been proven to prevent vision deterioration or that the statement "helps maintain a healthy prostate gland" means the product has been proven to prevent or reverse diseases such as prostate cancer. Be careful to avoid such misunderstandings; *do not assume that because a product claims to support or promote healthy body function that it prevents or reduces the risk of any disease, including cancer.* Recognize claims made by supplement manufacturers for what they are: untested, unproven, anecdotal reports.

References

About herbs, botanicals, & other products: Memorial Sloan-Kettering information resource database. Memorial Sloan-Kettering Cancer Center Web site. http://www.mskcc.org/aboutherbs. Accessed December 7, 2009.

Agus DB, Vera JC, Golde DW. Stromal cell oxidation: a mechanism by which tumors obtain vitamin C. *Cancer Res.* 1999;59(18):4555-4558.

American Cancer Society. *American Cancer Society Complete Guide to Complementary and Alternative Therapies.* 2nd ed. Atlanta, GA: American Cancer Society; 2009.

Claghorn K. Ask the experts: antioxidants during chemotherapy. Oncolink Web site. http://www.oncolink.com/experts/article.cfm?c=1&s=3&ss=3&id=1681. Published March 31, 2002. Accessed December 7, 2009.

D'Andrea GM. Use of antioxidants during chemotherapy and radiotherapy should be avoided. *CA Cancer J Clin.* 2005;55:319-321.

Doyle C, Kushi LH, Byers T, Courneya KS, Demark-Wahnefried W, Grant B, McTiernan A, Rock CL, Thompson C, Gansler T, Andrews KS; The 2006 Nutrition, Physical Activity and Cancer Survivorship Advisory Committee; American Cancer Society. Nutrition and physical activity during and after cancer treatment: an American Cancer Society guide for informed choices. *CA Cancer J Clin.* 2006;56(6):323-353.

de Souza Fête AB, Bensi CG, Trufelli DC, de Oliveira Campos MP, Pecoroni PG, Ranzatti RP, Kaliks R, Del Giglio A. Multivitamins do not improve radiation therapy-related fatigue: results of a double-blind randomized crossover trial. *Am J Clin Oncol.* 2007;30(4):432-436.

Hamilton KK. Antioxidant supplements during cancer treatments: where do we stand? *Clin J Onco Nurs.* 2001;5(4):181-182.

Harrison T. A guide to the new dietary supplement GMPs: reviewing the details, nuances, and potential impact of the new rule. NPICenter.com Web site. http://www.npicenter.com/anm/anmviewer.asp?a=19660. Posted September 15, 2007. Accessed January 4, 2010.

International Food Information Council Foundation. Functional foods fact sheet: antioxidants. Food Insight Web site. http://ific.org/publications/factsheets/antioxidantfs.cfm. Updated March 2006. Accessed December 8, 2009.

Jacobs EJ, Henion AK, Briggs PJ, Connell CJ, McCullough ML, Jonas CR, Rodriguez C, Calle EE, Thun MJ. Vitamin C and vitamin E supplement use and bladder cancer mortality in a large cohort of US men and women. *Am J Epidemiol.* 2002;156(11):1002-1010.

Labriola D, Livingston R. Possible interactions between dietary antioxidants and chemotherapy. *Oncology (Williston Park)*. 1999;13(7):1003-1008; discussion 1008, 1011-1012.

Lamson DW, Brignall MS. Antioxidants in cancer therapy: their actions and interactions with oncologic therapies. *Altern Med Rev.* 1999;4(5):304-329.

Meyskens FL Jr, Liu PY, Tuthill RJ, Sondak VK, Fletcher WS, Jewell WR, Samlowski W, Balcerzak SP, Rector DJ, Noyes RD, et al. Randomized trial of vitamin A versus observation as adjuvant therapy in high-risk primary malignant melanoma: a Southwest Oncology Group study. *J Clin Oncol.* 1994;12(10):2060-2065.

National Institutes of Health. Dietary supplement fact sheet: calcium. National Institutes of Health Web site. http://dietary-supplements.info.nih.gov/factsheets/calcium.asp. Accessed November 20, 2009.

National Institutes of Health. Dietary supplement fact sheet: iron. National Institutes of Health Web site. http://dietary-supplements.info.nih.gov/factsheets/iron.asp. Accessed November 20, 2009.

National Institutes of Health. Dietary supplement fact sheet: selenium. National Institutes of Health Web site. http://dietary-supplements.info.nih.gov/factsheets/selenium.asp. Accessed November 20, 2009.

National Institutes of Health. Dietary supplement fact sheet: vitamin E. National Institutes of Health Web site. http://dietary-supplements.info.nih.gov/factsheets/vitamine.asp. Accessed November 20, 2009.

National Institutes of Health. Dietary supplement fact sheet: zinc. National Institutes of Health Web site. http://dietary-supplements.info.nih.gov/FactSheets/Zinc.asp. Accessed November 20, 2009.

National Institutes of Health. Herbs at a glance fact sheets. National Institutes of Health Web site. http://nccam.nih.gov/health/herbsataglance.htm. Accessed December 9, 2009.

National Institutes of Health. NIH State-of-the-Science Conference statement on multivitamin/mineral supplements and chronic disease prevention. *NIH Consens State Sci Statements.* 2006;23(2):1-30.

National Institutes of Health. Vitamin and mineral supplement fact sheets. National Institutes of Health Web site. http://www.cc.nih.gov/ccc/supplements. Accessed December 9, 2009.

Penland JG. Dietary Reference Intakes (DRIs): new dietary guidelines really are new! United States Department of Agriculture, Agricultural Research Service Web site. http://www.ars.usda.gov/News/docs.htm?docid=10870. Updated October 23, 2006. Accessed December 9, 2009.

Prepared testimony of Joseph A. Levitt, Esq., Director, Center for Applied Food Safety and Nutrition, Food and Drug Administration, before the Senate Committee on Governmental Affairs: Dietary supplements and their use for weight-loss purposes. July 31, 2002.

Sarubin Fragakis A with Thomson C. *The Health Professional's Guide to Popular Dietary Supplements.* 3rd ed. Chicago, IL: American Dietetic Association, 2006.

Seattle Cancer Care Alliance. Adult and pediatric guidelines for the use of herbal and nutrient supplements during hematopoietic stem cell transplantation (HSCT) and high-dose chemotherapy. Seattle Cancer Care Alliance Web site. http://www.seattlecca.org/client/documents/practical-emotional-support/herbal_sup_2510_0.pdf. Accessed November 20, 2009.

Stankiewicz M, Migdalska A, Bankowska E, Jeska EL. Complement activation, phagocytosis, tumor growth and parasitic infection after magnesium supplementation in diet of mice. *Magnesium*. 1989;8(2):87-93.

US Food and Drug Administration. Dietary supplement health and education act of 1994. US Food and Drug Administration Web site. http://www.cfsan.fda.gov/~dms/dietsupp.html. Posted December 1, 1995. Accessed January 10, 2010.

US Food and Drug Administration. Illnesses and injuries associated with the use of selected dietary supplements. US Food and Drug Administration Web site. http://vm.cfsan.fda.gov/~dms/ds-ill.html. Published 1993. Updated August 29, 2005. Accessed May 19, 2009. Content no longer available.

US Food and Drug Administration. Overview of dietary supplements. US Food and Drug Administration Web site. http://www.fda.gov/Food/DietarySupplements/ConsumerInformation/ucm110417.htm. Updated May 7, 2009. Accessed December 9, 2009.

van Zandwijk N, Dalesio O, Pastorino U, de Vries N, van Tinteren H. EUROSCAN: a randomized trial of vitamin A and N-Acetylcysteine in patients with head and neck cancer or lung cancer. *J Natl Cancer Inst*. 2000;92(12):977-986.

Velicer CM, Ulrich CM. Vitamin and mineral supplement use among US adults after cancer diagnosis: a systematic review. *J Clin Oncol*. 2008;26(4):665-673.

World Cancer Research Fund. American Institute for Cancer Research. Food, nutrition, physical activity, and the prevention of cancer: a global perspective. Washington, DC: American Institute for Cancer Research; 2007.

Zeegers MP, Goldbohm RA, Bode P, van den Brandt PA. Prediagnostic toenail selenium and risk of bladder cancer. *Cancer Epid Bio Prev*. 2002;11(11):1292-1297.

Chapter Six

Diet and Nutrition Therapies Promoted as Treatments and Cures

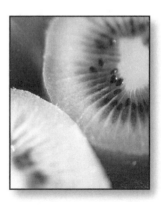

SCIENTIFIC EVIDENCE SUPPORTS eating a mostly plant-based diet that includes low-fat sources of protein, whole grains, vegetables and fruits as a way to prevent cancer or facilitate its treatment. In contrast, the health benefits of alternative diets are not supported by scientific evidence. Regimens that rely on enemas, fasting, or special dietary supplements, especially as meal replacements or in unnaturally large doses, can be harmful, especially during cancer therapy, when getting enough but not too much of the right nutrients is crucial. *There is no scientific evidence that a diet alone can treat or cure cancer*. In this chapter, the evidence and assertions behind some of the most asked-about diets promoted as cancer therapy will be explored.

Relying on any diet or food alone and avoiding or delaying conventional cancer treatment is likely to be detrimental to your health and may have serious health consequences. Talk to your health care team about making changes in your diet, and discuss how to make healthy changes a part of your care plan.

Please note: Some of the information in this chapter is also available in a more comprehensive form in the American Cancer Society Complete Guide to Complementary and Alternative Cancer Therapies, Second Edition. *Please refer to this publication for further reading on these and other diets of interest for people with cancer.*

Diet Therapy Promoted to Improve Immune Function

Livingston-Wheeler Therapy

Livingston-Wheeler therapy is an alternative cancer method that includes vaccines, antibiotics, vitamin and mineral supplements, digestive enzymes, cleansing enemas, support group therapy, and a vegetarian diet. The Livingston-Wheeler clinic that offered this therapy is no longer in operation, but there are private practitioners using the Livingston-Wheeler method who are still in practice in the United States.

The Claims

The therapy is promoted primarily as a form of biotherapy, or immunotherapy (a treatment that stimulates a person's immune system), to help a person fight off serious illnesses such as cancer. There is no evidence to support this claim.

The Evidence

Available scientific evidence does not support claims that Livingston-Wheeler therapy helps people with cancer. Few studies have evaluated the Livingston-Wheeler therapy. One investigation involving patients with advanced cancer compared survival and quality of life between patients receiving conventional treatment and those undergoing Livingston-Wheeler therapy. According to the 1991 report, there was no difference in survival between the two groups, but the patients treated with Livingston-Wheeler had significantly poorer quality of life. These results refuted the clinic's claim of an 82 percent cure rate, even for people with advanced cancer.

One report found that the bacterium *Progenitor cryptocides*, which Dr. Livingston-Wheeler claimed caused cancer, is actually a mixture of several different types of bacteria incorrectly labeled as one bacterium by Dr. Livingston-Wheeler. The other components of her therapy have also been criticized for lack of scientific evidence.

Possible Problems or Complications

The safety of Livingston-Wheeler therapy has never been firmly established. Some reported reactions to the vaccine given in the therapy include aching, slight fever, and tenderness at the injection site.

Diet Therapies Promoted to Remove Toxins and Strengthen the Body's Defenses

Metabolic Therapy Regimens

Metabolic therapy uses a combination of special diets, digestive enzymes, digestive supplements, and other measures in an attempt to remove "toxins" from the body and strengthen the body's defenses against disease. It is based on the theory that toxic substances in food and the environment build up in the body and create chemical imbalances that lead to diseases such as cancer, arthritis, and multiple sclerosis. Some claim that a special diet can cure serious illnesses, including cancer. Others claim that they can evaluate a patient's metabolism and diagnose cancer before symptoms appear and that they can locate tumors and learn the tumor's size and growth rate.

Metabolic therapy varies a great deal depending on the practitioner, but all types include special diets that usually emphasize ingesting fruits, vegetables, and vitamins and mineral supplements. Other components may include coffee enemas, digestive enzymes, visualization, stress-reduction exercises, and laetrile, a compound produced from almonds and apricot and peach pits.

The goal of metabolic therapy is to eliminate toxins from the body and enhance immune function so that the body can "fight off" cancer. Liver extract injections, pancreatic enzymes, and various supplements are said to stimulate metabolism. Proponents of metabolic therapy claim that it addresses the underlying cause of disease rather than treating the symptoms.

Among the better known types of metabolic therapy are Gerson Therapy, Kelley's Treatment, and the Gonzalez Regimen, as well as others such as Issels Whole Body Therapy, Contreras Therapy, and Manner Therapy. This section will cover Gerson Therapy, Kelley's Treatment, and the Gonzalez Regimen, three of the most common types of metabolic therapy.

Gerson Therapy

Gerson Therapy is a form of alternative cancer treatment involving coffee enemas, dietary supplements, and a special diet that is claimed to cleanse the body, boost the immune system, and stimulate metabolism. The therapy is based on the theory that disease is caused by the body's accumulation of toxic substances. Practitioners believe that fertilizers, insecticides, herbicides, and other chemicals contaminate food by lowering its potassium content and raising its sodium content. Food processing and cooking add more sodium, which they believe changes the metabolism of cells in the body and eventually causes cancer.

Gerson Therapy requires following a strict low-salt, low-fat, vegetarian diet, drinking juice from approximately twenty pounds of freshly crushed vegetables and fruits daily, and undergoing coffee enemas. Various other supplemental substances are injected or ingested to stimulate various organs, particularly the liver and thyroid. The fruit and vegetable diet that is part of Gerson Therapy is used to correct the person's imbalance of sodium and potassium and revitalize the liver so it can rid the body of cancer cells. Coffee enemas are claimed to relieve pain and eliminate liver toxins in a process called detoxification.

Kelley's Treatment and the Gonzalez Regimen

Kelley's Treatment and the Gonzalez Regimen are metabolic therapies that use a combination of special diets and nutritional supplements in an attempt to remove toxins from the body and strengthen the body's defenses against disease. Kelley's Treatment includes taking up to one hundred fifty dietary supplements daily (such as enzymes and large doses of vitamins, minerals, and amino acids), fasting, exercising, using laxatives or coffee enemas, eating a restricted diet, undergoing chiropractic adjustments, and praying. Practitioners classify people into different metabolic types that form the basis for specific dietary and supplement recommendations.

The Gonzalez Regimen is similar to Kelley's Treatment and includes extracts or concentrates from animal organs such as the thymus and liver (typically taken from a cow or lamb) and digestive enzymes. It focuses on detoxifying the body and bringing it into balance. Gonzalez Regimen was developed and used by a physician in New York, Dr. Nicholas Gonzalez, for the purpose of treating advanced cancer, particularly pancreatic cancer.

Metabolic Therapy Regimens Promoted as Treatments for Cancer

GERSON THERAPY OVERVIEW	KELLEY'S TREATMENT OVERVIEW	GONZALEZ REGIMEN OVERVIEW
•Involves coffee enemas, dietary supplements, and a special diet that is claimed to cleanse the body, boost the immune system, and stimulate metabolism •Mandates a strict diet, including drinking juice from approximately twenty pounds of fresh vegetables and fruits daily. Other substances are injected or ingested to stimulate organs. •Practitioners believe that chemicals create imbalances in food, which change the metabolism of cells in the body and eventually cause cancer.	•Includes taking up to one hundred fifty dietary supplements daily (such as enzymes and large doses of vitamins, minerals, and amino acids), fasting, exercising, using laxatives or coffee enemas, eating a restricted diet, undergoing chiropractic adjustments, and praying •Practitioners classify people into different metabolic types that form the basis for specific dietary and supplement recommendations.	•Similar to Kelley's Treatment •Includes extracts or concentrates from animal organs such as the thymus and liver and digestive enzymes •Focuses on detoxifying the body and bringing it into balance
THE EVIDENCE: •Retrospective analyses show no evidence of therapeutic efficacy. •Serious illness and death have occurred from some of the components of the treatment, such as coffee enemas.	**THE EVIDENCE:** •Records of patients who used the Kelley's Treatment have been reviewed by several groups of researchers to determine whether the therapy was beneficial. It was found to be ineffective, especially when compared with conventional cancer treatment.	**THE EVIDENCE:** •Small preliminary report from Dr. Gonzalez suggested regimen may prolong survival of pancreatic cancer patients by several months, but analysis involved only eleven patients. •National Center for Complementary and Alternative Medicine is conducting a much larger, seven-year study comparing chemotherapy with the Gonzalez Regimen in patients

Caution: Relying on a metabolic therapy alone and avoiding conventional medical care may have serious health consequences.

The Evidence

There is general agreement that there are differences in the cellular metabolism of people who have cancer compared with people who do not have cancer. There is also general agreement regarding the importance of attention to optimal nutrition as a component of conventional oncology care. Otherwise, there is no convincing clinical evidence that supports the claims made regarding metabolic therapy or any of its components. There have been no well-controlled studies published in the peer-reviewed medical literature showing that metabolic therapy is effective in treating cancer or any other disease, or that the therapy is safe. Some aspects of metabolic therapy may, in fact, be harmful.

An article on metabolic therapies on the Memorial Sloan-Kettering Cancer Center Web site concluded that "Retrospective analyses of the Gerson and Kelley therapies show no evidence of therapeutic efficacy" (2008). And a review article in the *Journal of Clinical Gastroenterology* concludes that "[c]offee enemas are a hazardous derivative of colon therapy.... Its proponents claim that caffeine is absorbed in the colon and leads to a vasodilation in the liver, which in turn enhances the process of elimination of toxins. None of this is proved, nor is there any evidence of the clinical efficacy of coffee enemas. Coffee enemas are associated with severe adverse reactions" (*J Clin Gastroenterol.* 1997;24:197).

In a 1990 report from the United States Congressional Office of Technology Assessment, three oncologists reviewed the "best cases" collected by Dr. Gonzalez. In the vast majority of these cases, they found claims of benefit from metabolic therapy to be unconvincing. In addition, they found a few cases to be "unusual" at best, meaning that these patients lived longer than typical people with the same type and stage of cancer, but concluded that this difference was probably due to statistical variation that occurs when "best cases" are selected from a large group of patients. A group of physicians who practiced alternative medicine (none of whom were cancer specialists) concluded that the alternative regimen was beneficial in some cases.

A small study of patients with pancreatic cancer—conducted by Dr. Gonzalez, who published the results in *Nutrition and Cancer* in 1999—found that patients treated with pancreatic enzymes survived longer than typical patients with pancreatic cancer. In a recent review of alternative cancer therapies, an expert in integrative oncology research methods noted that "The study was small and obviously prone to several biases. Not only is the comparison with national averages unadjusted for confounders (other factors that can affect outcome), but the principal results are based on patient selection; twelve patients who did not comply with treatment were excluded from analysis" (*CA Cancer J Clin.* 2004;54:115). The National Center for Complementary and Alternative Medicine is conducting a much larger, seven-year study comparing chemotherapy with the Gonzalez regimen in patients with pancreatic cancer, but results of this trial have not yet been published.

In a recent review of the medical literature, researchers from The University of Texas M. D. Anderson Cancer Center identified seven human studies of Gerson Therapy that have been published or presented at medical conferences. None of them were randomized controlled studies. One study was a retrospective review conducted by the Gerson Research Organization. They reported that survival rates were higher than would normally be expected for patients with melanoma, colorectal cancer, and ovarian cancer who were treated with surgery and Gerson Therapy, but they did not provide statistics to support the results. Other studies have been small, had inconclusive results, or have been plagued by other problems (such as a large percentage of patients not completing the study), making it impossible to draw firm conclusions about the effectiveness of treatment.

Several sets of researchers have reviewed the records of patients who used the Kelley's Treatment to determine whether the therapy was beneficial. It was found to be ineffective, especially when compared with conventional cancer treatment.

There is very little scientific evidence to support the use of the other components of metabolic therapies, such as consuming only fresh, raw juices prepared in a certain way, eliminating salt from the diet, and "detoxifying" the liver through coffee enemas and injected liver extracts. Some ideas put forth as part of metabolic therapy, such as eating large amounts of vegetables and fruits limiting fat intake, can be part of a healthy diet if not taken to the extreme. Researchers are continuing to study the potential anticancer properties of different substances in fruits and vegetables, but their actual effects are not well understood at this time.

Possible Problems and Complications

Some aspects of metabolic therapy are considered dangerous. Serious illness and death have occurred from some of the components of the treatment. There have been reports of complications related to liver cell injections, as well as nutritional deficiencies due to restricted diets. Several deaths have been directly linked to injecting live cells from animals, a practice known as cell therapy. The drug laetrile may cause nausea, vomiting, headache, dizziness, and even cyanide poisoning, which can be fatal. Care should be taken to make sure that any diet containing raw meat or juices from raw meat is free from contamination, given the increasing number of diseases that are known to be transmitted from animals to humans. Serious infections may result from poorly administered liver extracts. Thyroid supplements may cause severe bleeding in patients with who have cancer that has spread to the liver.

Reports of illness and even deaths linked to colonic irrigation have been published in several medical journals. People with diverticulitis, ulcerative colitis, Crohn's disease, severe hemorrhoids, or rectal or colon tumors, or who are recovering from bowel surgery, may be at higher risk of bowel injury when using enemas. Coffee enemas remove potassium from the body and can lead to electrolyte imbalances. People with kidney or heart failure may be more likely to experience fluid overload or electrolyte imbalances. Enemas can also cause discomfort and cramps. Continued home use of enemas may cause the colon's normal function to weaken, worsening constipation problems and colitis. Some metabolic diets used in combination with enemas cause dehydration.

Other Diets Promoted to Treat or Cure Cancer

Some treatments rely on certain foods and special methods of cooking—or not cooking food at all—to try to improve health. Diets that contain many vegetables and fruits can be healthy, but people who omit animal products from their diets need to consume other protein sources and get a balance of nutrients such as B12, vitamin D, calcium, zinc, and iron.

Vegetarian Diets

Vegetarian diets consist mainly or entirely of food that comes from plant sources such as vegetables, fruits, legumes, and grains. Vegetarian diets vary widely in the types of foods they include. Many proponents of vegetarianism believe the diet promotes health because it contains less fat, protein, and cholesterol and more fiber, vitamins, minerals, antioxidants, and phytochemicals than a diet containing meat.

All vegetarian diets include plant-based foods, such as grains, legumes, seeds, nuts, vegetables, and fruits, but they vary according to the kinds of animal products consumed.

There are many different types of vegetarian diets:
- vegan—no animal products, such as dairy or eggs
- lacto-ovo—includes dairy products and eggs
- lacto—includes dairy foods but no eggs
- pesca—includes fish and possibly shellfish
- fruitarian—raw fruits and fruit vegetables (such as tomatoes) only. This diet is extremely limited in nutrients.
- "Twinky vegetarians"—moniker for people who avoid all meat and dairy but eat large amounts of processed and convenience foods and snacks. They are more likely to have chosen a vegetarian diet based on animal preservation rather than value to health.

Currently, the American Cancer Society's nutrition guidelines recommend a mostly plant-based diet that includes five or more servings a day of vegetables and fruits, along with whole grain products, nuts and seeds, and beans. The Society recommends limiting your intake of red and processed meats, but notes that it is not necessary to avoid eating meat altogether.

The Evidence

Observational epidemiologic studies have linked vegetarian diets with a decreased risk of heart disease, diabetes, high blood pressure, obesity, and colon cancer. A review of research on the effects of vegetarian diets among Seventh-Day Adventists, whose religious doctrine advises against eating animal flesh, found that Seventh-Day Adventists experienced less heart disease and fewer cases of some types of cancer than the general population. On average, Seventh-Day Adventist males had lower-than-average serum cholesterol levels and blood pressure, and their overall cancer death rate was about half that of the general population. The overall cancer death rate of females was also lower. A couple of studies indicated an increased risk of colon and prostate cancer with increased animal fat intake. An increase in the consumption of beans and lentils appeared to decrease the risk of colon cancer and prostate cancer. The report cautioned that abstinence from tobacco and alcohol may have contributed to some of the health effects associated with vegetarian diets in the Seventh-Day Adventist community.

An observational study in Germany found the death rate for colon cancer was lower among moderate and strict vegetarians compared with that of the general population. However, the authors of the study also noted vegetarians tend to be more health conscious than the average person. In Great Britain, a seventeen-year observational study that followed eleven thousand vegetarians and health-conscious people concluded that the daily consumption of fresh fruit was linked to a significant reduction in deaths from ischemic heart disease, stroke, and all causes of death combined. Another population study found men who ate a diet rich in grains, cereals, and nuts had a lower risk of prostate cancer.

In 1991, two nutritionists studying the benefits and risks of vegetarian diets reported that vegetarians are not necessarily healthier than nonvegetarians and that well-planned omnivorous diets can provide health benefits as well. They also pointed out that many vegetarians adopt a healthier lifestyle, including more exercise and no smoking, which would likely improve their overall health and account for part of the health benefit that was first thought to be due to their diet.

A study published in 2005 compared more than one thousand German vegetarians with nearly seven hundred health-conscious nonvegetarians over a twenty-one-year period, and found that there were no major differences between the groups in terms of death and disease, although the vegetarians had slightly less heart disease. Both groups were healthier than the general population, in part due to less smoking and more exercise.

The majority of human evidence regarding vegetarianism consists of observational studies of the risk for various diseases such as cancer. Very few clinical studies of people with cancer have been reported. A few studies of men with prostate cancer have reported that comprehensive lifestyle changes including vegetarianism, exercise, and stress reduction can slow the rate increases in blood levels of prostate-specific antigens (PSA). The contribution of maintaining a vegetarian diet to these benefits remains unproven.

Possible Problems or Complications

Strict vegetarians, such as vegans, who eat no animal products at all, must be careful to consume adequate amounts of protein. Other nutrients that may be missing from a vegetarian diet include vitamin B12, vitamin D, calcium, zinc, and iron. Vegan diets must be carefully planned to ensure adequate amounts of required nutrients are consumed.

Vegan women who breastfeed their infants may want to take supplements containing sufficient vitamin B12. Severe B12 deficiencies in breastfed infants of vegan mothers have caused failure to thrive, poor brain development, and other serious problems.

Switching to a vegetarian diet may increase the amount of dietary fiber consumed, which can cause temporary problems such as bloating, discomfort, and gas. Registered dietitians suggest a gradual rather than quick change when adopting a vegetarian diet.

NO EVIDENCE: THE WHEATGRASS DIET

Wheatgrass is a tall grass commonly found in temperate regions of Europe and the United States. The roots and rhizomes (underground stems) are used in herbal remedies. Proponents claim that a dietary program based on wheatgrass, commonly called "the wheatgrass diet," can cause cancer to go into remission and extend the life of people with cancer. They believe that the wheatgrass diet strengthens the immune system, kills harmful bacteria in the digestive system, and rids the body of toxins and waste matter.

Wheatgrass is a natural source of vitamins and minerals, particularly B vitamins. However, available scientific evidence does not support the idea that wheatgrass or the wheatgrass diet alone can treat, cure, or prevent disease. One small early study found that wheatgrass juice, when used along with standard medical care, seemed to help control symptoms of chronic inflammation of the large intestine, a condition called ulcerative colitis. Although there are anecdotal reports that describe tumor shrinkage and extended survival among people with cancer who followed the wheatgrass diet, there are no clinical trials in the available scientific literature that support this claim.

The American Cancer Society's nutrition guidelines recommend eating a balanced diet that includes five or more servings a day of vegetables and fruit, choosing whole grains over processed and refined foods, and limiting red meats and processed meats. Choosing foods from a variety of fruits, vegetables, and other plant sources such as nuts, seeds, whole grain cereals, and beans is healthier than consuming large amounts of one particular food.

Macrobiotic Diet

A macrobiotic diet is generally vegetarian and consists largely of whole grains, cereals, and cooked vegetables. Whereas the macrobiotic diet was originally created to promote health, some of its proponents claim that it can prevent and cure disease, including cancer, and enhance spiritual and physical well-being.

Some vegetables are excluded. Fruits that do not grow locally, such as tropical fruits, are avoided. Eating dairy products, eggs, coffee, sugar, stimulant and aromatic herbs, red meat, poultry, and processed foods is discouraged. Macrobiotic principles also prescribe specific ways of cooking food using pots, pans, and utensils made only from materials such as wood, glass, ceramic, stainless steel, and enameled pieces. People who practice the diet do not usually cook with microwaves or electricity, nor do they consume vitamin or mineral supplements. In a macrobiotic diet, food is chewed until it is fluid to help with digestion.

The Evidence

There have been no randomized clinical studies published in the available medical literature to show the macrobiotic diet can be used to prevent or cure cancer. One of the earlier versions of the macrobiotic diet that involved eating only brown rice and water has been linked to severe nutritional deficiencies and even death. However, low-fat, high-fiber diets that consist mainly of plant products are believed to reduce the risk for cardiovascular disease and some forms of cancer. The National Institutes of Health's National Center for Complementary and Alternative Medicine has funded a study to determine whether a macrobiotic diet may prevent cancer.

Possible Problems or Complications

One of the earlier macrobiotic diets, which called for eating all grains, is severely deficient and has been linked to severe malnutrition and even death. Strict macrobiotic diets that include no animal products can result in nutritional deficiencies, such as inadequate intake of protein, vitamin D, zinc, calcium, iron, and vitamin B12. The risk may be more significant for people with cancer, who may have to contend with unwanted weight loss and often have increased nutritional and caloric requirements.

What we eat affects our bodies and our health and can even help prevent certain illnesses. But modern alternative therapies can be harmful if they require abandoning the nutrients your body needs, especially during cancer therapy, when your immune system needs to be strengthened. Although the studies and testimonials shared by proponents of some modern alternative therapies may sound tempting and even miraculous, purported nutritional treatments for cancer are not based in scientific evidence. Follow the healthy eating guidelines recommended in this book to build and maintain a stronger, healthier body.

Fasting and Juicing

Juicing and fasting are sometimes combined into one therapy. Juicing therapy requires drinking the juice from vegetables and fruits rather than eating the vegetables and fruits themselves. Fasting involves not eating for a period of time, although drinking liquids, such as water, tea, or juice, is permitted.

Fasting

Fasting is believed by some people to be an effective way of enabling the body to rid itself of toxins while promoting healing. Proponents of fasting for health rely on periods of not eating for several days to a month or more. By allowing the body to avoid the work of breaking down foods, those who fast hope the body will focus on healing and cleansing itself of toxins. Those who fast in hopes of treating cancer aim to improve the immune system by reducing its work of removing pathogens and allowing it to fight cancer.

When people fast, water and fat are lost, but toxins actually remain. Although fasting has been associated with reduced inflammation when done for a short period of time (a few days), long-term fasting depletes the immune system of essential nutrients and can lead to immunosuppression. Proponents claim that those who fast feel sick because toxins are being released, but the nausea actually occurs because the brain and other organs are deprived of the nutrients they need to work properly. Prolonged fasting (more than twenty-four to forty-eight hours) can result in ketosis (the rapid breakdown of fat to fuel the brain) as well as low blood sugar levels and loss of lean muscle mass. Particularly during cancer treatment, fasting can be problematic.

Fasting can place people with cancer at risk, especially those who are malnourished. Researchers have found that the body cannot distinguish between fasting and starvation. Studies related to cancer suggest that fasting could actually lead to the promotion of tumors. No evidence supports fasting as a healthy habit during cancer therapy or at any other time.

Juicing

In juice therapies, the primary sources of nourishment are fresh fruit and vegetable juices. Advocates of juice therapy believe that it stimulates the immune system and helps detoxify the body.

The many health benefits of vegetables and fruits are well documented, but juice therapy is not specifically recommended. Juices are not sufficient as a sole food source, although they are great sources of nutrients and phytochemicals when part of a healthful diet.

Juices may be less filling than whole vegetables and fruits and may contain less fiber; also, fruit juice, in particular, can provide lots of calories. Commercially juiced products should be 100 percent juice and should be pasteurized.

Commercially prepared, nonpasteurized juices and ciders may contain bacteria, which can be dangerous for people going through cancer treatment.

Juicing can add variety to the diet and can be a good way to consume vegetables and fruits, especially if chewing or swallowing are a problem or if your appetite is poor. Juicing also improves the absorption of some of the nutrients in vegetables and fruits. However, juices alone will not improve the immune system.

References

About herbs, botanicals, & other products: Memorial Sloan-Kettering Information Resource Database. Memorial Sloan-Kettering Cancer Center Web site. http://www.mskcc.org/aboutherbs. Accessed December 7, 2009.

American Cancer Society. *American Cancer Society Complete Guide to Complementary and Alternative Cancer Therapies.* 2nd ed. Atlanta, GA: American Cancer Society; 2009.

American Cancer Society. Questionable methods of cancer management: 'nutritional' therapies. *CA Cancer J Clin.* 1993;43(5):309-319.

American Cancer Society. Unproven methods of cancer management: Livingston-Wheeler therapy. *CA Cancer J Clin.* 1991;41(3):A7-A12.

American Cancer Society. Unproven methods of cancer management. The metabolic cancer therapy of Harold W. Manner, Ph.D. *CA Cancer J Clin.* 1986;36(3):185-189.

Associated Press. AP World Stream. *Cancer Research News.* Dutch authorities prosecuting a macrobiotic diet practitioner. March 1, 2000.

Barrett S, Herbert V. Manner metabolic therapy. Quackwatch Web site. http://www.quackwatch.org/01Quackery RelatedTopics/Cancer/manner.html. Posted July 1, 2001. Accessed December 9, 2009.

Barrett S, Herbert V. Questionable cancer therapies. Quackwatch Web site. http://www.quackwatch.org/01Quackery RelatedTopics/cancer.html. Updated July 6, 2001. Accessed December 9, 2009.

Caderni G, Perrelli MG, Cecchini F, Tessitore L. Enhanced growth of colorectal aberrant crypt foci in fasted/refed rats involves changes in TGFbeta1 and p21CIP expressions. *Carcinogenesis.* 2002;23(2):323-327.

Cassileth B. *The Alternative Medicine Handbook: The Complete Reference Guide to Alternative and Complementary Therapies.* New York, NY: W.W. Norton; 1998.

Cassileth BR, Lusk EJ, Guerry D, Blake AD, Walsh WP, Kascius L, Schultz DJ. Survival and quality of life among patients receiving unproven as compared with conventional cancer therapy. *N Engl J Med.* 1991;324(17):1180-1185.

Centers for Disease Control (CDC). Amebiasis associated with colonic irrigation— Colorado. *MMWR Morb Mortal Wkly Rep.* 1981;30(9):101-102.

Centers for Disease Control and Prevention (CDC). Neurologic impairment in children associated with maternal dietary deficiency of cobalamin — Georgia, 2001. *MMWR.* 2003;52(4);61-64.

Chang-Claude J, Hermann S, Eiber U, Steindorf K. Lifestyle determinants and mortality in German vegetarians and health-conscious persons: results of a 21-year follow-up. *Cancer Epidemiol Biomarkers Prev.* 2005;14(4):963-968.

Colonic irrigation. Aetna InteliHealth Web site. http://www.intelihealth.com/IH/ihtIH?d=dmtContent&c=358752. Accessed December 9, 2009.

Dingott S, Dwyer J. Vegetarianism: healthful but unnecessary. Quackwatch Web site. http://www.quackwatch.org/03HealthPromotion/vegetarian.html. Updated March 17, 2000. Accessed December 9, 2009.

Doyle C, Kushi LH, Byers T, Courneya KS, Demark-Wahnefried W, Grant B, McTiernan A, Rock CL, Thompson C, Gansler T, Andrews KS; The 2006 Nutrition, Physical Activity and Cancer Survivorship Advisory Committee; American Cancer Society. Nutrition and physical activity during and after cancer treatment: an American Cancer Society guide for informed choices. *CA Cancer J Clin.* 2006;56(6):323-353.

Eisele JW, Reay DT. Deaths related to coffee enemas. *JAMA.* 1980;244(14):1608-1609.

Elliott L, Molseed LL, McCallum PD, Grant B. *The Clinical Guide to Oncology Nutrition.* 2nd ed. Chicago, IL: American Dietetic Association; 2006.

Ernst E. Colonic irrigation and the theory of autointoxication: a triumph of ignorance over science. *J Clin Gastroenterol.* 1997;24(4):196-198.

Ernst E, ed. *The Desktop Guide to Complementary and Alternative Medicine: An Evidence-Based Approach.* New York: Mosby; 2001.

Eyre HJ, Lange DP, Morris LB. *Informed Decisions: The Complete Book of Cancer Diagnosis, Treatment, and Recovery.* 2nd ed. Atlanta, GA: American Cancer Society; 2001.

Fasting. PDRhealth Web site. http://www.pdrhealth.com/content/natural_medicine/chapters/201200.shtml. Accessed August 4, 2005. Content no longer available.

Frentzl-Beyme R, Chang-Claude J. Vegetarian diets and colon cancer: the German experience. *Am J Clin Nutr.* 1994;59(5 Suppl):1143S-1152S.

Gemcitabine compared with pancreatic enzyme therapy plus specialized diet (Gonzalez Regimen) in treating patients who have stage II, stage III, or stage IV pancreatic cancer. National Institutes of Health, ClincialTrials.gov Web site. http://clinicaltrials.gov/ct/show/NCT00003851. Accessed December 9, 2009.

Gerson regimen. Memorial Sloan-Kettering Cancer Center Web site. http://www.mskcc.org/mskcc/html/69233.cfm. Updated October 6, 2009. Accessed December 9, 2009.

Gonzalez NJ, Isaacs LL. Evaluation of pancreatic proteolytic enzyme treatment of adenocarcinoma of the pancreas, with nutrition and detoxification support. *Nutr Cancer.* 1999;33(2):117-124.

Green S. A critique of the rationale for cancer treatment with coffee enemas and diet. *JAMA.* 1992;268(22):3224-3227.

Green S. Nicolas Gonzalez treatment for cancer: gland extracts, coffee enemas, vitamin megadoses, and diets. Quackwatch Web site. http://www.quackwatch.org/01QuackeryRelatedTopics/Cancer/kg.html. Updated April 20, 2000. Accessed December 9, 2009.

Hebert JR, Hurley TG, Olendzki BC, Teas J, Ma Y, Hampl JS. Nutritional and socioeconomic factors in relation to prostate cancer mortality: a cross-national study. *J Natl Cancer Inst.* 1998;90(21):1637-1647.

Hikita H, Nuwaysir EF, Vaughan J, Babcock K, Haas MJ, Dragan YP, Pitot HC. The effect of short-term fasting, phenobarbital and refeeding on apoptotic loss, cell replication and gene expression in rat liver during the promotion stage. *Carcinogenesis.* 1998;19(8):1417-1425.

Hikita H, Vaughan J, Pitot HC. The effect of two periods of short-term fasting during the promotion stage of hepatocarcinogenesis in rats: the role of apoptosis and cell proliferation. *Carcinogenesis.* 1997;18(1):159-166.

Hildenbrand G, Hildenbrand L. Defining the role of diet therapy in complementary cancer management: prevention of recurrence vs. regression of disease. Proceedings of the 1996 Alternative Therapies Symposium: Creating Integrated Healthcare. San Diego, CA: January 18-21, 1996.

Hildenbrand GL, Hildenbrand LC, Bradford K, Cavin SW. Five-year survival rates of melanoma patients treated by diet therapy after the manner of Gerson: a retrospective review. *Altern Ther Health Med.* 1995;1(4):29-37.

Istre GR, Kreiss K, Hopkins RS, Healy GR, Benziger M, Canfield TM, Dickinson P, Englert TR, Compton RC, Mathews HM, Simmons RA. An outbreak of amebiasis spread by colonic irrigation at a chiropractic clinic. *N Engl J Med.* 1982;307(6):339-342.

Key TJ, Thorogood M, Appleby PN, Burr ML. Dietary habits and mortality in 11,000 vegetarians and health conscious people: results of a 17 year follow up. *BMJ.* 1996;313(7060):775-779.

Kushi LH, Byers T, Doyle C, Bandera EV, McCullough M, McTiernan A, Gansler T, Andrews KS, Thun MJ; American Cancer Society 2006 Nutrition and Physical Activity Guidelines Advisory Committee. American Cancer Society guidelines on Nutrition and Physical Activity for cancer prevention: reducing the risk of cancer with healthy food choices and physical activity. *CA Cancer J Clin.* 2006;56(5):254-281.

Kushi LH, Cunningham JE, Hebert JR, Lerman RH, Bandera EV, Teas J. The macrobiotic diet in cancer. *J Nutr.* 2001;131(11 Suppl):3056S-3064S.

Legro RS, Finegood D, Dunaif A. A fasting glucose to insulin ratio is a useful measure of insulin sensitivity in women with polycystic ovary syndrome. *J Clin Endocrinol Metab.* 1998;83(8):2694-2698.

Livingston-Wheeler therapy. Memorial Sloan-Kettering Cancer Center Web site. http://www.mskcc.org/mskcc/html/69283.cfm. Updated July 21, 2008. Accessed December 9, 2009.

Maritess C, Small S, Waltz-Hill M. Alternative nutrition therapies in cancer patients. *Semin Oncol Nurs.* 2005;21(3):173-176.

Metabolic therapies. Memorial Sloan-Kettering Cancer Center Web site. http://www.mskcc.org/mskcc/html/69299.cfm. Accessed December 9, 2009

Molassiotis A, Peat P. Surviving against all odds: analysis of 6 case studies of patients with cancer who followed the Gerson therapy. *Integr Cancer Ther.* 2007;6(1):80-88.

Murphy GP, Morris LB, Lange D; American Cancer Society. *Informed Decisions: The Complete Book of Cancer Diagnosis, Treatment, and Recovery.* New York: Viking; 1997.

National Institutes of Health. *Alternative Medicine: Expanding Medical Horizons: A Report to the National Institutes of Health on Alternative Medical Systems and Practices in the United States.* Washington, DC: US Government Printing Office; 1994. NIH publication 94-066.

Ornish D, Weidner G, Fair WR, Marlin R, Pettengill EB, Raisin CJ, Dunn-Emke S, Crutchfield L, Jacobs FN, Barnard RJ, Aronson WJ, McCormac P, McKnight DJ, Fein JD, Dnistrian AM, Weinstein J, Ngo TH, Mendell NR, Carroll PR. Intensive lifestyle changes may affect the progression of prostate cancer. *J Urol.* 2005;174(3):1065-1069.

Saxe GA, Major JM, Nguyen JY, Freeman KM, Downs TM, Salem CE. Potential attenuation of disease progression in recurrent prostate cancer with plant-based diet and stress reduction. *Integr Cancer Ther.* 2006;5(3):206-213.

Sesca E, Premoselli F, Binasco V, Bollito E, Tessitore L. Fasting-refeeding stimulates the development of mammary tumors induced by 7,12-dimethylbenz[a]anthracene. *Nutr Cancer.* 1998;30(1):25-30.

Singh PN, Fraser GE. Dietary risk factors for colon cancer in a low-risk population. *Am J Epidemiol.* 1998;148(8):761-764.

US Congress, Office of Technology Assessment. *Unconventional Cancer Treatments: OTA-H-405.* Washington, DC: US Government Printing Office; 1990.

Vegetarian lifestyle. American Dietetic Association Web site. http://www.eatright.org/Public/content.aspx?id=6372. Accessed December 9, 2009.

Vickers A. Alternative cancer cures: "unproven" or "disproven"? *CA Cancer J Clin.* 2004;54(2):110-118.

Chapter Seven

Preparing for Cancer Treatment

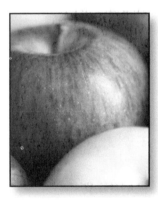

DURING YOUR TREATMENT, you will be concentrating on staying strong and minimizing side effects. Eating well is key to supplying your body with the nutrients it needs to stay well. This chapter explores some ideas to help you prepare for cancer treatment and its effects.

Not everyone undergoing cancer treatment experiences side effects, and for those who do, not everyone experiences the same side effects or experiences them in the same way. No one can predict how cancer treatment will affect you, and you will not know what your experience will be until you begin your therapy. Many factors influence side effects and their severity, including the type of cancer you have, your age, the part of your body being treated, the type and length of treatment, the treatment dose, and your current health. Your health care team will be able to tell you more about your likelihood of having side effects and what you might expect.

There are no hard and fast rules about nutrition during cancer treatment. You are simply encouraged to eat as healthfully as possible. Some people being treated for cancer continue to enjoy eating and have a normal appetite throughout most of their treatment. Others have days when they do not feel like eating at all. For many people, side effects come and go. Not eating enough can lead to weight loss, and weight loss can lead to weakness and fatigue. Eating as well as you can during treatment and recovery is an important part of taking care of yourself and managing your body's changing needs.

In this book, the terms "eating well" and "eating healthfully" are used to mean taking in a variety of nourishing foods that provide enough nutrients for optimal health during your cancer treatment. Eating healthfully provides you with distinct advantages:

- Eating a balanced diet allows you to enter and undergo treatment with body reserves of needed nutrients, such as protein, vitamins, and minerals. These reserves help to maintain strength, prevent body tissue from breaking down, rebuild tissue, and provide defense against infection.
- People who eat well are better able to cope with side effects and have a greater likelihood of receiving their treatment without unscheduled breaks or reduced doses. If you are well nourished and taking in enough calories and protein, health care professionals know that some cancer treatments are actually much more effective. Assuming you are not accumulating fluid in your abdomen, arms, or legs, your body weight is a great "barometer" to gauge your calorie intake. If you are losing weight, you are not getting enough calories!
- Eating well is crucial to helping your body stay healthy. As you undergo cancer treatment, it is more important than ever that you eat as healthfully as possible. However, do not be too hard on yourself on days when your appetite is poor. Take advantage of the times you feel well by eating as nutritiously as you can on those days.

Cancer and cancer treatment can cause changes in appetite and taste; you may be surprised by some of the foods that appeal to you during treatment. Do not be afraid to try new things—

foods you never liked before may taste good to you during treatment.

With your doctor's permission and guidance, be as physically active as possible. Whether it's walking around your neighborhood or doing light chores around your home, physical activity can help stimulate your appetite and improve feelings of physical well-being. Begin slowly, and gradually increase physical activity as you feel stronger. If you exercise outside, pick a time of day when the weather is most comfortable, remember to wear good shoes, and drink plenty of water.

Planning Ahead—Meal Preparation

Planning ahead will help you take advantage of time savers like food delivery, preplanned menus, and friends' help with cooking or shopping. On days when you are feeling well, you may want to focus on eating meals with more nutrients so your body can store them for later use. If you have more energy than usual, consider cooking nutritious meals that can be divided into portions and frozen. The stored portions can be reheated and eaten on days when you do not feel up to preparing a meal from scratch.

When Others Offer to Help

Friends and loved ones may offer to pitch in with cooking duties, or they may offer to get you out of the house for a meal on your feel-good days. Do not be too stubborn or embarrassed to accept help. Others want to help and need to feel useful. Let them pitch in; it makes them feel good, too. Thinking about specific tasks that you need help with or letting people know your food preferences beforehand can make it easier for others to support and care for you:

- For helpful ideas and recipes for cooking for people undergoing cancer treatment, refer to the companion cookbook from the American Cancer Society, *What to Eat During Cancer Treatment* (see the next page for more information).
- Keep a standby grocery list on hand so it is easy to send a friend or family member to the store or to order over the phone or Internet.
- Have someone go with you to the grocery store so that they can help you carry and put away your purchases.
- Take others up on offers to help prepare meals—and offers to clean up afterward.
- Offer menu ideas or favorite healthy recipes to friends and family members who want to cook for you and ask for your preferences.
- Ask your friends not to prepare or purchase too many high-calorie, low-nutrition "comfort" foods. There is nothing wrong with eating these foods in moderation. Remember that when your treatment is over, you will want to resume healthy habits. If you eat unhealthfully now, it may make it more difficult to change later.
- Keep a list of foods that appeal to you during treatment and recovery so those helping

you will know what you can tolerate.

- Do not be hesitant to let others take you out to eat when you feel up to it. Do not be afraid to ask the wait staff about exact ingredients in a dish, the method used to prepare it, or to ask for half portions.
- When you do not feel like going out, order from restaurants that offer take-out and let friends or family pick up your order and eat with you.
- Select restaurants with which you are familiar, that are clean, and that provide healthy meal options.
- If your cancer treatments have caused low white blood cell counts that put you at risk for food-borne infection, be sure to provide your friends and family with information on how to safely prepare foods. Refer to chapter 10 for tips on food safety at home or when eating out.

Food Shopping

Food shopping during treatment can be difficult if you are tired, not feeling well, or bothered by the smell of food. Friends and family may be able to pick up a few items for you as they do their own grocery shopping. If others are not able to take over shopping duties, consider ordering groceries online if it's an option in your area or phoning in an order to a grocery store that delivers. A number of online retailers sell and deliver groceries—try an Internet search for "online grocery delivery" or a similar phrase to find out whether any retailers deliver to your town.

WHAT TO EAT DURING CANCER TREATMENT

The American Cancer Society's companion cookbook, *What to Eat During Cancer Treatment: 100 Great-Tasting, Family-Friendly Recipes to Help You Cope* offers recipes adapted to meet the needs of people undergoing cancer treatment. Written by Jeanne Besser and registered dietitians Kristina Ratley, Sheri Knecht, and Michele Szafranski, the book is designed to be an easy-to-use tool for people experiencing side effects of treatment. Recipes are organized by side effect: Nausea, Diarrhea, Constipation, Sore Mouth and Difficulty Swallowing, Taste Alterations, and Unintentional Weight Loss, and include cross-reference tabs to indicate recipes that are appropriate for more than one symptom. The book also includes helpful advice for the caregiver, tips to make eating out easier, tips on assembling a take-along food "survival kit," advice on avoiding excess weight gain during treatment, and a kitchen staples list. For more information, visit cancer.org/bookstore or call 800-227-2345.

When you do need to go to the store, get the most out of your trip by following these steps:

- Write out a grocery list in the rough order of the aisles you'll pass so you don't get side-tracked and forget things.
- If possible, shop in a small local grocery store so you can get through the store and lines more quickly and easily.
- Visit an outdoor farmer's market if possible. You may feel better in the open air than in an enclosed store, where food odors are trapped.
- Buy multiples of items that won't go bad so you can reduce your trips to the store.
- Ask for help taking groceries to the car if you need it. If possible, shop when friends or family members will be available to bring in the groceries and put them away.

Ask your registered dietitian or health care team to help you plan meals and develop a grocery list of appropriate foods to rely on in case you have side effects such as constipation or nausea. Coping with eating- and digestion-related side effects is discussed further in chapter 12.

Stocking the Refrigerator and Pantry

On days when you are feeling well, ready your kitchen and pantry with items you will need for meals during treatment. Stock the pantry and freezer with your favorite foods so you will not need to shop as often. Include mild, easy-to-digest foods like gelatin, soup, broth, or hot cereal that you know you can eat even when you aren't feeling well.

- Purchase family-size or multiple individual portions in the freezer section of your grocery store. Warehouse stores like Sam's Club, BJ's Wholesale Club, and Costco have a wide variety of preprepared dishes in the refrigerator and freezer sections.
- Take advantage of preprepared foods like frozen entrées or soups, containers of hummus, individually wrapped cheeses, and ready-to-eat baby carrots and snap peas.
- Although eating a lot of processed foods is not the best choice in the long run, during treatment you may wish to opt for shelf-stable foods that are easy to prepare, including ready-to-serve canned soups or stews, packaged fish or poultry, and nut butters. These foods will not spoil and can be a quick meal.
- Choose a variety of fresh, frozen, and canned vegetables and fruits. Frozen vegetables are typically more nutritious and lower in salt than canned. Many packaged vegetables are picked and frozen at their peak so that they retain flavor and nutrients. For extra nutrition, add vegetables to salads, soups, and stews; add fruits to your cereal, salads, and smoothies.
- Keep the refrigerator, freezer, and pantry organized so that friends and family members not accustomed to your kitchen can easily find things.

In general, select meals with adequate protein, vegetables, fruits, pastas, rice and other grains. Be aware that some prepared foods are not the healthiest—they might contain more saturated fat or trans fats than are recommended. Look for the most nutritious choices.

Cooking for Yourself or Others

After a cancer diagnosis, some home routines may need to change to accommodate appointments, treatment, and recovery. If you enjoy cooking for yourself or others, continue doing so as long as it does not interfere with your nutritional intake and enjoyment of food. Just be sure to make it easy on yourself by saving time and energy. Here are some ways to make cooking more pleasurable and efficient:

Simplify

Use kitchen appliances and gadgets to save time at the counter or stove. Food processors, slow cookers (Crock-Pots), and microwaves help you cook more efficiently. In addition, cooking in a microwave does not spread cooking smells throughout the house, and a slow cooker can be moved to a garage or back porch to cut down on smells. Using prepared foods, mixes, and frozen foods can cut preparation time as well. Stir-fried meals can also save time and energy and are a great way to use up leftovers.

Label and Date Perishable Foods and Leftovers

Use masking tape, which is easy to remove, to label and date perishable foods. Note the date and dish name on each container, and see the table below for limits for food storage. Refer to chapter 10 for more tips on safe food storage.

Limits for Food Storage		
	REFRIGERATOR (34–40°F)	**FREEZER (0–2°F or below)**
Red meats—cooked	3 days	2 to 3 months
Red meats—raw	3 days	4 to 12 months
Poultry—cooked	3 days	4 months
Poultry—raw	1 to 2 days	9 to 12 months
Casseroles	3 days	2 to 3 months
Frozen dinners	3 days	3 to 4 months

Stay Flexible

When treatment begins, try to remain flexible. Plan to adjust your routine and usual diet to allow for potential changes in taste, smell, energy level, or appetite. Keep in mind the nutritional advice in this book, and try to have a variety of nutrients in each meal.

Work Together

If you cook and eat with friends or family, plan menus together so that everyone's tastes and nutritional needs are met. Share or delegate the grocery shopping, preparation, or cleanup duties—your friends and family will likely be glad to help. Set priorities, especially if you are fatigued; concentrate on what you enjoy.

Make Meals Enjoyable

Set the stage, relax, and view your mealtime as an opportunity to wind down, talk with others, or simply reflect. Keep your eating area uncluttered, well ventilated, and visually pleasing. Try eating in different locations: the backyard, front porch, on the lawn with a picnic blanket, at the dining room table with cloth napkins, or even in the bathtub. Spruce things up with linens, flowers, candles, and music. In addition, plan to use your favorite flavors and, if necessary, add extra spices or seasonings to your portion if others do not enjoy the same tastes.

Consider having meals delivered to your home or eating a meal at a community center or senior center. To learn more about meal delivery and other services, click on the "Contact Us" link at cancer.org or call 800-227-2345 for resources in your community. You might also look into support from local government agencies, area churches, and social services.

Personal chef businesses are cropping up around the nation. This service, which may include preparing meals on site or delivering premade meals, can be expensive but can help you meet specific dietary requirements when your energy is low and nutrition needs are high. Additional information on available services in your area can be found at www.personalchef.com; click through the "Find a Personal Chef" link to locate someone in your area.

Meals on Wheels Association of America is a membership association of programs that provide home-delivered and group meals for senior citizens and homebound individuals. The goal of the organization is to improve the quality of life for those in need. Some programs provide other health and social services such as transportation, recreation, nutrition information, education, resource information, referrals, and case management. Contact the social worker in your health care facility or contact Meals on Wheels directly at 703-548-5558 or www.mowaa.org.

Planning Ahead for Cancer Treatment and Related Side Effects

Many people have few or no side effects that keep them from eating. Those who do have eating problems usually do not have them every day. In addition, most eating-related side effects go away after cancer treatment is complete. Even if you do have side effects, they should be manageable and your health care team will work with you to relieve them using both medications and diet modifications. Talk to your health care team about the medication options that are appropriate for your situation. If you are already taking medications as prescribed by your doctor and you still have side effects such as nausea or diarrhea, ask your doctor whether a different medication might be more beneficial.

Because treatment methods differ in their approaches to treating cancer, their side effects can vary. Before your treatment begins, it is a good idea to have some information on the potential effects of treatment on your body, your eating habits, and your digestion. Ask members of your health care team for strategies to manage side effects should you encounter them. Planning ways to cope with possible side effects can make you feel more in control of your situation.

Conventional methods of cancer treatment—including surgery, radiation therapy, chemotherapy, hormonal therapy, biotherapy (also called immunotherapy or biologic therapy), or a combination of any of these treatments—target the fast-growing cancer cells in your body. However, these treatments can also damage healthy cells. The cells most affected by cancer treatment are those that grow and divide rapidly, such as blood cells, hair cells, and the cells lining your mouth and digestive tract.

Bone marrow transplantation is an intensive therapy used to treat cancers and diseases of the bone marrow. It involves high-dose chemotherapy and, in some instances, radiation therapy. Because of its complexity and the very specific treatment regimens that are used, this book will not present information regarding side effects or diet and nutrition management suggestions for this type of cancer treatment. If you are undergoing a bone marrow transplant, ask to work with the registered dietitian where you are receiving your bone marrow transplant. If you are interested in general information about nutrition and side effect management of bone marrow transplant, call the American Cancer Society at 800-227-2345 or visit the Web site, cancer.org. Information is also available through the Web sites of the National Cancer Institute, Memorial Sloan-Kettering Cancer Center, or The University of Texas M. D. Anderson Cancer Center. See chapter 14 for more information about these and other organizations.

The pages that follow will describe some of the side effects that can occur as a result of conventional cancer treatment. Later in this book, you will read more about specific side effects and what to expect, how to cope with them, and what to eat if you encounter them.

KEEPING TRACK OF SIDE EFFECTS

Here's a form to help you keep track of eating-related side effects you may experience while you are undergoing cancer treatment. Feel free to copy this form and keep your own record. You can also share it with the health care professional who is keeping track of side effects with you during this time.

Your Name: _____ **Week of:** _____

Write the type and date of your *last* treatment(s):

Type of Treatment: _____ **Date(s):** _____

_____ _____

Your Weight: _____lbs. (measure once a week)

In the list below, check the box next to any side effect that you experience this week. Next to each one you check, write a number from 1 to 3 indicating how severe each side effect was, where **1 = mild**; **2 = moderate**; and **3 = severe**.

Side Effect	M	T	W	T	F	S	Sun
Loss of Appetite	☐	☐	☐	☐	☐	☐	☐
Sore/Dry Mouth	☐	☐	☐	☐	☐	☐	☐
Nausea	☐	☐	☐	☐	☐	☐	☐
Vomiting	☐	☐	☐	☐	☐	☐	☐
Constipation	☐	☐	☐	☐	☐	☐	☐
Diarrhea	☐	☐	☐	☐	☐	☐	☐
Fatigue	☐	☐	☐	☐	☐	☐	☐
Other:	☐	☐	☐	☐	☐	☐	☐

Other Questions or Concerns (Use this space to write down questions or concerns you may want to talk about with your health care provider.)

_____

_____

_____

_____

Adapted from the National Cancer Institute. *Eating Hints for Cancer Patients: Before, During and After Treatment* (Bethesda, MD: National Institutes of Health, 2006).

Do not be afraid to talk with the members of your health care team about your feelings and any concerns you have about the side effects of treatment. Your doctor, nurse, and registered dietitian have helped many other individuals receiving cancer treatment. When you understand your diagnosis and treatment plan, you are less likely to encounter side-effect surprises along the way.

However, even the best laid nutrition and eating plans might not be enough, and nutritional support measures in the form of parenteral or enteral nutrition feeding might be necessary to help you get through cancer treatment. Enteral nutrition (liquid nutrition) is given directly into the gastrointestinal tract, and parenteral nutrition is special nutrition given intravenously (into a vein). These methods of nutrition support are discussed more on pages 257–261, in chapter 12. It is important to view these measures not as a failure to eat enough, but as tools to help you through your cancer treatment and to help maintain your body's nutrition stores and a healthy weight.

Surgery

Surgery to remove cancer cells and surrounding tissue is often combined with radiation therapy and chemotherapy to treat cancer. After surgery, the body needs extra calories and protein for healing and recovery. Many people have some pain and fatigue after surgery, and they may be unable to eat their usual diet because of surgery-related side effects. These side effects can last for weeks or months if the gastrointestinal tract is involved. The body's ability to digest and absorb nutrients can also be altered if any part of the mouth, esophagus, stomach, pancreas, small intestine, colon, or rectum is surgically removed. Before surgery, discontinue any dietary supplements and herbal products that can interact with anesthesia or affect the formation of red blood cells, thin the blood, or increase blood clots. Examples of these dietary and herbal supplements include vitamin E, vitamin K, omega-3 fatty acids (fish oil), garlic pills, flaxseed pills, St. John's wort, ginko biloba, and ginger pills. If you have been taking dietary supplements or herbal products, let your surgical team know what you have been using. Your surgeon or anesthesiologist will most likely ask you to stop taking these products for one to two weeks before your scheduled surgery. Once you have recovered from your surgery, check with your doctor before resuming their use.

Nutrition Suggestions Before, During, and After Cancer Surgery

The day or night before surgery, you may not be allowed to eat or drink anything. After your surgery, it may be several hours or even one or two days before you can eat normal foods and liquids. If you have not eaten for more than a day or two, your doctor may advise you to start with easy-to-digest foods and beverages. Your surgeon will provide you with specific diet information depending on your surgery. However, most people will begin with a clear liquid diet and transition slowly back to their usual diet. (See the information on special diets in the appendix for more details.)

These suggestions may be helpful to you if you have had cancer surgery:

- When reintroducing your digestive system to food after surgery, start with bland, easy-to-digest foods and beverages.
- Foods and beverages that are low in fat and easy to digest and absorb are easier to tolerate than high-fat items such as fried or greasy foods. For example, begin with clear juices, broth-type soups, and fruit ices. Once you can tolerate these foods, slowly begin adding back your usual foods and beverages.
- As you recover, make sure to take in plenty of fluids to prevent dehydration. Sip water, juices, or decaffeinated clear liquids throughout the day.
- Eat as well as you can on the days when your appetite is good. It may be easier to eat small, frequent meals or snacks. Begin with a goal of half of a presurgery portion. Do not be too hard on yourself if side effects make it difficult to eat.
- Eat by the clock rather than waiting for hunger. Try to eat small, frequent meals and snacks every three to four hours, or try to eat four to six small meals a day.
- Before surgery, ask family and friends for help with shopping for groceries and preparing meals. Do not be shy about asking for regular help with grocery store trips and cooking meals after surgery as well.
- Try to resume your normal, day-to-day activities as soon as possible, with the guidance of your health care team. Ease carefully into more vigorous exercise. Remember, you probably will not be able to resume your usual level of physical activity immediately after surgery. Most individuals need to slowly increase the duration and intensity of their physical activities and exercise.
- Protein helps rebuild strength and create new cells. Include high-protein foods in your diet each day. See chapter 8 for more information about protein-rich foods.
- After surgery, make sure you eat plenty of foods that are good sources of vitamin C, iron, calcium, magnesium, and potassium to aid in healing. Examples of these foods include vegetables and fruits (juice, cooked, canned, frozen, or raw), dairy foods, iron-fortified breakfast cereals, and lean proteins. If you are struggling with a poor appetite after surgery, speak with your health care provider about whether you should take a "one-a-day" type vitamin and mineral supplement to ensure adequate intake of micronutrients. Look for supplements that contain no more than 100 percent of the Recommended Daily Values.
- Refer to chapters 8–12 for tips to manage surgery-related side effects.

The type and duration of any side effects you have after surgery will depend on where in the body the surgery was performed and on your overall health. Medication, good hygiene, physician-approved physical activity, and changes in diet can help lessen side effects. If side effects persist, be sure to alert your doctor, nurse, registered dietitian, or another member of your health care team and ask about ways to cope.

Radiation Therapy

In radiation therapy, high-energy rays, known as ionizing radiation, are used to cure, control, or palliate cancer. Types of radiation therapy used in cancer treatment include radiotherapy, brachytherapy, stereotactic radiosurgery, and radiopharmaceutical therapy. The goal of radiation therapy is to prevent cells from growing and dividing. Radiation therapy is directed at the part of the body with cancer. While all cells exposed to radiation therapy are affected by it, most of the body's normal cells can heal and recover.

- *Radiotherapy* precisely delivers radiation into the body in fractionated doses with external beam megavoltage machines. Examples of radiation therapy machines include linear accelerators that generate x-rays or photons and electrons; cyclotrons that generate protons or neutrons; or cobolt-60 units that produce gamma rays.
- *Stereotactic radiosurgery* (SRS) or Gamma Knife therapy uses intensity-modulated radiation therapy (IMRT) and delivers it with extreme accuracy to cancer cells and thus limits exposure to normal cells. Examples of SRS include treatment of small tumors in defined areas in the brain or prostate gland.
- *Brachytherapy* delivers highly localized doses of radiation through use of sealed radioactive sources or implants placed directly in or near the cancer cells. Examples of brachytherapy are removable intercavitary implants for women with gynecologic cancer or interstitial implants of permanent radioactive seeds for men with prostate cancer.
- *Radiopharmaceutical therapy* involves injecting or ingesting unsealed liquid radioactive sources into the body. Examples of radiopharmaceuticals include oral iodine-131 to treat thyroid cancer or strontium-89 to treat painful bone metastases.

External beam radiation treatment for cancer is usually given five days a week for two to nine weeks. The types of side effects the therapy causes depend on the specific area of the body receiving radiation, the size of area being treated, the total dose of radiation, and the number of treatments (daily fractions).

- *Head and neck.* Radiation therapy to the head and neck can cause several changes to the mouth, including internal and external redness, irritation, dryness, oral secretions of thick mucus, pain, difficulty with chewing and swallowing, and changes in or loss of taste.
- *Chest.* Radiation therapy to the chest may cause difficulty or soreness when swallowing, heartburn, or esophageal reflux.

- *Abdomen.* Radiation therapy to the stomach or part of the abdomen, such as the liver or pancreas, can cause nausea with or without vomiting. Diarrhea can result from radiation to the lower abdomen.
- *Pelvis.* Radiation therapy to any part of the pelvis may cause changes in normal bowel habits and might cause diarrhea, bowel cramping, upper or lower abdominal gas or bloating, or intolerance for dairy products.

Do not expect to have the same side effects as someone else being treated for cancer in a different area of the body. In fact, even people undergoing the same type of treatment might have very different experiences and side effects.

With radiation therapy, side effects typically begin around the second or third week of treatment. Individuals who have a history of sensitive stomach or irritable bowel might experience side effects earlier. Regardless of what area of the body is treated, the most commonly reported side effect of radiation therapy is fatigue, usually increasing in intensity as the weeks of treatment progress. After radiation therapy ends, most acute side effects last two to three more weeks. However, some people can experience long-lasting effects, such as dry mouth after radiation to the oral cavity or difficulty swallowing coarse foods if the esophagus was irradiated. If side effects develop, ask your radiation oncologist, nurse, or registered dietitian whether medicines, changes in diet, or other changes can help you manage your eating-related concerns.

Nutrition Suggestions During and After Radiation Therapy

Eating well during the time that you are undergoing radiation therapy may be difficult. Receiving daily radiation therapy treatments often involves being away from home for long periods each day, especially if you are also receiving chemotherapy. Plan ahead and take snacks and beverages with you for car trips and long days in the clinic. If you have access to a kitchen or microwave in the clinic, you can bring along easy-to-prepare, prepackaged foods, or ready-to-eat soups or stews for meals or snacks. Remember to keep cold things cool in an ice-packed cooler or lunch box.

Sometimes, people temporarily relocate to a hotel or motel near the treatment center because the daily travel becomes too much. If there is no kitchen where you are staying, keep foods on hand that do not need refrigeration, such as single servings of canned fruit, gelatin, puddings, cheese or peanut butter and crackers, granola bars, or cereal. Beverages such as juice packs, water, and canned nutritional supplements are also safe to keep in the room. Once they are opened, however, they need to be consumed immediately; whatever you do not finish eating or drinking should be thrown away. Refer to chapters 8–12 for tips on managing treatment-related side effects.

Chemotherapy

Chemotherapy involves taking strong medications or chemical agents designed to kill rapidly dividing cells. These agents are most commonly given by infusion into the bloodstream or taken by mouth. Chemotherapy can damage both healthy cells and cancerous cells. Normal cells most likely to be affected are bone marrow, hair, and any part of the lining of the gastrointestinal tract, from the mouth to the anus.

Side effects will depend on what kind of chemotherapy you take and how often it is given. Common side effects of chemotherapy that can interfere with the ability to eat include loss of appetite, changes in taste and smell, mouth tenderness or sores, nausea, vomiting, changes in bowel habits, fatigue, and low white blood cell counts (which increase the chance for infection).

Myelosuppression (suppression of the bone marrow) is a common effect of chemotherapy. When production of the bone marrow is altered by chemotherapy, the following conditions may occur and affect the body's ability to fight infection:

- leukopenia—a decrease in the number of white blood cells
- neutropenia—a decrease in the number of neutrophils

As the white blood cell count falls, the risk for infection rises. Chemotherapy can also cause anemia (a decrease in the number of red blood cells) and thrombocytopenia (a decrease in the number of platelets). When white blood cell counts are low, you will need to take extra care when handling, preparing, and storing food so as to reduce your risk of a food-borne illness. See chapter 10 for information on the safe handling of food.

If you are having side effects from chemotherapy, tell your doctor, registered dietitian, or nurse. They will most likely recommend medicines, daily self-care practices, and changes in diet to lessen eating-related side effects you are having.

Nutrition Suggestions Before, During, and After Chemotherapy

Most people receive chemotherapy at an outpatient facility. A chemotherapy session can take anywhere from minutes to several hours or can even require hospital admission.

Fatigue is very common during chemotherapy. It usually does not happen during or right after chemotherapy administration but several days later. Dehydration, which can result from vomiting or diarrhea, can make chemotherapy-related fatigue more significant. Ask your health care team about medications or other possible methods to combat fatigue. Unless you are given other instructions, eat a balanced diet that includes protein (meat, poultry, fish, dairy products, eggs, or plant-based protein) to help increase your energy. Other suggestions to reduce fatigue are to prioritize your activities, doing the most important when you have the most energy, and to balance daytime rest so that it does not interfere with nighttime sleep. For more information about coping with fatigue, see chapter 9.

The following strategies may make eating during chemotherapy easier:

- Plan ahead, and bring a light meal or snack with you to treatment in an insulated bag or small cooler. Find out whether your facility has a refrigerator or microwave you can use. As a courtesy to others undergoing treatment, avoid bringing foods that have strong odors. These foods, while they may be tasty, could ruin someone else's appetite.
- Make sure you eat something before receiving your treatment. Most people find that a light low-fat meal or snack before chemotherapy is well tolerated even if it is just a few salted crackers and a clear juice.
- Do not be too hard on yourself if side effects make it difficult to eat. Try eating small, frequent meals or snacks. Go easy on fried or greasy foods, which can be hard to digest. On days when you're feeling well and your appetite is good, try to eat regular meals and snacks and regain any weight you lost during the days immediately after chemotherapy.
- Don't be afraid to ask loved ones for help with grocery shopping and preparing meals.
- Try canned nutritional supplements to add to the nutrients you are getting through food.

Some side effects of chemotherapy go away within hours of receiving treatment. If your side effects persist, tell your health care team. Prompt attention to nutrition-related side effects can help you maintain your weight and energy level and help you feel better. Keeping notes about your experience, especially in the days immediately after a chemotherapy treatment or cycle, will help jog your memory in preparation for conversations with health care team members. Their job is to make chemotherapy the most manageable experience possible, and if you had side effects, they may be able to change some things the next time around. Do not hesitate to talk to them or ask if there are other options should a medicine not work. You can use either the "Keeping Track of Side Effects" worksheet provided on page 148 of this book or a simple spiral notebook. Refer to chapters 8–12 for tips on managing treatment-related side effects.

Biotherapy

Biotherapy (sometimes called immunotherapy, biologic therapy, or biologic response modifiers) is treatment to stimulate the natural defenses of your immune system to fight cancer. Biotherapy is sometimes used by itself, but it is most often used as an adjuvant therapy (something used with or after another type of therapy) to add to the anticancer effects of a main therapy.

Researchers and doctors have designed different types of biotherapies to help the immune system recognize cancer cells and strengthen its ability to destroy them:

- *Monoclonal antibodies* bind to proteins on cancer cells and target them for destruction. Monoclonal antibodies are produced in large quantities in a laboratory rather than by a person's own immune system. This type of therapy can be effective even if the person's immune system is weakened.

- *Cancer vaccines* contain cancer cells, parts of cells, or pure antigens (anything that causes the immune system to produce a response). The vaccines increase the immune system's response to cancer cells that are already present in the body.
- *Nonspecific biotherapies* stimulate the immune system in a very general way. The overall increase in immune system activity can result in more activity against any cancer cells present.

Nutrition Suggestions During Biotherapy

Potential side effects vary from treatment to treatment, but biotherapy can cause fever, tiredness, muscle aches, and weakness, and it can lead to loss of appetite and an increased need for protein, calories, and liquids. Depending on their severity, these symptoms can cause gradual or drastic weight loss if they are ignored, which can lead to malnutrition (loss of body reserves, especially muscle). Malnutrition can complicate or delay the cancer treatment plan and the healing and recovery process.

If you are experiencing a loss of appetite when receiving biotherapy, eat small, frequent meals of high-calorie, high-protein foods. Eating a nutritious diet that includes plenty of liquids can help prevent significant weight loss and reduce treatment-related fatigue. If you are coping with nausea and vomiting, do not force yourself to eat or drink. But to prevent dehydration, do try to sip water or other clear liquids or eat ice chips, Popsicles, or sorbet. Talk to your health care team about the common side effects of your specific biotherapy, medicines for managing side effects, and strategies to meet your nutritional needs. For more information about coping with specific side effects of treatment, see chapters 8–12.

Hormonal Therapy

Hormones are chemical substances that are released by glands and travel through the bloodstream and regulate body functions. Certain hormones influence the development and progression of some types of cancer, such as breast and prostate cancer. Hormonal therapy involves treatment with medications that interfere with hormone production or activity or the surgical removal of the body's hormone-producing glands. Hormonal therapy helps kill cancer cells or slow their growth.

Nutrition Suggestions During Hormonal Therapy

Some hormonal therapies can cause fluid retention, increased appetite, hot flashes, decreased libido, mood swings, or weight gain. Other hormone treatments can cause mild nausea and fatigue. Talk to your health care team about the side effects commonly experienced by people undergoing your specific therapy, and take medications as directed by your doctor to deal with any side effects. For more information about coping with specific side effects of treatment, see chapters 8–12.

Hormonal therapies are common treatments for breast or prostate cancer. This type of treatment can alter estrogen and/or testosterone levels and may have a negative affect on the cardiovascular health of cancer survivors. People who are prescribed these therapies should be even more diligent about following a healthful eating plan to reduce their risk for heart disease.

Suggestions for Managing Hot Flashes

Women receiving hormonal agents, such as tamoxifen (Nolvadex), letrozole (Femara), anastrozole (Arimidex), exemestane (Aromasin), or toremifene (Fareston), for treatment of hormone-sensitive cancer (breast, ovarian, or endometrial cancers) and men receiving hormone ablation therapy, such as leuprolide (Lupron), goserelin (Zoladex), or bicalutamide (Casodex), for treatment of prostate cancer frequently experience treatment-related hot flashes. Controlling hot flashes can be challenging! People having hot flashes often experience difficulty sleeping, fatigue, and irritability. The following diet and lifestyle suggestions can make it easier to cope:

- Drink plenty of cool, hydrating fluids throughout the day.
- Be aware of foods that may "trigger" or intensify hot flashes:
  - alcoholic beverages
  - hot soups or hot beverages, such as coffee and tea
  - spicy, highly seasoned foods
  - high-fat, greasy foods
- Avoid over-heated rooms whenever possible.
- Avoid tight-fitting clothes.
- Wear clothing made of cotton or other natural fibers, especially at night. Avoid synthetic fabrics such as polyester, nylon, and spandex.
- Use bedding made of natural fibers, such as cotton or flannel sheets and cotton or wool blankets. Avoid sheets and blankets made of synthetic materials.
- Try complementary therapies such as acupuncture, meditation, and relaxation training.
- Check with your doctor or registered dietitian before taking any popular herbal or dietary supplements promoted as hot flash remedies, such as soy, vitamin E, dong quai, evening primrose, or black cohosh.
- Ask your doctor whether medication might be right for you. Studies show some people have fewer or less-intense hot flashes when they use prescription medications such as paroxetine (Paxil), gabapentin (Neurontin), or venlafaxine (Effexor).

The following strategies can be helpful in coping with common side effects of hormonal therapy:

- If you are experiencing treatment-related fluid retention, cut down on salt used in cooking and at the table.
- Pay attention to portion sizes and try to monitor your caloric intake to avoid excessive weight gain.
- If you are risk for osteoporosis, talk to your health care team about how to increase your intake of calcium-rich foods and whether calcium supplements might help you retain bone mass and density during your hormonal therapy.
- Consider adding doctor-approved physical activity to your daily schedule. This activity will help develop muscle, burn calories, and promote bone health and a sense of well-being.
- If you have an estrogen receptor–positive cancer like breast, ovarian, or endometrial cancer, talk to your doctor before using dietary supplements containing high amounts of soy isoflavones. See chapter 3 for more in-depth guidance regarding soy.
- If you are experiencing hot flashes, talk to your doctor, nurse, and registered dietitian on ways to manage them. See the box on page 156 for more information.
- Keep in mind that most of the side effects of hormonal therapy are usually temporary and persist only a short time during treatment.

Cancer, Healthy Eating, and the Family

Family, friends, and caregivers are often eager to help people with cancer feel better and regain their health. They focus, and sometimes obsess, on a person's diet and weight—as well as that person's strength or physical activity level—since these are aspects of health over which people have some control. Open and honest discussions of these topics can help prevent frustration about eating-related issues.

For people experiencing the side effects of cancer treatment, simply eating, keeping up their strength, and maintaining a somewhat normal schedule can be a challenge. Disinterest in food can clash with a caregiver's need to provide nourishment, care, and comfort. Misunderstanding and lack of appreciation for the emotional and physical challenges each party faces can cause an unnecessary divide, especially at a time when support for both the cancer survivor and caregiver is so crucial.

People with cancer often feel a loss of control and resent being treated as helpless, and this might cause them to appear less than motivated. The caregiver might feel that the survivor is not trying hard enough to feel and eat better. Communicating with each other and possibly consulting a member of the cancer center's psychosocial team (such as a social worker, counselor, or chaplain) can help overcome these common bumps in the road through treatment and recovery.

Nutrition-Related Coping Tips for Caregivers

Cancer can cause role changes that require individuals and family members to be flexible and sensitive to each other's needs. If the head of the household or the person who traditionally took care of the grocery shopping, meal planning, and food preparation is ill, he or she may now be more reliant on other family and friends.

Anyone preparing food or meals for a person with cancer can keep these perspectives and ways of coping in mind:

- Many people who undergo cancer treatment eat less frequently and select fewer nutritious foods than they did prior to treatment.
- Most people going through treatment are not comfortable eating large quantities at one time. Therefore, it is essential to plan for small, frequent (every two hours or so) meals or snacks. Make each bite count by choosing calorie- and nutrient-dense snacks, such as peanut butter, cheese, or egg salad.
- Have food within easy reach at home, and have meals and snacks ready so the person can have something to eat when he or she is ready.
- Be prepared for times when the person is able to eat only one or two foods for a few days in a row, until side effects diminish. Even if he or she can't eat at all, encourage drinking plenty of fluids.
- If the caregiver needs to work outside the home and the person undergoing treatment is staying home alone, prepare food and beverage possibilities and store things in the refrigerator and on the countertop in easy sight. Call home periodically throughout the day to remind your loved one to eat and drink, as treatment often takes away the appetite and people forget to do either.
- Be prepared for the person undergoing treatment to experience taste changes from day to day. Some days, favorite foods will no longer taste good. Other days, they will be able to eat a food that did not appeal to them even the day before.
- Talk with the person being treated for cancer about nutrition and physical activity strategies that might promote healing and well-being. A willingness to be flexible, supportive, and accepting of differences will help everyone involved feel in control of the situation.
- Practice safe handling, preparation, and storage of food as discussed in chapter 10. Your loved one's immune system may be compromised, and it is important that you ensure safety guidelines are followed.

For more information on caregiving and cooking for a person undergoing cancer treatment, consult the American Cancer Society's companion cookbook, *What to Eat During Cancer Treatment: 100 Great-Tasting, Family-Friendly Recipes to Help You Cope*. See page 143 for more information about this publication.

References

Besser J, Ratley K, Knecht S, Szafranski M. *What to Eat During Cancer Treatment: 100 Great-Tasting, Family-Friendly Recipes to Help You Cope*. Atlanta, GA: American Cancer Society; 2009.

Biological therapies for cancer: questions and answers. National Cancer Institute Web site. http://www.cancer.gov/cancertopics/factsheet/Therapy/biological. Updated June 13, 2006. Accessed December 9, 2009.

Bone marrow transplantation and peripheral blood stem cell transplantation. National Cancer Institute Web site. http://www.cancer.gov/cancertopics/factsheet/Therapy/bone-marrow-transplant. Updated October 29, 2008. Accessed December 9, 2009.

Chemotherapy and you: support for people with cancer. National Cancer Institute Web site. http://www.cancer.gov/cancertopics/insides-chemotherapy-and-you.pdf. Updated October 2008. Accessed December 9, 2009.

Elliott L, Molseed LL, McCallum PD, Grant B. *The Clinical Guide to Oncology Nutrition*. 2nd ed. Chicago, IL: American Dietetic Association; 2006.

Grant B, Hamilton KK. *Management of Nutrition Impact Symptoms in Cancer and Educational Handouts*. Chicago, IL: American Dietetic Association; 2004.

Managing side effects. American Cancer Society Web site. http://www.cancer.org/docroot/MBC/content/MBC_2_1x_Managing_Side_Effects_of_Chemotherapy.asp. Accessed December 9, 2009.

National Cancer Institute. Eating hints: before, during, and after cancer treatment. National Cancer Institute Web site. http://www.cancer.gov/cancerinfo/eatinghints. Published September 2009. Accessed November 20, 2009.

National Cancer Institute. Eating hints for cancer patients: before, during, and after treatment. National Cancer Institute Web site. http://www.cancer.gov/cancerinfo/eatinghints. Published July 16, 2003. Accessed May 13, 2009. Content no longer available.

Nutrition for the Person with Cancer During Treatment: A Guide for Patients and Families [booklet]. Atlanta, GA: American Cancer Society; 2006.

Nutrition in cancer care (PDQ®). National Cancer Institute Web site. http://www.cancer.gov/cancerinfo/pdq/supportivecare/nutrition/HealthProfessional#Section_157. Updated May 1, 2009. Accessed December 9, 2009.

Radiation therapy effects. American Cancer Society Web Site. http://www.cancer.org/docroot/MBC/MBC_2x_RadiationEffects.asp. Accessed December 9, 2009.

Radiation therapy and you: support for people with cancer. National Cancer Institute Web site. http://www.cancer.gov/cancertopics/insides-radiation-therapy-and-you.pdf. Updated September 2009. Accessed December 9, 2009.

Surgery. American Cancer Society Web site. http://www.cancer.org/docroot/MBC/content/MBC_6_2X_When_You_Have_Cancer_Surgery.asp. Accessed December 9, 2009.

United States Department of Agriculture. Fact sheets: freezing and food safety. United States Department of Agriculture Web site. http://www.fsis.usda.gov/Fact_Sheets/Focus_On_Freezing/index.asp. Accessed November 20, 2009.

Yarbo CH, Goodman M, Frogge MH. *Cancer Symptom Management*. 3rd ed. Sudbury, MA: Jones and Bartlett Publishers; 2003.

Chapter Eight

Maintaining a Healthy Body Weight

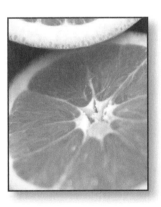

PEOPLE UNDERGOING TREATMENT FOR CANCER often lose or gain weight. It is becoming more widely accepted that being underweight or overweight may negatively influence cancer outcomes. Therefore, paying attention to weight is very important for people undergoing cancer treatment. Body weight also has been shown to play a role in the occurrence of cancer (primary prevention) and possibly the recurrence of cancer (secondary prevention). This chapter focuses on maintaining a healthy weight and lean body mass (muscle stores) during cancer treatment. In chapter 13, recommendations for achieving a healthy body weight after cancer treatment will be discussed.

Why Body Weight Is Important

It can be hard both for people undergoing cancer treatment and their health care providers to tell the difference between healthy and unhealthy weight loss. Whereas steady, mild weight loss in overweight or obese individuals is not a significant concern during treatment, sudden or rapid weight gain or loss may indicate a health problem. Generally, all people in cancer treatment should aim to maintain their weight during therapy unless otherwise advised by their health care team. Exceptions might be for overweight or obese individuals who have an early-stage, obesity-associated cancer, such as breast, colon, or prostate cancer, in which reasonable weight loss (not more than 5 percent of their body weight) would not be harmful. It is particularly important for individuals receiving radiation therapy to try to maintain their body weight. Treatment plans are based on starting body shape and weight. If you lose more than ten pounds during radiation therapy, your doctor may need to recalculate your radiation treatment plan.

Many people with cancer lose their appetite. Cancer treatment also can cause loss of appetite and make it difficult for you to eat enough to maintain your weight. Decreased eating can lead to weight loss, which can lead to malnutrition and loss of lean muscle mass. For these reasons, people undergoing cancer treatment who are experiencing rapid or undesirable weight loss are often advised to eat a high-calorie, protein-rich diet.

In contrast, some people gain weight while undergoing treatment for cancer. This can happen for a number of reasons:

- You might be eating larger portions or eating more often, consuming more calories than your body needs.
- You might not be able to exercise or be as physically active as usual, which results in not burning enough calories.
- You might be eating more because you are taking medications that stimulate your appetite, such as corticosteriods (steroids).
- You might be retaining fluid in your legs, arms, or belly because of your cancer or your cancer treatment.

With your doctor's permission, you can alter your food and beverage intake or increase your physical activity to help counteract these concerns. If you are gaining weight for reasons you cannot control, talk to your health care team about your concerns.

What Is a Healthy Weight?

Maintaining a healthy weight is important for your overall physical health and well-being. A variety of methods can be used to evaluate health related to your body weight. The most common and simplest methods to evaluate body weight are calculating body mass index (BMI) and waist circumference.

The BMI is a mathematical formula that uses your height compared to your weight to estimate whether you are underweight, overweight, or obese. BMI is used as an indicator of disease risk and to screen for possible health problems. Waist circumference is simply a measurement of the distance around (the circumference) your waist. A measurement is

BMI	
Below 18.5	Underweight
18.5 to 24.9	Normal weight
25.0 to 29.9	Overweight
30.0 to 39.9	Obese
40.0 and above	Extremely obese

also taken around the hip. A waist circumference of more than forty inches in men or thirty-five inches in women signifies a risk for obesity and heart disease. Neither of these measures gives any direct estimate of body fat, although larger waist circumference is directly linked with increased abdominal fat.

For an online BMI calculator for adults and children, visit the Centers for Disease Control and Prevention's Web site at www.cdc.gov/bmi. BMI can also be calculated according to the following formula: (weight in pounds x 703) ÷ (height in inches²).

A more accurate health indicator is to measure your body composition. Body composition can be estimated by taking skin fold measurements at different places on your body (such as your abdomen or upper arm), or it can be measured using bioelectrical impedance (BIA) or Dual X-Ray Absorptiometry (DXA) tools. These measurement tools provide an estimate of your body fat and lean body mass (muscle). This measurement is important because loss of body fat if you are overweight or obese is considered a good thing—even during cancer treatment—as long as you do not lose muscle as well. Maintaining a healthy lean body mass while losing fat requires a diet rich in protein, with only modest caloric reductions and ongoing physical activity. BIA is quick, easy, and a cost-effective way to measure body composition during treatment, but it is sensitive to fluid shifts. DXA is an alternative but is generally only useful when comparing changes over longer periods (six to twelve months or more).

Weight Loss

Having an accurate scale for home can help you monitor changes in your weight. You do not need to weigh yourself every day, just once or twice a week. In fact, you should expect day-to-day fluctuations in weight and should not be alarmed by these daily changes. Weight loss can result from any of the following factors:

- *the effect of the cancer*, for example, a growth in the head or neck area that results in discomfort and inability to eat;
- *psychological reasons*, such as depression and a resulting lack of appetite;
- *cancer treatment*, for example, a surgery that causes weight loss for a few weeks or biotherapy that causes severe weight loss;
- *side effects from treatment*, especially from radiation therapy or chemotherapy, which can cause nausea, diarrhea, dehydration, or changes in appetite, taste, or how the body processes nutrients.

Weight loss can cause fatigue, lengthen recovery, suppress your immune system, make you more susceptible to infection, and negatively affect your quality of life.

Coping with Weight Loss

If you have lost weight before beginning treatment or if you are losing weight during treatment, try eating small, frequent meals and snacks every one to two hours. Keep handy high-calorie, high-protein snacks and foods that are easy to take along when you go out. Also keep in mind these tips:

- Some people going through cancer treatment may develop a distaste or intolerance for fats. If this happens, try eating foods high in protein but low in fat, such as yogurt, cottage cheese, eggs, and lean beef, poultry, or pork.
- To increase calories and still get nutrients from fruits and vegetables, try dried fruits; 100 percent fruit or vegetable juice; higher-calorie produce like sweet potatoes, corn, and peas; or add fats such as butter, margarine, or cheese sauce to vegetables.
- Moderate levels of physical activity can help reduce stress and increase appetite.

Consult your doctor if you experience any of the following symptoms:

- inability to eat for more than a day
- inability to drink or drinking much less than usual
- weight loss of more than three pounds in a week
- persistent nausea, despite taking anti-nausea medication as prescribed
- vomiting for more than twenty-four hours

- diarrhea for more than forty-eight hours, despite taking anti-diarrhea medication as prescribed
- pain while eating
- inability to urinate for an entire day or infrequent urination accompanied by pungent or very yellow urine
- lack of bowel movement for two days or more

How to Increase Calories

The following information on how to increase calories was adapted from the National Cancer Institute publication, *Eating Hints Before, During, and After Cancer Treatment.*

Cancer and its treatment often place extra demands on the body, and you may need to take in more calories than in the past just to maintain your weight. Carbohydrates and fats supply the body with the bulk of the calories it needs. Fats have more than twice as many calories per gram than do carbohydrates or protein, so they are a more efficient way to increase total calorie intake. Here are some suggestions to add calories to your daily diet. Avoid products containing trans fats, and use lactose-free dairy products if necessary. Lactose intolerance is discussed in chapter 12.

Butter and Margarine
- Add to mashed and baked potatoes, hot cereals, grits, rice, noodles, and cooked vegetables.
- Combine with herbs and seasonings and spread on cooked meats, poultry, fish, and egg dishes.
- Use melted butter or margarine as a dip for bread or seafood such as shrimp, scallops, crab, or lobster.

Whipped Cream
- Use sweetened whipped cream on hot chocolate, desserts, gelatin, puddings, fruits, pancakes, and waffles.
- Fold unsweetened whipped cream into mashed potatoes, soups, or vegetable purées.

Milk and Cream
- Use in cream soups, sauces, egg dishes, batters, puddings, and custards.
- Put on cold cereal. Use in place of water in cooked cereals.
- Mix with noodles, pasta, rice, and mashed potatoes.
- Pour on chicken and fish while baking.
- Use as a binder in hamburgers, meatloaf, and croquettes.
- Use whole milk or half-and-half instead of low-fat milk.

- Use cream instead of milk in recipes.
- Make hot chocolate with cream and add marshmallows.

Cheese

- Melt cheese on top of casseroles, potatoes, rice, soups, noodles, and vegetables.
- Add cheese to meat dishes, omelets, and sandwiches, or melt on toast.

Cream Cheese

- Spread on breads, muffins, fruit slices, and crackers.
- Add to vegetable or egg dishes.
- Roll into balls and coat with chopped nuts, wheat germ, or granola.

Sour Cream

- Add to cream soups, baked potatoes, macaroni and cheese, vegetables, sauces, salad dressings, stews, baked meat, and fish.
- Add to nachos (along with melted cheese, chili, olives, and guacamole).
- Use as a topping for cakes, fruit, gelatin, desserts, breads, muffins, and blintzes.
- Use as a dip for fresh fruits and vegetables.
- Scoop onto fresh fruit, add brown sugar, and refrigerate until cold before eating.

NUTRITIONAL SUPPLEMENTS

During treatment, you may find it difficult to meet your nutritional needs by eating solid food alone. High-calorie, nutrient-rich drinks and snacks can help pick up where your meals leave off.

Nutritional supplements, some of which are similar to milk shakes, puddings, or candy bars, come in different flavors. Some products offer high-calorie or high-protein options. Examples of these include Ensure (Abbott Nutrition) and Boost (Nestle Nutrition). If the supplements are too sweet, try a plain or vanilla flavor and then experiment with syrups, blended fruits, decaffeinated coffee crystals, or other taste enhancers. Other nutritional drinks are similar to fruit juice and can be mixed with ginger ale for variety. If you experience diarrhea, try lactose-free or clear, fruit-flavored nutritional drinks.

Instant Breakfast–type drinks, are another liquid nutrition option. These consist of powders mixed with milk or other products, such as ice cream, to add calories and protein. However, if you are sensitive to milk or know that you are lactose intolerant, substitute with lactose-free milk, soy milk, or rice milk. Nutritional products also come in other forms such as meal replacement bars and puddings.

Salad Dressings and Mayonnaise

- Use with sandwiches.
- Add to eggs for egg salad, tuna for tuna salad, and whitefish for whitefish salad.
- Use as a dip for raw vegetables.
- Use as a binder in croquettes.
- Use in sauces and gelatin dishes.

Granola

- Use in cookie, muffin, and bread batters.
- Sprinkle on vegetables, yogurt, ice cream, pudding, custard, and fruit.
- Layer with fruits and bake.
- Mix with dry fruits and nuts for a snack.
- Substitute for bread or rice in pudding recipes.
- Add to cereal, especially hot cereal.

Dried Fruits (Raisins, Prunes, Apricots, Dates, Figs)

- Try stewing dried fruits; serve for breakfast or as a dessert or snack.
- Add to muffins, cookies, breads, cakes, cereals, puddings, stuffing, and rice and grain dishes.
- Bake in pies and turnovers.
- Combine with cooked vegetables, such as carrots, sweet potatoes, yams, and acorn and butternut squash.
- Combine with nuts or granola for snacks.

Eggs

- Add chopped, hard-boiled eggs to salads and dressings, vegetables, casseroles, and creamed meats.
- Make a rich custard with eggs, milk, and sugar.
- Add extra hard-boiled yolks to deviled-egg filling.
- Beat eggs into mashed potatoes, vegetable purées, and sauces. (Be sure to keep cooking these dishes after adding the eggs, as raw eggs may contain harmful bacteria.)
- Add extra eggs or egg whites to custards, puddings, quiches, scrambled eggs, omelets, and to pancake and French toast batters before cooking.

Food Preparation

- Add breading to meat and vegetables.
- Sauté and fry foods if you can tolerate these cooking methods. Sautéing and frying add

more calories by adding oils such as olive or canola than do baking or broiling.
- Add sauces or gravies.

Adapted from the National Cancer Institute. *Eating Hints Before, During, and After Cancer Treatment.* (Bethesda, MD: National Institutes of Health, 2009).

How to Increase Protein

The following information on how to increase protein was adapted from the National Cancer Institute publication, *Eating Hints Before, During, and After Cancer Treatment.*

During and after cancer treatment, your body usually needs additional protein to heal tissues, maintain muscle, and help prevent infection. Good sources of protein include meat, fish, poultry, dairy products, nuts, dried beans, peas, lentils, and soy foods. Use lactose-free dairy products if necessary. Lactose-free whey powder can be substituted for nonfat instant dry milk. Incorporating the following foods into your diet can help ensure that your body gets enough protein:

Hard or Semisoft Cheese
- Melt on sandwiches, bread, muffins, tortillas, hamburgers, hot dogs, other meats or fish, vegetables, eggs, desserts, stewed fruit, or pies.
- Grate and add to soups, sauces, casseroles, vegetable dishes, mashed potatoes, rice, noodles, or meatloaf.

Cottage Cheese and Ricotta Cheese
- Mix with or use to stuff fruits and vegetables.
- Add to casseroles, spaghetti, noodles, and egg dishes such as omelets, scrambled eggs, and soufflés.
- Use in gelatin, pudding-type desserts, cheesecake, and pancake batter.
- Use to stuff crepes and pasta shells or manicotti.
- Add to salsa for a high-protein dip.

Milk
- Use milk instead of water in beverages and in cooking.
- Use in hot cereal, soups, cocoa, and pudding.
- Add cream sauces to vegetables and other dishes.
- Look for high-protein milk in the dairy case and add to foods and beverages where you would normally use regular milk.
- Add to coffee or tea.

Nonfat Instant Dry Milk (*Use lactose-free whey powder, if necessary.*)

- Add to regular milk and milk drinks, such as pasteurized eggnog and milk shakes.
- Use in casseroles, meatloaf, breads, muffins, sauces, cream soups, mashed potatoes, puddings, custards, and other milk-based desserts.

Commercial Products

- Use Instant Breakfast powder or canned nutritional supplements in milk drinks and desserts, or mix with ice cream, milk, and fruit for a high-protein milk shake.
- Use protein-containing meal replacement bars as quick meals or easy between-meal, on-the-go snacks.

Ice Cream, Yogurt, and Frozen Yogurt

- Add ice cream or frozen yogurt to carbonated beverages, such as ginger ale or cola.
- Add ice cream to milk drinks, to make milk shakes.
- Add yogurt to cereal, fruit, gelatin desserts, and pies; blend or whip with soft or cooked fruits.
- Sandwich ice cream or frozen yogurt between cake slices, cookies, or graham crackers.
- Make breakfast drinks with yogurt and fruit to make fruit smoothies.

Eggs

- Keep hard-boiled eggs in the refrigerator for quick snacks.
- Add chopped, hard-boiled eggs to salads, dressings, vegetables, casseroles, and creamed meats.
- Add extra eggs or egg whites to quiches and to pancake and French toast batters.
- Add extra egg whites to scrambled eggs and omelets.
- Make a rich custard with eggs, high-protein milk, and sugar.
- Add extra hard-cooked yolks to deviled-egg filling.
- Avoid raw eggs, which may contain harmful bacteria, because your treatment makes you susceptible to infection. Make sure all eggs you eat are well cooked or baked; avoid eggs that are undercooked or uncooked, such as those in eggnog. Alternatively, use refrigerated or frozen egg substitute made from egg whites.

Nuts, Seeds, and Wheat Germ

- Add to casseroles, breads, muffins, pancakes, cookies, waffles, and ice cream.
- Sprinkle on fruit, cereal, ice cream, yogurt, vegetables, salads, and toast as a crunchy topping; use in place of bread crumbs.
- Blend with spinach, parsley, or other herbs and cream for a noodle, pasta, or vegetable sauce.

- Roll bananas in chopped nuts.
- Make trail mix using assorted nuts, dried fruit, and maybe even a little chocolate, such as M&Ms.
- Sprinkle seeds on desserts such as fruit, ice cream, pudding, and custard.
- Serve seeds on vegetables, salads, and pasta.

Nut Butters

- Look for a variety of nut butters, such as peanut butter, almond butter, or hazelnut butter, in the grocery store. Do not eat freshly ground nut butter as it might have harmful bacteria; instead, purchase it commercially prepared.
- Spread nut butter on sandwiches, toast, muffins, crackers, waffles, pancakes, and fruit slices.
- Use nut butter as a dip for raw vegetables, such as carrots, cauliflower, and celery.
- Blend nut butter with milk drinks, shakes, and smoothies.
- Swirl nut butter through soft ice cream and yogurt.

Meat, Poultry, and Fish

- Add chopped, cooked meat and poultry or fish to vegetables, salads, casseroles, soups, sauces, and biscuit dough.
- Use in omelets, soufflés, quiches, or sandwich fillings.
- Wrap in pie crust or biscuit dough with vegetables to make pot pies or turnovers.
- Add to stuffed baked potatoes.
- Mix diced and shredded meat with sour cream and spices to make a dip.

Beans and Legumes

- Cook and use peas, legumes, beans, and tofu in soups or add to casseroles, pastas, and grain dishes that also contain cheese or meat.
- Mash cooked beans with cheese and eat on crackers, tortilla chips, or flatbread.
- Use hummus (a spread made from ground chickpeas) on pitas, crackers, and vegetables.

Protein Powder Supplements

- Add whey or soy powders to milk and milk drinks, smoothies, and shakes.
- Add whey or soy powders to hot cereals and soups.
- Try commercially available protein supplements, such as Nestle Nutrition's Beneprotein, Abbott Nutrition's Pro-Mod, or Medical Nutrition USA's Pro-Stat.

Adapted from the National Cancer Institute. *Eating Hints Before, During, and After Cancer Treatment.* (Bethesda, MD: National Institutes of Health, 2009).

HEALTHY SNACK IDEAS

A healthy snack provides nutrients to optimize health when meals alone are not enough to reach daily nutrient goals. Healthy snack choices vary, depending on individual nutrient needs.

If you need more protein, select these types of snacks:
- peanut butter
- nuts
- seeds
- dairy products such as cheese, cottage cheese, or milk
- hard-boiled eggs
- rolled, thin slices of lean meat or poultry

If you need more calories, try these options:
- drink high-calorie nutritional supplements
- eat whole-fat dairy products
- add extra cheese, meat, or avocado to sandwiches
- dip fruit in commercially prepared peanut or nut butters

If you need more potassium, try these suggestions:
- eat bananas, dried apricots, oranges, or tangerines
- put molasses in tea, coffee, or hot cereal
- eat a serving of yogurt
- drink a serving of vegetable juice, such as V8 or V8 Splash

If you need more calcium, think about these options:
- add cheese to vegetables
- select low-fat dairy products
- drink calcium-fortified soy milk
- drink calcium-enriched orange juice
- snack on low-fat dairy products
- snack on canned fish with edible bones

Weight Gain

Some people, especially those with hormone-sensitive cancers such as breast cancer, have a tendency to gain weight during and after treatment. Weight gain is often difficult to control during treatment. It can result from side effects of treatment (such as increased appetite or water retention), treatment itself (such as chemotherapy, corticosteroids, or hormonal therapies), reduced activity, lack of or frequently interrupted sleep, eating in response to stress, treatment-induced menopause, or a combination of these factors.

Weight gain can contribute to fatigue, lowered self-esteem, depression, high blood pressure, and increased blood cholesterol or blood glucose levels. It may also increase your risk for a cancer recurrence or for another cancer. Weight management is important for all cancer survivors, but especially if you have a diagnosis of breast, colorectal, or prostate cancer.

Coping with Weight Gain

Healthy eating is an essential part of successful weight management. A healthy eating plan meets caloric needs but does not include many excess calories. Reduce your salt intake if you are experiencing fluid retention or if you have high blood pressure. With your doctor's permission, increase physical activity as you are able. Even moderate physical activity (such as ten-minute walks around the block) can help improve your strength and sense of well-being and can help you maintain a stable weight.

Obesity is a risk factor for some of the most prevalent cancers in the United States, including postmenopausal breast cancer and colorectal cancer. For this reason, and because obesity is increasingly common, many people are overweight or obese when their cancer is diagnosed.

If you are interested in losing weight, talk to your health care team. They may want you to wait to pursue weight loss until after you have recovered from treatment, or they may advocate a program of modest weight loss (with a goal of losing no more than two pounds per week) and carefully monitor any potential interference with treatment.

Women treated for breast cancer who gain weight during treatment typically gain fat tissue but have either no change or a decrease in their lean body mass. Many are able to cope with this type of weight gain with exercise, especially physical activity that emphasizes resistance training or weight lifting. While there has been concern about a link between exercise, particularly weight training, and increased risk for lymphedema in women who have had a standard (nonsentinel node) lymph node resection, recent studies have not confirmed an increased risk.

Obesity has been associated with poorer prognoses for breast and colon cancers. There is also increasing evidence that being overweight increases risk for cancer recurrence. If you want to lose weight during or after treatment, discuss your health and weight with your doctor and also with a registered dietitian, who can discuss your weight-loss goals and evaluate your body fat percentage and your BMI. Refer to page 164 for information about BMI.

A safe weight-loss plan for those in treatment or those who have completed treatment includes a healthy, well-balanced diet and appropriate physical activity. Refer to chapter 13 for recommendations for healthy eating and physical activity for cancer survivors.

WHAT A NORMAL PORTION LOOKS LIKE

How do you know a reasonable portion of food when you see it? It may be smaller than you think. Try to visualize the objects mentioned below when eating out, planning a meal, or grabbing a snack. For example, the amount of meat recommended as part of a healthy meal is three to four ounces, which is about the size of a deck of cards. Results from one study suggest that the typical portion size of food items on the market is at least twice as large as the United States Department of Agriculture (USDA) standard for portions, sometimes eight times as large. Aiming to lower your portion sizes is a positive step even if you do not always reach the goals listed in the table below. Supplementing with other healthy choices may help satisfy your appetite.

Portion	Size
Meat	
1 ounce	Matchbox
3 ounces (recommended for a meal)	Deck of cards or bar of soap
8 ounces	Thin paperback book
Fish	
3 ounces	Checkbook
Cheese	
1 ounce	Four dice
Potato	
Medium	Computer mouse
Peanut butter	
2 tablespoons	Ping-Pong ball
Pasta	
1 cup	Tennis ball
Bagel	
Average	Hockey puck

Ways to Cut Back on Calories

If you feel hungry between meals, drink water or low-calorie drinks or have a piece of fruit. Choose lower-calorie, higher-fiber foods for snacking, and order healthful meals when you go out.

Smart Snacks at Home

These healthy snack ideas are good for you and convenient. But even with healthy snacks, do not consume large volumes or too many portions. Even low-calorie items add up when eaten in large amounts:

- sticks of carrots and celery
- bite-sized portions of other vegetables
- low-fat cottage cheese
- low-fat cheese sticks or slices
- lean slices of meats or poultry
- apple slices
- raisins or other dried fruit
- orange sections
- rice cakes
- low-salt sunflower seeds
- unsalted walnuts or almonds
- low-salt or unsalted pretzels
- unsalted air-popped popcorn
- flavored decaffeinated coffee
- fruity or herbal teas
- water with added fresh citrus (slices or juice)
- one-hundred–calorie prepackaged snacks
- a bite-sized piece of chocolate

Eat Out Without Overdoing It

- Look for "heart-healthy" meals. Many restaurants now offer entrees that follow heart-healthy guidelines for preparation.
- Order a vegetable plate, but avoid the casseroles and opt for "straight" steamed, baked, or boiled vegetables instead. Alternately, order a lean piece of meat or poultry with steamed vegetables as a side.
- Choose salad as your main meal with dressing served on the side. Watch out for too many high-fat add-ons, such as cheese, eggs, meat, nuts, or avocado.
- Choose calorie-free beverages.
- Share an entrée with a friend; get a small salad on the side for more vegetables.

- Request that sauces and dressings be served on the side so you can control how much you use.
- Ask for half of the entrée to be served and half to be wrapped for home.

Ways to Be More Physically Active

The American Cancer Society recommends at least thirty minutes of activity on five or more days of the week.

- Walk around the track, the neighborhood, or the local mall or grocery store.
- Purchase a pedometer and keep track of your steps. Begin with a goal of five thousand steps per day, then gradually increase to ten thousand per day.
- Walk up and down the stairs.
- Swim or take a gentle water aerobics class at your local pool.
- Gently ride a bicycle or stationary bike.
- Take exercise classes at your local gym or recreation center.
- Garden or do yardwork.
- Dance.
- Do yoga or pilates at home or in a class.
- Practice martial arts; kickboxing is a great way to relieve stress!

Other Causes for Weight Fluctuations

Fluid Retention and Weight Gain

Fluid retention can increase your body weight, but it is not "true" weight gain. Fluid retention can be a sign of several things of concern that could be related to your cancer or your treatment. Weight gain caused by fluid retention is often accompanied by a feeling of heaviness and/or the collection of fluid in your chest, abdomen, arm(s), or in your leg(s) or ankle(s). Be on the lookout for the following signs of fluid retention, and contact your doctor immediately if you experience any of them:

- weight gain of three or more pounds in one week or ongoing weight gain
- shortness of breath
- swollen ankles or feet
- swollen abdomen
- swollen arm(s)
- swelling accompanied by warmth to the touch, pain, and/or redness

Dehydration and Weight Loss

Sudden weight loss is also a concern for people undergoing cancer treatment, especially if you are experiencing diarrhea or vomiting. If these side effects of treatment are not controlled, they can lead to dehydration, which is a serious condition. Be on the lookout for the following symptoms of dehydration, and consult a doctor if you experience any of them:

- weight loss of three or more pounds in one week or ongoing weight loss
- dry skin or skin that "tents" when pinched or pulled up slightly
- excessive thirst
- dark or strong-smelling urine
- dizziness or lightheadedness

When to Call the Doctor

Report weight changes of more than three pounds in a week or continuing weight loss of even one pound a week for more than two weeks in a row to your doctor.

Remember that weight loss over time may affect your ability to function, leaving you weak and unable to participate in daily activities. In addition, unintentional weight loss or rapid weight loss usually reflects a loss of muscle rather than fat, which can place you at higher risk for malnutrition or depressed immune function and can affect your ability to carry out normal daily activities. On the other hand, weight gain over time can result in a serious health condition such as diabetes or high blood pressure.

Are You Getting Enough Calories and Protein?

If you are eating a balanced diet and maintaining your weight, you are most likely getting the calories and protein you need each day. However, if you are losing weight or gaining weight, you may need to more carefully examine the amount of calories and protein you need each day. These quick and easy calculations can help you determine your daily calorie and protein needs. For individualized help, see a registered dietitian.

First, calculate how much you weigh in kilograms by dividing your weight in pounds by 2.2. For example, for a 120-pound woman, divide 120 by 2.2, which equals 54.5 kilograms.

To determine your daily caloric needs, follow the guidelines below:

- If you need to maintain your weight, multiply your weight in kilograms by thirty.
- If you want to lose weight, multiply your weight in kilograms by twenty-five.
- If you need to gain weight, multiply your weight in kilograms by thirty-five.

To determine how much protein you need each day, follow these guidelines:

- If your goal is to gain weight or you are undergoing cancer treatment, multiply your body weight in kilograms by 1.2 or 1.5 grams of protein, depending on your situation. A daily protein intake of 1.2 grams per kilogram of body weight is recommended for people who are experiencing moderate weight loss (nutritionally depleted). A daily protein intake of 1.5 grams per kilogram of body weight is recommended for people who are experiencing significant weight loss (seriously depleted). For example, for a woman weighing 132 pounds (60 kilograms), her weight multiplied by 1.2 or 1.5 would equal 72 or 90 grams of protein.

- If your goal is to maintain your weight, multiply your weight in kilograms by 0.8 or 1.0 grams of protein per kilogram of body weight, depending on your situation. If you are experiencing minimal cancer treatment–related side effects or you did not lose weight before starting treatment, multiply your weight in kilograms by 0.8 to determine your daily protein needs. If you are experiencing treatment-related side effects that are causing changes in your appetite or ability to eat, you would benefit from consuming additional protein each day. To determine your daily protein needs, multiply your body weight in kilograms by 1.0 grams of protein. For example, for a man weighing 176 pounds (80 kilograms), his weight multiplied by 0.8 or 1.0 would equal 64 or 80 grams of protein.

SOURCES OF PROTEIN

1 ounce of meat, fish, or poultry	7 grams
8 ounces of milk	8 grams
8 ounces of soy milk	6 grams
1 ounce of cheese	6 grams
1 egg	6 grams
½ cup of oatmeal	4 grams
½ cup of beans, lentils, or peas	6 grams
½ cup of hummus	6 grams
½ cup of firm tofu	14 grams
2 tablespoons of peanut butter	7 grams
¼ cup of nuts	9 grams
½ cup plain pasta or white rice	2 grams
½ cup whole grain pasta or rice	3 grams

Books that list the nutritional content of food are available at the public library and bookstores. A free, easy-to-use, and reliable Internet resource is available at www.nutritiondata.com.

References

Besser J, Ratley K, Knecht S, Szafranski M. *What to Eat During Cancer Treatment: 100 Great-Tasting, Family-Friendly Recipes to Help You Cope.* Atlanta, GA: American Cancer Society; 2009.

Claghorn K. Ask the experts: liquid nutrition supplements. Oncolink Web site. http://www.oncolink.com/experts/article.cfm?c=1&s=3&ss=3&id=1053. Published November 21, 2001. Accessed December 9, 2009.

Doyle C, Kushi LH, Byers T, Courneya KS, Demark-Wahnefried W, Grant B, McTiernan A, Rock CL, Thompson C, Gansler T, Andrews KS; 2006 Nutrition, Physical Activity and Cancer Survivorship Advisory Committee; American Cancer Society. Nutrition and physical activity during and after cancer treatment: a guide for informed choices by cancer survivors. *CA Cancer J Clin.* 2006;56(6):323-353.

Elliott L, Molseed LL, McCallum PD, Grant B. *The Clinical Guide to Oncology Nutrition.* 2nd ed. Chicago, IL: American Dietetic Association; 2006.

Grant B, Hamilton KK. *Management of Nutrition Impact Symptoms in Cancer and Educational Handouts.* Chicago, IL: American Dietetic Association; 2004.

National Cancer Institute. Eating hints: before, during, and after cancer treatment. National Cancer Institute Web site. http://www.cancer.gov/cancerinfo/eatinghints. Published September 2009. Accessed November 20, 2009.

Obesity and cancer: questions and answers. National Cancer Institute Web site. http://www.cancer.gov/cancertopics/factsheet/Risk/obesity. Updated March 13, 2004. Accessed December 9, 2009.

Physical activity and cancer. National Cancer Institute Web Site. http://www.cancer.gov/cancertopics/factsheet/prevention/physicalactivity. Updated July 22, 2007. Accessed December 9, 2009.

World Cancer Research Fund. American Institute for Cancer Research (AICR). Food, nutrition, physical activity, and the prevention of cancer: a global perspective. Washington, DC: AICR; 2007.

Yarbo CH, Goodman M, Frogge MH. *Cancer Symptom Management.* 3rd ed. Sudbury, MA: Jones and Bartlett Publishers; 2003.

Chapter Nine

Coping with Treatment-Related Fatigue

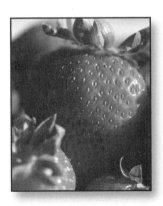

FATIGUE IS THE MOST COMMON SIDE EFFECT OF CANCER and its treatment. It is a recognized side effect of surgery, chemotherapy, radiation therapy, biotherapy, and even hormonal therapy. In fact, some estimates suggest that nine of ten people experience some fatigue during or after treatment.

Understanding Fatigue

Fatigue that occurs during cancer treatment is different from the tiredness you might feel from the activities of everyday life. This lack of energy can appear suddenly or develop slowly over time, but either way, it can be overwhelming. Cancer-related fatigue is generally not relieved by rest or sleep. The following can be signs of fatigue:

- feeling like you have no energy
- sleeping more than usual, either during the night or day
- not wanting to do normal activities
- lack of interest in personal hygiene or appearance
- feeling tired even after sleeping your usual nighttime rest period
- having difficulty concentrating
- lack of sexual desire
- feeling irritable or impatient

Once cancer treatment ends, fatigue will lessen over time, but some individuals can feel fatigued for as long as several months or even years afterward. Treatment-related fatigue can affect many aspects of life, including your ability to take part in your usual daily activities.

Reasons for Fatigue

Fatigue during treatment can be related to the cancer itself or to side effects of treatment, such as neutropenia (low white blood cell count) or anemia (low red blood cell count). Sometimes, however, it is difficult to pinpoint the exact reason for fatigue. During treatment, cells are rapidly growing and dying. Healing after surgery or between treatments or cycles can drain your reserves of energy. Treatment can cause fatigue in a number of ways:

- Many chemotherapy drugs cause fatigue because they destroy rapidly dividing cells, such as those in the bone marrow. When red blood cells (which are made in the bone marrow) are destroyed, you can develop anemia, and fatigue is the most common symptom of anemia. When anemia resolves, fatigue usually lessens as well. When your blood cell counts reach a certain level, your anemia can be managed with an injection of medications (epoetin alfa or darbepoetin alpha) or a transfusion packed with red blood cells. Epoetin alpha (examples are Epogen and Procrit) or darbepoetin alpha (for example,

Aranesp) are prescribed by doctors in very specific situations. These medicines function like hormones in your body in that they help the bone marrow produce more red blood cells. Bone pain can be a side effect of these medications.

- Neutropenia, another common side effect of chemotherapy, can also cause fatigue. Neutropenia is a low white blood cell count, and just like anemia, this side effect results from chemotherapy's effect on the bone marrow. Neutropenia can put you at risk for infection. If your fatigue is related to neutropenia, it might resolve over time as your body recovers. Or, when your blood cell counts reach certain levels, your neutropenia can be managed with an injection of granulocyte colony-stimulating factor, known as G-CSF (examples are filgrastim [Neupogen] and pegfilgrastim [Neulasta]). Because this medication also stimulates the bone marrow to work harder and produce more blood cells, bone pain is also a possible side effect of G-CSF.

- Fatigue is a common side effect of radiation therapy. Fatigue increases gradually over a five-to-six-week course of radiation therapy and then gradually declines. If you are receiving radiation therapy to bony areas you may also experience anemia and anemia-related fatigue.

- When chemotherapy and radiation therapy are given together, you can have fatigue for all of the reasons stated above. The therapies are given together for a better treatment outcome, but side effects can begin sooner and be more pronounced.

- Chemotherapy-induced menopause is associated with fatigue. This may be related to changes in sleep patterns, loss of lean muscle mass, or even an increase in body fat and inflammatory cytokines.

- Biotherapy, which is used to stimulate the body's immune response to fight cancer, can lead to ongoing physical and mental fatigue.

- Some types of hormonal therapy cause short-term or longer-lasting fatigue, which is related to changes in estrogen, progesterone, or testosterone levels.

Side effects of treatment also can contribute to fatigue:

- Eating less, not getting enough nutritious foods, and losing weight because of treatment side effects, such as loss of appetite, nausea, vomiting, mouth sores, taste changes, diarrhea, or constipation, can cause fatigue.

- Dehydration, diarrhea, or vomiting can lead to an imbalance in electrolytes, which can cause weakness. Electrolytes, such as sodium, potassium, magnesium, and calcium, are involved in the body's metabolism and help cells function normally.

- Cancer cells may be competing with normal cells for nutrients, thus slowing the growth of normal cells and causing fatigue, decreased appetite, and weight loss. Do not be tempted to try to "starve" the cancer; it does not work. Eat enough to maintain a healthy weight, fight fatigue, and tolerate anticancer treatments.

- Chronic pain can disrupt sleep and leave you feeling fatigued.
- Medications for coping with cancer treatment–related side effects such as pain and nausea can also make you fatigued.
- Stress, feeling depressed, or not getting enough sleep during treatment can contribute to fatigue.
- Interrupted sleep, whether from frequent urination, insomnia, or conditions like restless leg syndrome, can make treatment-related fatigue worse. If you experience any of these problems or cannot sleep for more than two hours at a time, speak to your health care team.

Coping With Fatigue

It is important to determine the cause of fatigue so your health care team can offer you appropriate treatment. Some ways to decrease and manage your fatigue include adjusting your diet, reducing stress, and increasing physical activity. Other ways to cope with fatigue include the following:

- Plan short rest periods to conserve energy for important things.
- Use light stretching and exercise (such as yoga, qigong, or tai chi) to counter the effects of fatigue. See page 188 for ideas.
- Schedule necessary activities during the time of the day when you have the most energy. Do the most important things first and the least important last. Space out activities, allowing time to rest, if needed.
- Get enough continuous sleep (at least eight hours). Most people need a block of time, not just cat naps here and there. It may be necessary to modify your sleeping room to block out light, noises, and other interruptions (such as animals, a snoring spouse, etc.).
- Get a good night's sleep. Consider making an appointment with a professional counselor or social worker who specializes in techniques for relaxation or meditation.
- Ask your doctor for a sleep evaluation. Your fatigue could be related to sleep apnea or other breathing issues that can lead to sleep interruption.
- Remember that fatigue due to anemia is temporary. Your energy level will slowly improve when blood counts return to normal.
- Let others help you with meals, housework, or errands.
- Do not force yourself to do more than you can manage.
- With your doctor's approval, gradually incorporate a daily routine of walking.
- Drink small amounts of caffeine-containing beverages.

Call your doctor if you are unable to get out of bed for more than twenty-four hours, if you are confused, or if your fatigue gets progressively worse.

Using Nutrition to Your Advantage

Treatment-related fatigue can be made worse by poor nutrition choices but can be helped by choosing nutritious foods and beverages. Keep these goals in mind:

- **Get enough calories**. An important part of any nutrition plan to combat fatigue includes sufficient calories and protein. (See "How to Increase Calories" on page 166.)

- **Include protein**. Protein helps heal and rebuild tissues. Protein from animal sources like milk, eggs, and meat or from plant-based sources like legumes and nuts can help you get the amount you need. (See "How to Increase Protein" on page 169 for specific protein sources.)

- **Get enough vitamins and minerals**. Getting nutrients through food is ideal, but if you are not consuming enough food and beverages because of eating or digestion-related treatment side effects, ask your doctor about taking a simple multiple vitamin/mineral supplement that provides approximately 100 percent of the Recommended Daily Value of many nutrients. To maximize absorption, do not take your multiple vitamin/mineral supplement with coffee or tea in the morning. Supplements are better digested and absorbed by your body when taken with food. Taking supplements with food also helps decrease the chance of nausea. (See chapter 5 for more information on dietary supplements during cancer treatment.)

- **Stay hydrated**. Try to drink at least eight cups of healthy liquids each day to help keep you hydrated. If you have side effects like vomiting or diarrhea, you will need more liquids than normal. The rule of thumb is one cup of healthy fluid after every bout of vomiting or diarrhea. Water, fruit juices, small amounts of milk, and broth count as good choices. Coffee and caffeinated beverages can be dehydrating, so stay away from caffeinated coffee, sodas, and teas. (See chapter 11 for more information on the importance of proper hydration.)

- **Avoid sweets**, which may drive up blood sugar levels only to have them drop a few hours later. Peaks and valleys in blood sugar likely contribute to fatigue.

- **Talk to a registered dietitian**. A registered dietitian can help identify the nutrients your diet is lacking and can help you create a balance in your diet that may alleviate fatigue. A registered dietitian can also help you cope with side effects that may be making it hard for you to eat and digest enough food to maintain a healthy weight.

- **Ask for help**. If you are so exhausted that you do not have the energy to eat, ask friends or family members to help with purchasing food, making meals, and cleaning. Ask your health care team about caregiver to-do lists and organizations or services that might help during these difficult times.

Other Ways to Cope with Fatigue

You can help conquer fatigue through nondietary methods as well. The two ways of coping listed here, being physically active and managing stress, complement each other.

Physical Activity

You may not feel like being very physically active during treatment, and there may be times when you are temporarily confined to a comfortable chair or bed. But decreased activity itself can cause a lack of energy and a tired feeling. In fact, studies assessing the effect of activity on fatigue show that being more physically active reduces fatigue in cancer patients.

Exercise slows down the release of stress-related hormones. Studies have shown that moderate physical activity on most or all days can help you cope with anxiety and depression, improve mood, boost self-esteem, and lessen symptoms of fatigue as well as nausea, pain, and diarrhea. Even light physical activity can improve your appetite, aid digestion, and regulate bowel movements. There is good evidence that physical activity during treatment can help people cope with common side effects of treatment such as fatigue, pain, or nausea; improve physical and functional well-being; and improve overall quality of life. Moving your muscles, even if in a limited fashion, is essential for maximizing your strength and energy level. See the "Types of Physical Activity" chart on the next page.

If you are considering beginning an exercise program, keep these points in mind:

- Talk to your health care team first about whether exercise is a possibility for you during treatment. Ask about any limitations or boundaries you should keep in mind.
- Don't overdo it. Start with activities that are not too strenuous, and set small goals. Then, build up to moderate exercise.
- Over time, commit to exercising regularly, five or more times a week, for at least thirty minutes—or with the frequency and duration your health care team recommends.
- Swimming, walking, practicing gentle yoga, and riding stationary bicycles are safer than other high-impact physical activities and may pose less of a risk of injury.

Managing Stress and Depression

Fatigue can also be a side effect of something more significant, like depression. A cancer diagnosis, treatment, and learning to live with cancer can cause depression, anxiety, and fear. These are normal responses to a life-altering experience. Fear of the unknown, additional stress at home or work, and the potential loss of control over some parts of your life can lead to sadness and feeling blue. If you are already experiencing treatment-related fatigue, feelings of anxiety and depression can worsen your symptoms and make you even more tired.

TYPES OF PHYSICAL ACTIVITY			
	LIGHT ACTIVITIES	**MODERATE ACTIVITIES**	**VIGOROUS ACTIVITIES***
Exercise and Leisure	Mild stretching; walking slowly on a level, firm surface; pushing a stroller and walking; walking around the house or school; walking from house to car	Walking, dancing, bicycling, iceskating or rollerskating, horseback riding, canoeing, yoga	Jogging or running, fast bicycling, circuit weight training, aerobic dance, martial arts, jump rope, swimming
Home Activities	Sitting and playing with children, light housework, walking while playing with animals, bathing, dressing or undressing	Mowing the lawn, general lawn and garden maintenance	Digging, carrying and hauling, masonry, carpentry
Occupational Activities	Walking around the office, working at the computer/typing	Walking and lifting as part of a job (custodial work, farming, auto repair)	Heavy manual labor (forestry, construction, fire-fighting)
Sports		Volleyball, golfing, softball, baseball, badminton, doubles tennis, downhill skiing	Soccer, hockey, lacrosse, tennis, racquetball, basketball, cross-country skiing

* **Caution:** Take part in these types of activities only with your doctor's approval.

Consider these options as you cope with stress or depression:

- Talk about your feelings and fears with your cancer center's psychosocial support personnel.
- Talk about your feelings and fears with loved ones.
- Remember that it is okay to feel sad or worried or frustrated.
- Seek help and advice through private counseling and support groups.
- Use prayer or other types of spiritual support.
- Try to be more physically active as a method of coping.
- Take part in activities to distract you and keep you engaged both at home or outside the home.
- Try deep breathing and relaxation exercises several times a day.
- Consider guided imagery or meditation to help promote more positive thoughts and decrease anxiety. Ask your health care team about programs in your area.
- Consider activities such as reiki, yoga, or pilates as ways to be active and relax at the same time.
- Consider music therapy to help decrease anxiety and promote relaxation. Contact your health care team for help in locating a local music therapist that specializes in this type of therapy.
- Talk with your doctor about using anti-anxiety or antidepressant medications.

DEEP BREATHING AND GUIDED IMAGERY EXERCISE

Close your eyes. Breathe deeply. Concentrate on each body part and relax it, starting with your toes and working up to the head. When you are relaxed, try to think of a pleasant place such as a beach in the morning or a field on a spring day.

Do not keep your feelings inside or blame yourself for feeling worried or blue. Your health care team can recommend someone who has experience helping people with cancer cope with their complex feelings. Feelings of sadness are normal when you have cancer. But sadness or emotional upset that lasts weeks or months or gets in the way of day-to-day functions might be clinical depression.

When to Call the Doctor

Depression does not just go away, and it can be a serious ongoing condition. Talk to your doctor if five or more of the following symptoms last for two weeks or longer or are severe enough to interfere with your daily activities. You may need to be evaluated for clinical depression by a qualified health or mental health professional.

- persistent sad or "empty" mood almost every day for most of the day
- loss of interest or pleasure in ordinary activities
- loss of appetite or overeating
- significant weight loss or gain
- inability to sleep, early waking, or oversleeping
- restlessness or feeling "slowed down" almost daily
- profound fatigue, almost every day
- feelings of guilt, worthlessness, or helplessness
- difficulty concentrating, remembering, or making decisions
- thoughts of death or suicide

References

Coping with cancer-related fatigue. WebMD Web site. http://www.webmd.com/cancer/fatigue-cancer-related. Updated August 20,2009. Accessed December 12, 2009.

The complete guide—nutrition and physical activity. American Cancer Society Web site. http://www.cancer.org/docroot/PED/content/PED_3_2X_Diet_and_Activity_Factors_That_Affect_Risks.asp. Updated March 19, 2008. Accessed December 12, 2009.

Doyle C, Kushi LH, Byers T, Courneya KS, Demark-Wahnefried W, Grant B, McTiernan A, Rock CL, Thompson C, Gansler T, Andrews KS; 2006 Nutrition, Physical Activity and Cancer Survivorship Advisory Committee; American Cancer Society. Nutrition and physical activity during and after cancer treatment: a guide for informed choices by cancer survivors. *CA Cancer J Clin.* 2006;56(6):323-353.

Eyre HJ, Morris LB, Lange D. *Informed Decisions: The Complete Book of Cancer Diagnosis, Treatment, and Recovery.* 2nd ed. Atlanta, GA: American Cancer Society; 2002.

Grant B, Hamilton KK. *Management of Nutrition Impact Symptoms in Cancer and Educational Handouts.* Chicago, IL: American Dietetic Association; 2004.

"I get tired easily." University of Michigan Comprehensive Cancer Center Web site. http://www.cancer.med.umich.edu/support/nutrtired.shtml. Accessed May 19, 2009.

Kushi LH, Byers T, Doyle C, Bandera EV, McCullough M, McTiernan A, Gansler T, Andrews KS, Thun MJ; American Cancer Society 2006 Nutrition and Physical Activity Guidelines Advisory Committee. American Cancer Society Guidelines on Nutrition and Physical Activity for cancer prevention: reducing the risk of cancer with healthy food choices and physical activity. *CA Cancer J Clin.* 2006;56(5):254-281; quiz 313-314.

Nutrition and exercise important after treatment. American Cancer Society Web site. http://www.cancer.org/docroot/NWS/content/update/NWS_2_1xU_Nutrition_and_Exercise_Important_After_Treatment_.asp. Published July 18, 2001. Accessed December 12, 2009.

Nutrition in cancer care (PDQ®). National Cancer Institute Web site. http://www.cancer.gov/cancerinfo/pdq/supportivecare/nutrition/HealthProfessional#Section_157. Updated August 11, 2009. Accessed December 12, 2009.

Yarbo CH, Goodman M, Frogge MH. *Cancer Symptom Management*. 3rd ed. Sudbury, MA: Jones and Bartlett Publishers; 2003.

Chapter Ten

Strengthening Your Immune System

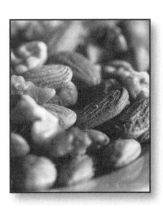

THE IMMUNE SYSTEM IS MADE UP OF THE ORGANS AND CELLS that defend your body against infection or disease. Lymph nodes are bean-sized collections of immune system cells that are scattered throughout your body. Immune system cells are also found in the spleen (an organ found underneath the left rib cage), in the bone marrow (the soft inner part of bones where blood cells are produced), and in the digestive and respiratory systems. Your immune system responds to toxins and germs (bacteria and viruses) by producing antibodies. These antibodies recognize and kill some toxins and germs and mark others, so that immune system cells and blood cells can destroy them. In other cases, toxins and germs are killed directly by the immune system cells working alone or together with blood cells. The major function of white blood cells is to defend your body against infections.

During the course of your treatment for cancer, there may be times when your body will not be able to protect itself from infection as well as usual. Cancer or cancer treatment can cause immunosuppression, a weakening of the immune system. Cancer treatments, such as some chemotherapy or biotherapy agents and radiation therapy to large areas of bone marrow such as the hip bone, breast bone, or vertebrae, can also cause myelosuppression. Myelosuppression refers to the suppression of bone marrow, the place where blood cells are formed in your body. Myelosuppression can cause a reduction in the number of white blood cells (neutropenia), platelets (thrombocytopenia), and red blood cells (anemia). The term "nadir" refers to the point at which your blood counts are the lowest. The nadir usually occurs seven to fourteen days after chemotherapy, depending on which chemotherapy agent is used. White blood cells attack and destroy invading bacteria, viruses, and fungi and protect you against infection, foreign organisms, and food-borne illness. As the number of neutrophils, a type of white blood cell, decreases, your risk of infection increases.

You may have heard about supplements promoted to boost the immune system and help fight cancer. The term "boost" may lead you to believe that a substance will increase the function of the immune system. But the word "boost" does not identify what a product does, and claims for "boosting the immune system" often are not supported by evidence. No such product has had proven benefits. Whether in active treatment or recovery, people with cancer who are considering taking any product that makes this claim should first talk with their doctor or health care team. The following herbal supplements are often claimed to "boost" the immune system:

- **Astragalus.** Available scientific evidence does not indicate that astragalus can kill cancer cells or stave off illness.
- **Echinacea.** Available scientific evidence does not prove that echinacea increases resistance to cancer or alleviates the immune suppression resulting from chemotherapy.
- **Cat's claw, Essiac tea, mistletoe, pau d'arco, and Siberian ginseng (eleuthero).** All of these herbs are promoted as immune boosters that help fight cancer. Available scientific evidence has not proven a benefit from any of these herbs, and some might even

have harmful side effects for people undergoing cancer treatment. See page 111.

- *Medicinal mushrooms (such as reishi, maitake, shiitake, and others).* Whereas several cancer-fighting properties have been found in mushrooms, available scientific research does not support claims that mushroom-containing supplements and food products can affect immune function in people during cancer treatment.

Cancer Treatments' Effects on Your Immune System

All cancer treatments have an effect on the immune system, and nutrition is an important part of keeping your immune system strong. All cells need nutrients to grow and function. If your cells do not have adequate nutrients because your intake of vitamins, minerals, fat, calories, and protein has decreased, their immune function can be altered. Poor nutrition makes your immune system less effective at recognizing and destroying germs. If you are malnourished, you are at greater risk for developing infections. Making sure you are consuming enough calories, protein, and vitamins and minerals can help keep your immune system functioning properly.

Surgery

Any type of major surgery can cause immunosuppression, but the reason for this change is not totally clear. Researchers have noted decreases in immune function within hours of surgery. Anesthesia may play a role in reducing immunity. After surgery, complete immune system recovery may take ten days to several months. Also, surgery often disrupts the skin and mucous membranes and exposes internal tissues to germs, thereby placing you at increased risk for infection. It is for those reasons and more that you should allow time for rest and recovery following procedures.

Surgery is commonly used to diagnose, stage, and treat cancer. Factors that increase the risk of infection after surgery include the length of hospitalization, the extent of the surgery, the duration of the operation, the amount of bleeding during surgery, your nutritional status, prior cancer treatment such as chemotherapy or radiation therapy of the surgical area, and other medical conditions you may have, such as diabetes.

Because surgical wounds are common sites of infection, you will be given antibiotics before surgery to decrease your risk of infection. You will be monitored for signs of infection after surgery.

Chemotherapy

Chemotherapy is the most common cause of myelosuppression (the suppression of bone marrow) in people receiving cancer treatment. The severity of myelosuppression depends on the specific chemotherapy agents used, the dosage, the schedule, previous treatments for cancer, your age and nutritional status, type of cancer, and the stage of the cancer. Some agents have a greater effect on the bone marrow than others. When chemotherapy agents are said to be myelosuppressive, this usually means that the agent affects production of all blood cells. However, chemotherapy agents may have different effects on the production of white blood cells, red blood cells, and platelets. Generally, white blood cell production is most sensitive to chemotherapy drugs.

Biotherapy

Biotherapy (also called biologic therapy or immunotherapy) is intended to improve the immune system's ability to recognize and attack cancer cells. Although these treatments stimulate immune reactions against cancer cells, they sometimes interfere with immunity against infections. If you are receiving biotherapy, you are at risk for immunosuppression and low white blood cell counts.

Radiation Therapy

Unless you receive total body irradiation or radiation treatment to large areas of bone marrow production (hip bone, breast bone, or vertebrae), you will most likely not experience extremely low blood counts because of your radiation therapy. This is because radiation therapy is usually given to just one area of the body at a time (whereas chemotherapy is a systemic treatment, meaning it travels throughout the body). However, depending on the dose and type of radiation therapy, the skin and mucous membranes may become damaged, making them less effective in keeping germs away from internal organs. Today, radiation therapy treatments are given over many treatment sessions (fractions) rather than in one large dose. This technique has helped decrease the amount of myelosuppression and risk for infection.

If bony areas are in the radiation therapy treatment area, the effects on bone marrow cells are similar to the effects of chemotherapy. Specifically, you may develop anemia or a low white blood cell count, which will increase your risk for infections. The total radiation dose, the radiation schedule, and the number of bone marrow cells directly in the radiation field (in other words, how much of the bone marrow is irradiated) affect the degree of myelosuppression from radiation therapy.

Food Safety Guidelines and Your Immune System

When your immune system is weakened, the first step in staying free from infection is being aware of the bacteria and other organisms that could make you ill and avoiding or getting rid of them. The choices you make when buying and handling foods, preparing meals, and dining out can affect your exposure to infectious organisms. Following food safety guidelines reduces your risk of developing a food-related infection.

Food Safety Guidelines at Home

Look at the lists provided here and keep in mind these simple ways of staying healthy when your immune system is weakened because of your cancer treatment.

COOK IT SAFELY

- Wash hands and kitchen surfaces often.
- Use separate cutting boards and knives for raw meats and vegetables.
- Use a clean food thermometer to ensure that food is cooked to the proper internal temperature. This also applies to food cooked or reheated in a microwave. Keep the temperature chart on pages 207–208 in a handy place.
- Food thermometers come in several styles, including instant-read digital thermometers, which are recommended for measuring the temperature of thin food, such as hamburger patties and boneless chicken breasts.
- Oven-proof thermometers may be placed in food *at the beginning* of cooking and remain there throughout cooking. Instant-read thermometers are used to check internal temperature during cooking and *after* the food is cooked.
- As a general rule, insert the thermometer into the thickest portion of the food. For whole poultry, insert into the inner thigh near the breast, but not touching the bone. For thin food such as patties, insert an instant-read thermometer sideways or at an angle. To prevent cross-contamination, wash the thermometer probe (the part inserted into the food) with hot water and soap after each use.
- Do not partially cook food and then finish later—harmful bacteria will grow between the time you start and finish cooking—even if you refrigerate the food in between.
- Do not roast food at temperatures below 325°F—bacteria may grow while cooking at this low temperature. Never cook a turkey overnight in the oven below 325°F.
- When cooking food in a microwave oven, make sure there are no cold spots where bacteria can survive. Cover food, stir, and rotate for even cooking. If there is no turntable in your microwave, rotate the dish by hand once or twice. Stir food half-way through cooking, even if your microwave has a rotating turntable.
- Allow microwaved food to stand for a few minutes after cooking; this distributes the heat, cooking the food evenly. Check for doneness with a clean food thermometer.
- Reheat carry-out meals and leftovers to a minimum internal temperature of 165°F, and stir to cook evenly. Bring sauces, soups, and gravy to a boil when reheating.

Adapted from US Food and Drug Administration and United States Department of Agriculture. "Cook It Safely! It's a Matter of Degrees." www.foodsafety.gov.

The following food safety guidelines are adapted from guidelines created by the Seattle Cancer Care Alliance. They were developed for all people with cancer and for those receiving bone marrow transplants. Although these guidelines were created for people with weakened immune systems, they can be used as safe food practices for all people, not just people undergoing cancer treatment. Talk to your doctor about whether you should follow these guidelines during your treatment.

Personal Hygiene

- Wash hands frequently—before and after each step of food preparation—with plenty of soap and hot, running water for at least twenty seconds.
- Wash hands before eating and after using the restroom, handling garbage, answering the phone, or touching pets.

Preparing Foods

- Use different knives and cutting boards to cut meat, produce, and bread.
- Do not taste food with the same utensil used for stirring.
- Wash vegetables and fruits thoroughly under clean, cold running water just before use and scrub lightly with a vegetable brush to remove dirt and debris. Follow the directions provided on page 89 in chapter 4 for cleaning produce.
- Individually rinse the leaves of leafy vegetables such as lettuce or cabbage. Wash all packaged salads and other prepared produce under clean, cold running water, even when they are marked as prewashed. Keep track of the "use by" dates on packaged and prepared produce and do not eat items that have expired.
- Wash and softly scrub with a vegetable brush the outside of all vegetables and fruits (such as oranges, melons, and bananas), even if the produce will be peeled or cut. This will prevent any bacteria or debris on the outside of the fruit from being transferred to the fruit itself.
- Wash the tops of canned foods before opening, and clean the can opener after each use.

Thawing and Cooking Foods

- Thaw meat, fish, or poultry in the refrigerator away from raw vegetables and fruits and other prepared foods. Place on a dish to catch drips. Cook defrosted meat right away, and do not refreeze without first cooking it thoroughly. If you are in a hurry, you may thaw meat in the microwave, but cook it immediately after thawing.
- Cook eggs until the yolks and whites are firm. Cook egg dishes, custards, egg sauces, and casseroles that include eggs to a minimum internal temperature of 160°F, using a food thermometer as a guide.

- Cook meats until they are no longer pink and the juices run clear. The only way you can be sure that meat has been cooked to a safe temperature is by using a food thermometer and following the recommended minimum cooking temperatures that are specified in the table on pages 207–208.
- Heat leftovers to 165°F, using a food thermometer as a guide.
- When microwaving, rotate the dish a quarter turn once or twice during cooking if there is no turntable in the microwave oven. This prevents cold spots in food where bacteria can survive.
- Use a lid or vented plastic wrap to thoroughly heat leftovers in the microwave. Stir several times during reheating. When food is heated thoroughly (to a minimum of 165°F, using a food thermometer as a guide), cover and let sit two minutes before serving.
- Boil tofu, in half-inch cubes, for five minutes before using. (This process is not necessary if you are using tofu in shelf-stable packaging for which refrigeration is not needed until the product is opened.)

Refrigerating and Storing Foods

- Purchase and use a food and refrigerator thermometer (available at many grocery and hardware stores). After foods are prepared and/or heated to their recommended temperatures, hold foods at safe temperatures: cold food below 40°F and hot foods above 165°F, using a food thermometer as a guide. See pages 207–208 of this chapter for recommended food cooking temperatures.
- Never leave perishable food out of the refrigerator for more than two hours; throw away food left out longer than two hours.
- Never re-refrigerate or refreeze leftovers not eaten within the food safety guidelines listed on page 145 of chapter 7. Throw them out!
- Refrigerate vegetables and fruits. Discard vegetables and fruits that are slimy, mushy, or show mold.
- Throw out foods that look or smell strange. Never taste them! When in doubt—throw it out!

Drinking Water (Note: Water safety is discussed in greater detail in chapter 11.)

- Do not drink well water unless it is tested yearly for coliform bacteria.
- Do not drink water straight from lakes, rivers, streams, or springs.
- If using a water service other than the local city water service, drink bottled or distilled water.
- If using a home water-filtering system with city water, change the water filter regularly according to the manufacturer's instructions.

- When in doubt about your water's safety, simply bring the water to a rolling boil for one minute. After boiling, store the water in a clean covered container in the refrigerator, and throw out any unused water after seventy-two hours (three days).

Work Surfaces and Kitchen Equipment

- Use separate cutting boards for cooked foods and raw foods. Cut on plastic or glass cutting boards when cutting raw meat and poultry. Wooden boards used exclusively for raw meat and poultry are acceptable, but use a different board for cutting other foods, such as produce or bread.
- Wash cutting boards after each use in hot, soapy water; rinse and air dry or pat dry with fresh paper towels. Nonporous acrylic, plastic, glass, and solid wood boards can be washed in the dishwasher (laminated boards may crack and split).
- Make up a sanitizing solution for general use on kitchen work surfaces, cutting boards, and other utensils. Mix two teaspoons of household (chlorine) bleach in one quart (four cups) of water. After using the sanitizing solution, rinse with clean water, wipe with a paper towel, and allow to air dry. Alternatively, use a commercial sanitizing agent and follow the directions on the product.
- Clean food particles off of the microwave oven, toaster, can opener, and blender and mixer blades. Remove blender blades and the bottom ring when washing the blender container. Use a bleach solution of two tablespoons of household bleach to one quart (four cups) of water to sanitize these items.
- Keep the counter and kitchen surfaces free of food particles. Clean regularly with a bleach solution (as outlined above).

Sink Area

- Keep soap available for hand washing.
- Use paper towels for drying hands.
- Replace dishcloths and dishtowels daily.
- Replace sponges at least weekly.
- Sanitize sponges daily in a solution of two tablespoons of household bleach and one quart (four cups) of water or place in dishwasher. Or use paper towels instead of sponges while your immune system may be compromised.
- Do not store food supplies under the kitchen sink. Do not store chemicals and cleaning solutions near or over food supplies.
- Use liquid dish soap when hand washing dishes, pans, and utensils.
- Air dry dishes instead of towel-drying them.

Refrigerator and Freezer

- Keep the refrigerator clean: clean up spills immediately, discard food scraps, and sanitize shelves and doors regularly with a solution of two tablespoons of household bleach to one quart (four cups) of water.
- Keep the refrigerator temperature between 34°F and 40°F.
- Keep the freezer temperature below 0–2°F.
- Cool hot foods, uncovered, in the refrigerator in shallow containers; cover storage containers tightly after cooling. Freeze what you do not plan to use within the next two to three days.
- Throw away all refrigerated, cooked leftovers after seventy-two hours (three days). Label foods with the date to keep track of the age of leftovers.
- Throw out eggs with cracked shells or eggs with chicken feces on them.
- Throw out foods older than their "use by" expiration dates.
- Throw out entire food packages or containers with any mold present, including yogurt, cheese, cottage cheese, fruit, vegetables, jelly, and bread and pastry products.
- Throw out freezer-burned foods.

Cupboards and Pantry

- Throw out—without tasting or opening—any can with a bulge, leak, crack, or deep indentation in the seam area.
- Rotate food stock so older items are used first. Do not use foods older than their "use by" expiration dates.
- Keep food storage areas clean, and monitor for signs of insect or rodent contamination.
- Review the processing used in preparing home-canned foods to be sure it is appropriate for the acidity of the food, size of the container, and elevation above sea level. Look for mold and leaks. Check seals. If you suspect a home-canned food may not have been processed properly (for example, if the lid bulges, or if the food has any bad odor or unusual characteristics after opening), throw it away. Use home-canned foods within one year of canning, as chemical changes may occur.
- Shelf-stable refers to unopened canned, bottled, or packaged food products that can be stored at room temperature before opening. After being opened, the container may require refrigeration.

Food Safety Guidelines Outside the Home

It is easier to control bacteria and other organisms in your home than in other environments. But you can keep an eye on food safety when you are outside the home by following a few tips:

Grocery Shopping

- Wipe down the handle of the grocery cart or basket with a sanitary wipe (usually available at the entrance of grocery stores).
- Shop for shelf-stable items first, such as canned and boxed foods. Select frozen and refrigerated foods last, especially during the summer months.
- Check "sell by" and "use by" dates on dairy products, eggs, cereals, canned foods, and other goods. Purchase only the freshest products.
- Check the packaging and "use by" dates on fresh meats, poultry, and seafood. Do not purchase any products that are out of date.
- Reject damaged, swollen, rusted, or deeply dented cans. Make sure that packaged and boxed foods are properly sealed.
- Select unblemished vegetables and fruits that look and smell fresh. Avoid wilted produce.
- Avoid delicatessen foods, such as sliced meats and cheeses and premade sandwiches and salads.
- In the bakery, avoid unrefrigerated cream- and custard-containing desserts and pastries.
- Avoid foods from self-serve or bulk containers.
- Resist trying free food samples.
- Open egg cartons to be sure you do not buy cracked eggs.
- Do not buy unrefrigerated eggs.
- Ask that meat, poultry, and fish be placed in separate bags from fresh produce at the checkout stand.
- Use a "stay-cool" bag to transport refrigerated or frozen products for the trip home from the grocery store.
- Refrigerate or freeze perishables promptly, and never leave perishables in a hot car.

Dining Out

- Eat early to avoid crowds.
- Ask that fresh food be prepared in fast-food restaurants.
- Ask if fruit juices are pasteurized, and do not drink nonpasteurized juice.
- Avoid raw prepared vegetables and fruits, such as cut-up fruit or vegetables or ready-made fruit and vegetable trays. Eat these items at home where you can clean them thoroughly.
- Request single-serving condiment packages, and avoid self-serve bulk condiment containers. Do not eat salsa or other condiments that are unrefrigerated and/or used by multiple people at a restaurant.
- Avoid salad bars, delicatessens, buffets, smorgasbords, potlucks, and sidewalk vendors. These are high-risk food sources because of potentially improper food storage or holding temperatures and poor hygiene by those handling the food.

- Consider the general condition of the restaurant before eating there. Are the plates, glasses, and utensils clean? Are the restrooms clean and stocked with soap and paper towels? The cleanliness of the restaurant itself may indicate the cleanliness and care involved in food preparation.
- Avoid soft-serve ice cream, milk shakes, and frozen yogurt dispensed from a machine.
- Avoid self-serve ice cream and beverage and ice machines.

Nutrition Suggestions for People with Weakened Immune Systems

There are certain foods that all people should avoid, regardless of the state of their immune systems. These foods can harbor high levels of bacteria, and eating them can lead to contracting a food-borne illness:

- Uncooked vegetable sprouts (all types, including alfalfa, radish, broccoli, mung bean, etc.), because of a high risk of contamination with salmonella and E. coli.
- Raw or runny eggs, including nonpasteurized or homemade eggnog, Caesar salad dressing made with raw eggs, smoothies or drinks made with raw eggs, and unbaked meringues. To avoid bacterial contamination, substitute frozen pasteurized eggs or powdered egg whites for raw eggs in recipes for uncooked foods.
- Nonpasteurized vegetable and fruit juice, unless prepared at home with washed produce.
- Undercooked meat or poultry, especially ground meats.

Within seven to fourteen days after chemotherapy, white blood cell counts can drop to a dangerous level (the nadir, as discussed previously). During this time, you may be at a higher risk for infection and may need to avoid foods that are likely to harbor high levels of bacteria, including unwashed vegetables and fruits, nonpasteurized juices, and raw or undercooked fish, meats, and eggs.

Your doctor can determine your current neutrophil count and if you are neutropenic (meaning you would be more susceptible to infection). Your doctor will most likely monitor your blood counts at least weekly during chemotherapy to determine your neutrophil count. Consider avoiding the foods listed below when your immune system is extremely weak, such as when your absolute neutrophil count falls below one thousand per microliter:

- raw or undercooked tofu
- raw or undercooked animal products, including meat, pork, game, poultry, eggs, hot dogs, luncheon meats, deli meats, sausage, and bacon
- uncooked foods containing raw eggs, such as hollandaise sauce, raw cookie dough, or

homemade mayonnaise (Liquid pasteurized egg product may be used in recipes that call for raw eggs.)

- raw or lightly cooked fish, shellfish, lox, sushi, or sashimi
- nonpasteurized milk and dairy products. (You may eat products made from pasteurized milk, including grade A milk, hard cheeses, processed cheeses, cream cheese, cottage cheese, and yogurt.)
- soft cheeses such as feta, Brie, Camembert, blue-veined (Roquefort, Stilton, Gorgonzola, and blue), or Mexican-style (such as queso blanco fresco)
- fresh salad dressings and salsas found in the refrigerated section at the grocery store. Choose salad dressings and salsas that are shelf-stable.
- unwashed raw vegetables and fruits and those with visible mold
- raw honey (Instead, select commercial grade A or heat-treated honey.)
- unprocessed or raw peanut butter or other nut butters
- sun tea, meaning tea that is left to steep in sunlight (Instead, make tea with boiling water, using commercially packaged tea bags.)
- nonpasteurized beer
- uncooked brewer's yeast
- untested well water

People sometimes confuse low red blood cell counts with low white blood cell counts. Iron supplements can increase red blood cell counts but will not help raise your level of white blood cells. Unfortunately, there is no known dietary supplement that can increase the white blood cell count. However, the micronutrients zinc, selenium, iron, copper, folic acid, and vitamins A, C, E, and B6 have important influences on immune responses. Taking a daily multivitamin/mineral supplement that contains no more than 100 percent of the Recommended Daily Value is a good way to get enough vitamins and minerals without taking potentially harmful amounts. Talk to your health care team about an optimal plan for you.

Improving Immunity in Other Ways

Beyond avoiding bacteria and harmful organisms that could make you ill during treatment, how else can you improve your immune system? You may hear about ways people with cancer try to improve their immune systems, including fasting. But fasting and avoiding taking in nutrients actually causes the immune system to suffer, because the cells involved in providing an immune response need nutrients to run properly. (For more about fasting, see chapter 6.) Here are some medically sound suggestions that may help improve your immune system.

Coping with Stress

A cancer diagnosis is often overwhelming. Having to make decisions about your treatment and facing uncertainties about medical coverage, expenses, and the future can all be very stressful. Research has shown that some people with cancer experience higher-than-average levels of stress. These people tend to be at higher risk for infection. The relationship of psychological factors to risk of infection, however, is not clearly understood. Long periods of stress or depression can lead to poor nutrition, which can weaken your immune system and contribute to susceptibility for infection. Research also suggests that emotional stress can affect your body's hormones, which, in turn, can influence the immune system. Lack of sleep, loneliness, or depression can add to stress.

Take some time for yourself. Try relaxing and breathing deeply. Light exercise may help you cope as well. See pages 187–190 for more information about ways to cope with stress.

Physical Activity and Your Immune System

Being physically active has been shown to help the immune system fight off infections, and it may also help prevent illnesses such as heart disease, osteoporosis, and cancer. Physical activity can improve your immune system by stimulating antibodies and white blood cells to move through the body more quickly than normal. Faster-moving antibodies or white blood cells can find and attach to toxins and germs more quickly. Exercise also may reduce the levels of stress-related hormones.

If you are already exercising regularly, do not develop a more intense workout program in the hopes of increasing immune system benefits. Before you begin a physical activity regimen for the first time, talk to your doctor or health care team. The level of activity appropriate for you depends on where you are in the course of treatment, the type of treatment you are receiving, and your general health. Your doctor and physical therapist can advise you about the level of activity that would help you the most. See chapter 9 for ways to be more physically active.

Prescription Medications that May Help

The medications filgrastim (Neupogen) or pegfilgrastim (Neulasta) are similar to substances made by your body that stimulate the bone marrow to make more white blood cells and make them work better. Not everyone receives these medications. They are given only to people receiving chemotherapy agents that are known to be myelosuppressive to white blood cells or to people who are becoming neutropenic as result of cancer or its treatment.

Filgrastim and pegfilgrastim are injected under the skin. Either the person with cancer or a family member can be taught to give the injections. These medications are given at least twenty-four hours after chemotherapy and may be given until the neutrophils in the blood have reached a certain level. Pegfilgrastim is a long-acting form of filgrastim and only needs to be given once with each chemotherapy cycle. Side effects of filgrastim and pegfilgrastim include pain in the bones and flu-like symptoms. These symptoms are easily managed if they occur.

Cooking Guidelines for Eggs, Meats, Poultry, and Seafood		
	PRODUCT	**COOK UNTIL...**
Eggs, egg dishes, and casseroles	Eggs	Yolks and whites are firm
	Casseroles, egg dishes, custard, egg sauces	Internal temperature reaches 160°F
Beef, pork, veal, lamb, rabbit, goat, game	Whole pieces of meat, chops, ribs	Internal temperature reaches 160°F
	Ground beef, pork, veal, lamb, rabbit, goat, game	Internal temperature reaches 160°F
Poultry (chicken, turkey, duck, goose)	Chicken and turkey: whole bird and dark meat (thigh, wing)	Internal temperature reaches 180°F
	Breast, roast	Internal temperature reaches 170°F
	Ground chicken, turkey	Internal temperature reaches 165°F
	Stuffing (always cook in separate container outside of bird)	Internal temperature reaches 165°F
Ham	Fresh (raw)	Internal temperature reaches 160°F
	Precooked (to reheat)	Internal temperature reaches 160°F

Cooking Guidelines for
Eggs, Meats, Poultry, and Seafood (continued)

	PRODUCT	COOK UNTIL...
Seafood	Fin fish (such as salmon, cod, halibut, snapper, sole, bass, trout)	Opaque and flakes easily with a fork
	Shrimp, lobster, crab	Turns red and flesh becomes pearly opaque
	Scallops	Turns milk white or opaque and firm
	Clams, mussels, oysters	Shells open, and do not eat those that do not open during cooking. (Note: These foods may be high-risk for people with low white blood cell count or immunosuppression.)
Ready-to-eat meats*	Hot dogs, luncheon meats, cold cuts, deli-style meats	Heat thoroughly until steaming

* Keep your intake of processed meats to a minimum, if they are eaten at all. Choose more nutritious, leaner meats whenever possible.

Adapted from Saundra Aker and Polly Lenssen. *A Guide to Good Nutrition During Cancer Treatment, Fourth Edition.* (Seattle, WA: Fred Hutchinson Cancer Research Center, 2000).

What to Eat and Avoid When Your White Blood Cell Count Is Low

	RECOMMENDED	AVOID
Meat, poultry, fish, tofu, and nuts	• Ensure all meats, poultry, and fish are cooked thoroughly. • Use a food thermometer to be sure that meat and poultry reach the proper temperature when cooked. • When using tofu purchased from the refrigerated section (not shelf-stable), cut tofu into one-inch cubes or smaller and boil five minutes in water or broth before eating or using in recipes. This cooking process is not necessary if using aseptically packaged, shelf-stable tofu, such as Mori-Nu silken tofu. • Eat vacuum-sealed nuts and shelf-stable nut butters.	• Do not eat raw or lightly cooked fish, shellfish, lox, sushi, or sashimi. • Do not eat raw nuts or fresh nut butters.
Eggs	• Cook eggs until the yolks and whites are solid, not runny. • Cook with pasteurized eggs or egg custard.	• Do not eat raw or soft-cooked eggs. This includes over-easy, poached, soft-boiled, and sunny side up.

What to Eat and Avoid When Your White Blood Cell Count Is Low
(continued)

	RECOMMENDED	AVOID
Eggs	• Drink pasteurized eggnog.	• Do not eat foods that may contain raw eggs, such as Caesar salad dressing, homemade eggnog, smoothies, raw cookie dough, hollandaise sauce, and homemade mayonnaise.
Milk and dairy products	• Eat or drink only pasteurized milk, yogurt, cheese, or other dairy products.	• Avoid soft, mold-ripened or blue-veined cheeses, including Brie, Camembert, Roquefort, Stilton, Gorgonzola, and blue cheese. • Avoid Mexican-style cheeses such as queso blanco fresco, since they are frequently made from unpasteurized milk.
Bread, cereal, rice, and pasta	• Breads, bagels, muffins, rolls, cereals, crackers, noodles, pasta, potatoes, and rice are safe to eat as long as they are purchased as wrapped, prepackaged items, not sold in self-service bins.	• Avoid bulk-bin sources of cereals, grains, and other foods.

What to Eat and Avoid When Your White Blood Cell Count Is Low
(continued)

	RECOMMENDED	AVOID
Vegetables and fruits	• Raw vegetables and fruits and fresh herbs are safe to eat if washed carefully under running water and lightly scrubbed with a vegetable brush. Follow the directions listed on page 89 of chapter 4.	• Avoid fresh salsas and salad dressings found in the refrigerated section of the grocery store. Choose shelf-stable salsas and salad dressings instead. • Do not eat any raw vegetable sprouts (including alfalfa, radish, broccoli, or mung bean sprouts).
Desserts and sweets	• Fruit pies, cakes, and cookies, flavored gelatin; commercial ice cream, sherbet, sorbet, and Popsicles; and sugar, commercially-prepared and pasteurized jam, jelly, preserves, syrup, and molasses are safe to eat.	• Avoid unrefrigerated, cream-filled pastry products. • Do not consume raw honey or honeycomb. Select commercial, grade A, heat-treated honey instead.
Water	• Drink only water from city or municipal water services or commercially bottled water.	• Do not drink water straight from lakes, rivers, streams, or springs. • Do not drink well water, unless it is tested at least yearly and contains no coliform bacteria.

What to Eat and Avoid When Your White Blood Cell Count Is Low (continued)		
	RECOMMENDED	**AVOID**
Beverages	• Drink pasteurized fruit and vegetable juices, soda, coffee, and tea.	• Do not drink unpasteurized fruit and vegetable juices. • Avoid sun tea. Make tea with boiling water, by using commercially prepared tea bags. • Avoid vitamin- or herbal-supplemented waters. These beverages provide little, if any, health benefit.

References

Aker SN, Lenssen P. *A Guide to Good Nutrition during Cancer Treatment.* 4th ed. Seattle, WA: Fred Hutchinson Cancer Research Center; 2000.

American Cancer Society. *American Cancer Society Complete Guide to Complementary and Alternative Cancer Therapies.* 2nd ed. Atlanta, GA: American Cancer Society; 2009.

Biological therapies for cancer: questions and answers. National Cancer Institute Web Site. http://www.cancer.gov/cancertopics/factsheet/Therapy/biological. Updated June 13, 2006. Accessed December 9, 2009.

Bone marrow transplantation and peripheral blood stem cell transplantation. National Cancer Institute Web site. http://www.cancer.gov/cancertopics/factsheet/Therapy/bone-marrow-transplant. Updated October 29, 2008. Accessed December 9, 2009.

Chandra RK. Nutrition and the immune system: an introduction. *Am J Clin Nutr.* 1997;66(2):460S-463S.

Chemotherapy and you: support for people with cancer. National Cancer Institute Web site. http://www.cancer.gov/cancertopics/insides-chemotherapy-and-you.pdf. Updated October 2008. Accessed December 9, 2009.

Cody MM, for the American Dietetic Association. *Safe Food for You and Your Family: Up-to-Date Tips from the World's Foremost Nutrition Experts.* Chicago, IL: American Dietetic Association; 1996.

Doyle C, Kushi LH, Byers T, Courneya KS, Demark-Wahnefried W, Grant B, McTiernan A, Rock CL, Thompson C, Gansler T, Andrews KS; 2006 Nutrition, Physical Activity and Cancer Survivorship Advisory Committee; American Cancer Society. Nutrition and physical activity during and after cancer treatment: a guide for informed choices by cancer survivors. *CA Cancer J Clin.* 2006;56(6):323-353.

Elliott L, Molseed LL, McCallum PD, Grant B. *The Clinical Guide to Oncology Nutrition.* 2nd ed. Chicago, IL: American Dietetic Association; 2006.

FDA Center for Food Safety and Applied Nutrition. Cook it safely! It's a matter of degrees. FoodSafety.gov Web site. http://www.foodsafety.gov/~fsg/f99broch.html. Published September 1999. Accessed August 25, 2009. Content no longer available.

Foodborne illness: what consumers need to know. USDA Food Safety and Inspection Web site. http://www.fsis. usda.gov/Fact_Sheets/Foodborne_Illness_What_Consumers_Need_to_Know/index.asp. Posted April 3, 2006. Accessed December 7, 2009.

Food safety guidelines. Seattle Cancer Care Alliance Web site. http://www.seattlecca.org/food-safety-guidelines.cfm. Accessed December 7, 2009.

Grant B, Hamilton KK. *Management of Nutrition Impact Symptoms in Cancer and Educational Handouts.* Chicago, IL: American Dietetic Association; 2004.

Guidelines for herbal and nutrient supplements. Seattle Cancer Care Alliance Web site. http://www.seattlecca.org/client/documents/practical-emotional-support/herbal_sup_2510_0.pdf. Accessed December 7, 2009.

National Library of Medicine, National Institutes of Health. Exercise and immunity. Medline Plus Web site. http://www.nlm.nih.gov/medlineplus/ency/article/007165.htm. Updated May 5, 2008. Accessed December 7, 2009.

NIH funds botanical center in Iowa to study health effects of echinacea and St. John's wort [news release]. Bethesda, MD: National Institutes of Health; July 25, 2002. National Institutes of Health Web site. http://www.nih.gov/news/pr/jul2002/niehs-25.htm. Posted July 25, 2002. Accessed December 7, 2009.

Nutrition for the Person with Cancer During Treatment: A Guide for Patients and Families [booklet]. Atlanta, GA: American Cancer Society; 2006.

People with weak immune systems. American Cancer Society Web site. http://www.cancer.org/docroot/MBC/content/MBC_6_2X_Impact_of_Altered_Immune_Function.asp. Accessed December 9, 2009.

Radiation therapy and you: support for people with cancer. National Cancer Institute Web site. http://www.cancer.gov/cancertopics/insides-radiation-therapy-and-you.pdf. Updated September 2009. Accessed December 9, 2009

Sources for food safety. Seattle Cancer Care Alliance Web site. http://www.seattlecca.org/sources-for-food-safety.cfm. Accessed December 7, 2009.

Whitmire S. Water, electrolytes, and acid-base balance. In: Mahan LK, Escott-Stump S. *Krause's Food, Nutrition, and Diet Therapy.* 10th ed. Philadelphia, PA: W. B. Saunders and Company; 2000.

Yarbo CH, Goodman M, Frogge MH. *Cancer Symptom Management.* 3rd ed. Sudbury, MA: Jones and Bartlett Publishers; 2003.

Chapter Eleven

Staying Hydrated

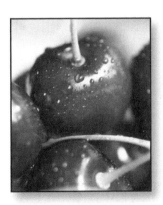

WATER IS ESPECIALLY IMPORTANT TO OUR BODIES, perhaps even more so than protein, carbohydrates, fats, and vitamins and minerals. Our bodies are primarily made of water, and we need water to survive. You need to drink plenty of healthy beverages every day to stay well-hydrated. A list of healthy beverages is provided on pages 218–219 of this chapter. Depending on age, body size, and health, normal fluid needs range from 25 to 30 milliliters (mL) of fluid per kilogram (kg) of body weight. For example, for a 132-pound (60 kg) woman, that would be 1.5 to 1.8 liters of fluid (about 6 to 7 cups) per day. For a 178-pound (80 kg) man, that would be 2.0 to 2.4 liters (8 to 10 cups) per day. (To convert pounds to kilograms, divide your weight in pounds by 2.2.) The amount of fluid you need could change when you are undergoing and recovering from cancer treatment. Your doctor or health care team will help you determine how much fluid is right for you during your treatment.

Adequate fluid intake is needed to keep your body in balance. When you take in enough fluid, it is spread throughout your body and helps each organ function. Fluid also helps with crucial processes like digestion, regulation of body temperature, and creation of new body tissue. In addition, adequate fluid intake helps flush your kidneys and bladder if you are taking medications that can affect kidney function. Because the human body can tolerate only moderate changes in fluid balance, changes in that balance affect the way a person feels. Swelling in the arms and legs indicates that the body is retaining too much water. Dehydration, the opposite of good hydration, means that the body has an inadequate amount of fluid or that the fluid is not in the right places.

Staying Hydrated

Good hydration, or maintaining adequate fluid levels in the body, is essential during and after cancer treatment. Staying well hydrated in the long term is important for overall good health. Depending upon your body's specific needs and your health care team's instructions, drinking an adequate amount of fluid each day will help keep you well hydrated. Emphasize fluid choices that are more nutritious, and limit beverages that contain empty calories and caffeine, such as caffeinated soft drinks and energy drinks, which provide little, if any, health benefit. If you have side effects from cancer treatment, such as diarrhea or vomiting, you will need to take in more fluid than normal. The rule of thumb is that one cup of fluid is needed to replace each cup of fluid lost from each episode of vomiting or diarrhea.

People who have preexisting renal disease or a condition such as edema (fluid retention), significant hypertension, or fluid overload that is worsened by their cancer or cancer treatment may need to restrict fluid intake. Talk to your health care team about how much fluid you need each day to stay well hydrated. Do not restrict your fluid intake unless you are given specific instructions to do so by your health care team.

Healthy Fluid Choices

What type of fluid is a healthy beverage? For most people water, milk, broth, and pasteurized 100 percent vegetable and fruit juices and nectars are all good choices. Caffeinated drinks are generally not as healthy because they can act as a diuretic—something that flushes fluid out of the body. Your doctor may advise you to limit your consumption of caffeine-containing beverages such as caffeinated coffee, soft drinks, black and green teas, and some energy drinks. Sports drinks such as Gatorade or Powerade are often recommended because they contain glucose (a simple sugar), which provides quick energy, and electrolytes (sodium and potassium) to replace the electrolytes lost through vomiting or diarrhea. You may, however, be asked to limit your intake of these and other sugar-sweetened beverages (such as sodas) because these types of drinks can lead to poorer hydration, especially if they cause an elevation in blood sugar, which can lead to excess urination. If sugar is a concern, try carbohydrate-free or low-sugar sports drinks, such as Isopure Zero Carb, Propel, or Crystal Light On the Go, which has added electrolytes.

Foods Containing Fluid

Liquid in food also counts toward the total amount of fluid you take in each day. Some fruits, such as melons, grapes, and tomatoes, naturally contain a lot of water. Other calorie-containing, fluid-type foods include:

- Popsicles and flavored ice pops
- flavored fruit ices made without fruit pieces or milk
- gelatin (regular or sugar-free)
- clear-liquid, high-protein beverages such as Isopure Company's Isopure Plus, Nestle Nutrition's Boost Breeze, or Abbott Nutrition's Enlive (Protein content varies from eight to fifteen grams per container.)

Water Alternatives

If you don't enjoy drinking water, or if you are experiencing taste aversions to plain water, try drinking a flavored water. With many brands and flavors available, these beverages have a little bit of flavor, and some are slightly sweetened with Splenda or NutraSweet, which makes them a good choice for people with diabetes. Carbonated water and seltzer waters, whether plain or flavored, are also good choices if you are not experiencing abdominal bloating and distention or bowel gas. Other suggestions for making water taste more pleasing include adding pieces of fruit, such as lemon, lime, or orange slices, or adding an ounce or two of fruit juice. You can also try other water alternatives:

- clear fruit juices
- clear, caffeine-free carbonated beverages
- fruit punch and other fruit-flavored drinks

- weak, caffeine-free hot or iced tea
- hot or iced herbal tea
- broth, bouillon, or consommé

Suggestions for Getting Enough Fluid

You may not become thirsty until after your body has lost precious water. By then, you need to drink even more fluid to replace what has been lost. Keep a glass or bottle of water with you at all times so you are reminded to sip throughout the day: while riding in the car, working, reading, or watching TV. Consider trying one of the following methods to achieve your daily fluid goals: keep a log of each glass of healthy fluid consumed, drink a specific number of bottles of water each day, or fill a plastic container of water with the needed amount of fluid.

How do you know when you're getting enough water? One simple way to tell is the urine test. When your urine is a pale color, you are likely getting enough water and fluid into your system; if it is dark-colored and concentrated, try increasing your intake of water and other healthy liquids. (Please note: multivitamin/mineral supplements and some prescription medications can make your urine bright yellow or different colors.)

Dehydration

Dehydration happens when the body loses too much water or does not get enough water to function properly. Symptoms can include the following:
- dry mouth
- thirst
- dizziness
- headache
- weakness
- low blood pressure
- inability to swallow dry food
- difficulty talking
- dry skin
- skin that "tents" when pinched
- swollen, cracked, or dry tongue
- fever
- weight loss
- production of little or no urine
- dark, strong-smelling urine
- fatigue
- muscle cramps

Loss of Body Fluid

Fever, diarrhea, or vomiting that is severe or long-lasting can cause loss of body fluid. Loss of body fluid can result in a loss of the body's electrolytes—including sodium, potassium, calcium, and magnesium—that are needed for proper body function. Other conditions that can result in dehydration include increased output in an ileostomy or colostomy bag, overuse of diuretics, ascites (fluid buildup in the abdomen), or edema. Acute and chronic pain can also lower the appetite for food and drink, which can contribute to or cause dehydration. Physical activity, while important, can contribute to dehydration. When active, be sure to drink even more fluids.

Fatigue and Dehydration

Fatigue can be one of the first signs of fluid depletion and dehydration. Because people being treated for cancer are often tired, this symptom can go unrecognized until it is very serious. You need to eat and drink enough each day to maintain strength and energy. Antiemetics, which are anti-nausea medications that provide relief from nausea and vomiting, can be very helpful in restoring appetite for food and beverages.

Coping with Dehydration

Your health care team can help you deal with any underlying causes of dehydration. While it is important to drink healthy fluids, do not force yourself to drink immediately after vomiting; wait approximately thirty minutes, and then sip room-temperature water or flat soda. You can also try clear liquids. Please refer to pages 307–308 for a list of beverages and foods you can consume on the Clear-Liquid Diet.

Drinking small amounts of water, juices, and other clear, calorie-containing liquids throughout the day will help keep your body hydrated and give you some energy. You might be able to tolerate cool or room-temperature liquids better than very hot or very cold fluids. But be sure to let your doctor know if you have only clear liquids for more than two days in a row. Consuming a diet of clear liquids alone does not provide you with the needed variety of nutrients and calories.

When you are feeling better and your appetite has returned, balance solid foods and beverages in your diet. Drink as much fluid as you need to help get food down during the meal, and drink more or most of your fluids in between meals. This strategy will help you get the nutrition and fluids you need.

Here are some ways to cope with dehydration:
- Suck on ice chips, frozen fruit pops, or Popsicles to relieve dry mouth.
- Drink healthy fluids, such as water, 100 percent vegetable or fruit juices, nectars, low-sugar sports drinks, or herbal teas.

- Try fluid-rich foods or foods that are liquid at room temperature, such as watermelon, sorbet, and gelatin.
- Apply wet cloths or clothing to your body—especially your neck, face, and the core of your body (your back, chest, and abdomen).
- Frequently apply unscented no-color-added lotion to dry skin.
- Treat and eliminate the cause of dehydration, such as vomiting, diarrhea, or fever.
- Apply lip balm or petroleum jelly to dry lips.
- Keep a small cooler with ice and healthy beverages near you to make drinking more convenient.

Call the doctor about any of the following symptoms:
- vomiting, diarrhea, or fever lasting more than twenty-four hours
- very dark urine
- inability to urinate much (or at all) for twelve hours or more
- dizziness or feeling faint when standing up
- disorientation or confusion
- increased heart rate

Water Safety Guidelines

Relying on safe water sources is essential when your immune system is suppressed. It is extremely important that you drink water that is safe and free of bacteria and other harmful organisms.

Public water quality and treatment varies throughout the United States, so always check with your local health department and water utility to confirm the safety of household and community tap water and ice. Also keep in mind the issues below:
- **Tap water.** Water from your home faucet is considered safe if your water source is a city water supply or is from a municipal well serving highly populated areas; such water is tested regularly for contamination. If you have concerns about your water supply, contact your local municipal water department or your county department of public works.
- **Private and small community wells**. The quality of water from these sources cannot be guaranteed. When your immune system is weak, use alternative recommended water sources, such as boiled water, bottled water, or distilled water (see the Safe Water Sources section below).

- **Filtration systems for well water.** Most water-filtration devices will not make the well water safe if it is not chlorinated.

Safe Water Sources

If your water is not from a city water or municipal well supply, you may want to rely on the following sources of water:

- **Boiled and distilled water.** At home, you can make water safe by bringing tap water to a rolling boil for one minute. Distilled water can be made by using a home distiller. After processing, the water should be stored in a clean, covered container in the refrigerator; discard water not used within seventy-two hours.
- **Bottled water.** Acceptable forms of bottled water have been processed to remove organisms known to cause stomach or intestinal infection. Bottled water labeled "well water," "artesian well water," "spring water," or "mineral water" is not guaranteed to be safe to drink. Bottled water with one of the following labels is considered safe:
  - treated with reverse osmosis
  - distilled
  - filtered through an absolute pore size of 1 micron or smaller
  - filter meets NSF/ANSI Standard 53 for cyst removal

To be sure that a brand of bottled water has undergone one of the above processes, contact the International Bottled Water Association (IBWA) at 800-WATER-11 (800-928-3711) or www.bottledwater.org. If IBWA does not have information on a specific brand, call the bottling company directly and ask about safety.

Water Filters

If you install water filters on household water taps, make sure they meet the following specifications:

- The filters must be designed to remove E. coli and *Cryptosporidium* species. Any of the following are acceptable:
  - reverse osmosis
  - absolute pore size of 1 micron or smaller
  - tested and certified by NSF/ANSI Standard 53 for cyst removal
- The water tap filter must be installed immediately above the water tap.
- Manufacturer directions must be followed for filter maintenance and replacement.

Most water-filtration devices will not make the water safe if the supply has not been previously chlorinated. Portable water filters, such as Brita filters, and refrigerator-dispensed water and ice machine systems may improve the taste or appearance of water, but they do not meet rigid filtration standards. Portable water systems filter for chemical impurities but not for bacteria. If you use a portable water system in combination with a safe water supply, change the system's filters frequently according to manufacturer's guidelines.

For a list of approved filtration systems, contact NSF International at 734-769-8010 or visit their Web site at www.NSF.org and search in the Consumer section.

References

Aker SN, Lenssen P. *A Guide to Good Nutrition during Cancer Treatment.* 4th ed. Seattle, WA: Fred Hutchinson Cancer Research Center; 2000.

Bullers AC. Bottled water: better than the tap? *FDA Consumer Magazine.* July/August 2000. US Food and Drug Administration Web site. http://www.fda.gov/fdac/features/2002/402_h2o.html. Accessed May 13, 2009. Content no longer available.

Elliott L, Molseed LL, McCallum PD, Grant B. *The Clinical Guide to Oncology Nutrition.* 2nd ed. Chicago, IL: American Dietetic Association; 2006.

Grant B, Hamilton KK. *Management of Nutrition Impact Symptoms in Cancer and Educational Handouts.* Chicago, IL: American Dietetic Association; 2004.

Institute of Medicine Panel on Dietary Reference Intakes for Electrolytes and Water. *Dietary Reference Intakes for Water, Potassium, Sodium, Chloride, and Sulfate.* Washington, DC: National Academies Press; 2004.

Kleiner SM. Water: an essential but overlooked nutrient. *J Am Diet Assoc.* 1999;99:200-206.

National Cancer Institute. Eating hints: before, during, and after cancer treatment. National Cancer Institute Web site. http://www.cancer.gov/cancerinfo/eatinghints. Published September 2009. Accessed November 20, 2009.

National Cancer Institute. Nutrition in cancer care (PDQ®). National Cancer Institute Web site. http://www.cancer.gov/cancerinfo/pdq/supportivecare/nutrition/HealthProfessional#Section_157. Updated August 11, 2009. Accessed December 12, 2009.

Water safety guidelines. Seattle Cancer Care Alliance Web site. http://www.seattlecca.org/water-safety-guidelines.cfm. Accessed December 7, 2009.

Yarbo CH, Goodman M, Frogge MH. *Cancer Symptom Management.* 3rd ed. Sudbury, MA: Jones and Bartlett Publishers; 2003.

Chapter Twelve

Coping with Changes in Eating and Digestion

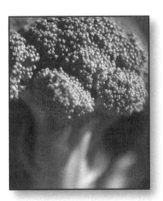

NOT EVERYONE WILL EXPERIENCE THE EATING- and digestion-related side effects discussed in this chapter. If you know a friend or family member who felt ill during treatment, remember that he or she is not you. Everyone reacts differently to treatment.

Some cancer- or treatment-related changes in eating and digestion can be embarrassing to talk about. Remember that thousands of others have experienced side effects at some point during their treatment. Your health care team's goal is to treat your cancer while helping you stay strong. Part of that mission includes helping you and your body cope with changes in eating and digestion so that you can eat foods that keep you well. Do not be afraid to talk about your experiences and concerns. This chapter will discuss common eating and digestion challenges, including nausea, vomiting, changes in bowel habits, difficulty with chewing and swallowing, changes in senses of taste and smell, and decreased appetite.

Digestion Challenges

If you do experience challenges with eating and digestion, remember that you may need to try various tactics before finding the ones that help you. There are many ways to successfully deal with the basic challenges of eating and digesting food during treatment. Keep in mind that what works for one person may not work for you. If you or your caregiver becomes frustrated or concerned about eating and digestion challenges, ask to speak with a registered dietitian for individualized help.

Nausea and Vomiting

Nausea and vomiting are most often caused by either chemotherapy or radiation therapy to the stomach, abdomen, or brain. These symptoms also may occur if you have an obstruction in your gastrointestinal tract. If you receive chemotherapy, the type of agent you receive may or may not make you feel ill. Many agents do not. Some people tolerate treatment more easily than others, so try not to compare your response to treatment to that of others. Chemotherapy agents can cause different kinds of nausea:

- *anticipatory*—occurs before receiving chemotherapy
- *acute*—occurs within the first twenty-four hours after receiving chemotherapy
- *delayed*—occurs one to four days after chemotherapy

Frequent or uncontrolled vomiting can make it difficult for you to eat or drink. If vomiting is not managed, it can lead to dehydration or loss of body fluids. Be sure to tell your doctor if you are having nausea and vomiting. Your doctor will prescribe a specific type of anti-nausea medicine to help control the type of nausea you are experiencing.

How to Cope with Nausea and Vomiting

Do not force yourself to eat or drink when you are nauseated and vomiting. Sips of water or other clear liquids will help you stay hydrated during this difficult period. If you are vomiting often, avoid eating solid food for two to four hours. Wait approximately thirty minutes after vomiting, and then try taking small sips of room-temperature water or flat soda. Refer to the tips for how to eat when you have nausea and vomiting on the next page. If the vomiting persists, call your doctor, especially if you are taking anti-nausea medications as prescribed. Your doctor may be able to prescribe another medicine that will be more effective for you. After the vomiting has stopped, you can move on to more clear liquids (see the Clear-Liquid Diet on page 307), but do not rely on clear liquids alone for more than two days in a row.

If you need to rest after eating, try sitting up or reclining with your head elevated for an hour or so. Food odors sometimes cause nausea; for more information about coping with food odors, see "Changes in Taste and Smell" on page 254 of this chapter.

If you are receiving a cancer treatment that is likely to cause nausea and vomiting, ask your doctor about antiemetics (anti-nausea medicines). Generally, a person with cancer begins taking antiemetics (intravenously or by mouth) before chemotherapy or treatment and continues taking them at home by mouth after treatment for as long as necessary. Some people may also take antiemetics right before their treatment if anticipatory nausea (feeling ill before your treatment) is a problem. Do not wait until you are vomiting to take antiemetics; these medicines are usually meant to be taken on a regular schedule to prevent vomiting. Your health care team might give you more than one anti-nausea medicine because certain types work differently.

These suggestions may help you cope with nausea and vomiting:
- Be sure to sip fluids before and during your chemotherapy treatment. Extra fluids can help your body get rid of chemotherapy byproducts.
- Eat a light meal before your chemotherapy treatment. Eat foods that are easy to digest, such as a bowl of soup with crackers, cottage cheese and fruit, yogurt, cheese and crackers, or cereal with milk. During treatment, sip on clear, cool fluids such as clear fruit juices, sports drinks, lemon-lime soda, ginger ale, or tea or iced tea. Salty foods, crackers, or pretzels are also well tolerated.
- If you are in bed, lie on your side with your head elevated. If you are vomiting, this will help make sure you do not inhale or swallow vomit.
- If you cannot swallow or are unable to keep fluids down, request that medications be prescribed in a melt-on-the-tongue form or suppository form (a glycerin suppository containing anti-nausea medication can be placed in the rectum if you are vomiting and unable to keep fluid or food down).
- Take liquids in the form of ice chips or frozen juice chips, which can be sucked on slowly.

Call the doctor about any of the following:

- inhaled or swallowed vomit
- vomiting more than three times an hour for three or more hours
- blood or material that looks like coffee grounds in vomit
- inability to consume more than four cups of liquid or ice chips in a day
- inability to eat food for more than two days
- inability to take medications
- weakness, lightheadedness, or dizziness

How to Eat When You Have Nausea and Vomiting

To avoid dehydration, try to drink as much liquid each day as you can. Drink one additional cup of liquid after each episode of vomiting. Try taking small sips of clear liquids at room temperature thirty minutes after vomiting. Often cool or room-temperature liquids are best tolerated. Sip on the clear liquids listed in the Clear-Liquid Diet on page 307.

Once you are able to keep down clear liquids, you can try the following foods:

- Nibble on dry foods, such as crackers, pretzels, toast, dry cereals, or bread sticks, when you wake up and every few hours during the day.
- Gradually add easily digested foods like gelatin, Popsicles, fruit ices, or sorbet. They provide some nourishment and also some fluid, as they are liquid at room temperature.

How to Eat When You Have Nausea Without Vomiting

Do not be afraid to experiment with recipes, flavorings, spices, types, and consistencies of food. Your likes and dislikes may change from day to day. Drink as much liquid as you can each day to stay hydrated. Sometimes nausea can be worse if you do not take in enough liquid. Refer to chapter 11 for tips on staying well hydrated.

Try these other suggestions for when and how to eat when coping with nausea:

- Eat small, frequent meals and snacks.
- Eat food cold or at room temperature to decrease its smell and taste. Cold or cool foods may be more soothing as well.
- Avoid eating in very warm rooms.
- Try taking a ginger supplement. New research shows that taking a ginger supplement just before and during chemotherapy treatment may help reduce treatment-related nausea. Ask a registered dietitian or your doctor whether ginger is right for you. If you are not interested in taking a ginger supplement, try adding fresh ginger or ginger tea to your diet.

- Rinse your mouth before and after meals. Avoid alcohol-containing commercial mouthwashes. Use instead a simple mixture of one teaspoon of baking soda and one teaspoon of salt in one quart of room temperature water. Rinse and then spit.
- Avoid lying flat after eating or drinking; if you need to rest, sit up or recline with your head raised for at least an hour.
- Suck on hard candy such as peppermints, lemon drops, or other tart candies if there is a bad taste in your mouth.
- Talk to your doctor if you have nausea, burping, and stomach pains while on chemotherapy, biotherapy, or radiation therapy. You may benefit from antacid therapy.

These suggestions may work for you if you are dealing with nausea:

- Slowly sip cool or room temperature clear liquids, such as ginger ale, juice, or broth. Refer to the Clear-Liquid Diet on page 307.
- Eat fish and chicken if you develop a distaste for red meat and meat broths, which commonly happens to people undergoing cancer treatment.
- Avoid foods that are greasy, fried, spicy, or overly sweet, such as french fries or rich desserts.
- Try bland, soft, easy-to-digest foods on scheduled treatment days.
- Avoid foods with strong odors.
- Avoid extremes in temperature. Foods served at room temperature, cool, or slightly chilled are often more easily tolerated and appealing.
- Avoid eating spicy or overly seasoned foods, unless well tolerated. These foods may be upsetting to your stomach or intestinal tract.
- Avoid your favorite foods when you are feeling nauseated to decrease the chance of food aversions in the future.

What to Eat During and Following Chemotherapy

Talk to your doctor about trying the eating guidelines on the next two pages on the days you receive chemotherapy and for a few days afterward. Keep in mind, however, that this diet does not supply adequate protein, calories, vitamins, or minerals. It should be followed for no more than three days. If you cannot keep down more foods after three days, tell your doctor.

What to Eat Before Chemotherapy

Before your chemotherapy infusion, eat a light meal or snack. Choose food and beverages that you know you can tolerate. If you will be spending the day in the infusion center, be sure to pack a light lunch, snacks, and favorite beverages. Some of these may work for you:

- Cereal with milk

- Vegetables with dip
- Cottage cheese and fruit
- Soup with crackers
- Cheese and crackers
- Half a sandwich and a glass of juice
- Hummus and pita chips
- Yogurt

What to Eat on the Day of Chemotherapy When Nausea and Vomiting <u>May Be</u> a Problem		
	RECOMMENDED	**MAY CAUSE DISTRESS**
Protein	Protein-rich liquid commercial supplements, such as Enlive (Abbott Nutrition) or Boost Breeze (Nestle Nutrition)	All others
Breads, cereals, rice, and pasta	Dry toast, saltines, rice	All others
Fruits and vegetables	Apple, cranberry, and grape juice	All others
Beverages, desserts, and other foods	Ginger ale; lemon-lime soda; decaffeinated, noncarbonated drinks such as fruit punch and sports drinks; Popsicles, fruit ice, sherbet; flavored gelatin; pretzels	All others

What to Eat on Other Days When Nausea and Vomiting Is a Problem

	RECOMMENDED	MAY CAUSE DISTRESS
Protein	Boiled or baked meat, fish, poultry; cold meat or fish salad; eggs; cream soups made with low-fat milk; peanut butter; lean ham; nonfat yogurt	Fatty and fried meats, such as sausage and bacon; fried eggs; milk shakes (unless made with low-fat milk or ice cream)
Breads, cereals, rice, and pasta	Saltines, soda crackers, bread, toast, cold cereal, English muffins, bagels plain noodles, rice	Doughnuts, pastries, waffles, pancakes, muffins
Fruits and vegetables	Potatoes (baked, boiled, or mashed), juices, canned or fresh fruits, vegetables as tolerated (omit if appetite is poor or nausea is severe)	Potato chips, french fries, hash browns; breaded, fried, or creamed vegetables; vegetables with strong odor
Beverages, desserts, and other foods	Cold fruit drinks, decaffeinated soft drinks, iced tea, sports drinks, sherbet, fruit-flavored gelatin, angel food cake, sponge cake, vanilla wafers, pudding (made with low-fat milk), Popsicles, juice bars, fruit ices, pretzels, butter or margarine in small amounts, fat-skimmed gravy, salt, cinnamon, spices as tolerated	Alcohol, coffee, pie, ice cream, rich cakes, spicy salad dressings, olives, cream, pepper, chili powder, onion, hot sauce, seasoning mixtures

Adapted from the American Dietetic Association. Grant B and Hamilton KK. *Management of Nutrition Impact Symptoms in Cancer and Educational Handouts.* (Chicago, IL: American Dietetic Association, 2004).

Constipation

Constipation (stooling) is when the bowels move less frequently and stools become more difficult to pass. It can be caused by changes in eating habits, general weakness, not drinking enough liquid, and decreased physical activity. Constipation may be a symptom of cancer, a result of tumor growth, or a result of cancer treatment. Dehydration and not eating enough also can contribute to constipation, as can other changes in the body, such as organ failure, decreased ability to move, or depression.

Constipation may also be a side effect of medications used to treat cancer or pain. Certain types of chemotherapy and some anti-nausea medications can cause constipation. Chemotherapy agents can often intensify an existing problem with constipation, especially in the elderly and those who eat a low-fiber diet and do not drink enough liquid or get enough physical activity. Pain medications, medications for anxiety and depression, stomach antacids, diuretics, anti-nausea medications, multivitamin/mineral supplements containing iron and calcium, sleep medications, or general anesthesia can also cause constipation. Ask your doctor, registered dietitian, or pharmacist for help in identifying whether any of your medications could cause constipation.

Talk to your health care team if you have any of the following symptoms:
- no bowel movement for three days
- cramps or stomach pain
- gas and/or bloating
- vomiting or nausea
- any other pain or discomfort
- hard bowel movements followed by diarrhea-like stool may be a sign of bowel obstruction

How to Cope with Constipation

To help your doctor develop a plan to cope with constipation, keep a record of all bowel movements. If you are constipated, try to stimulate your bowels to move by following these tips:
- Drink plenty of healthy fluids to keep your digestive system moving.
- Try to have a bowel movement at the same time each day to establish regularity.
- Avoid using extreme force or straining in trying to move your bowels.
- Try to eat and snack at the same times each day.
- To lessen the amount of air you swallow while eating, try reducing the amount you talk at meals, and drink without using a straw. Also avoid chewing gum.
- Get as much physical activity as possible. If you are not able to walk, you can try abdominal exercises in bed or moving from the bed to a chair.
- Use stool softeners or laxatives as instructed by your doctor or nurse.

- Use a soluble fiber–containing product such as Benefiber, Citrucel, FiberCon, or Metamucil as instructed by your health care team. Be sure to drink plenty of fluid if using any of these products. If you do not take in enough fluid, these products could make your constipation worse.
- Ask your registered dietitian to recommend a high-calorie, high-protein, fiber-containing liquid supplement if you need more calories, protein, or fiber.

Call the doctor if you experience any of the following symptoms:
- no bowel movement in three days
- blood in or around the anal area or in the stool
- no bowel movement within two days of taking a laxative
- persistent abdominal cramps or vomiting

How to Eat When You Are Constipated

Stay away from foods that have caused you to be constipated in the past. Some possible examples include chocolates, cheese, and eggs.

Unless instructed by your doctor, do not use over-the-counter laxatives or enemas, especially if your white blood cell count or platelet count is low. In people with cancer, these products could lead to bleeding, infection, or other harmful side effects. Instead, try the following:
- Increase your intake of high-fiber and bulky foods, such as whole grain breads and cereals, fresh raw or cooked fruits with skins and seeds, fresh raw vegetables, fruit juices, dried fruits, seeds, dates, apricots, prunes, popcorn, dried beans, and nuts. Refer to the High-Fiber diet on page 315.
- When increasing dietary fiber, drink more liquid, or your constipation could worsen.
- If excessive gas is a problem, you may need to avoid gas-producing foods and beverages (such as cabbage, broccoli, cauliflower, cucumbers, dried beans, peas, onions, and carbonated drinks).
- Drink more liquid to help prevent dehydration— eight to twelve glasses of liquid each day, if it is all right with your doctor. Try water, warm prune juice, or other warmed juices. In the morning, try warm or hot fluids, such as teas, juices, and hot lemonade.
- Eat a breakfast that includes a hot drink and high-fiber foods.
- Talk to your health care team about using a soluble fiber-containing product, such as Benefiber, Citrucel, FiberCon, or Metamucil.
- A moderate amount of caffeine may also help stimulate bowel function and alleviate constipation.

Tips for Managing Constipation for People with Special Situations

If you have low blood counts (for example, neutropenia or thrombocytopenia), do not use over-the-counter laxatives or enemas without your doctor's permission. Use of these products may lead to infection or bleeding.

If you have a bowel obstruction, *or* if you have undergone a recent bowel surgery such as bowel resection, *or* if you have a newly placed ileostomy or colostomy, do not eat a high-fiber diet. Talk to your health care team about whether a high-fiber diet is appropriate for you. Sometimes constipation can be made worse if you add too many high-fiber foods to your diet. Consider these guidelines:

- Avoid eating high-fiber, high-residue foods.
- Avoid eating gas-producing foods and beverages, such as cabbage, broccoli, dried beans, peas, onions, melons, and carbonated beverages.
- Drink plenty of liquids to keep your digestive system moving and to keep stools soft and easy to pass.
- Eat small, frequent meals and snacks throughout the day to stimulate bowel function.
- Eat foods containing soluble fibers, such as applesauce, bananas, canned peaches and pears, white rice, and pasta.
- Speak with your health care provider about using a soluble fiber–containing product, such as Benefiber, Citrucel, FiberCon, or Metamucil.
- Ask to work with a registered dietitian for individualized help.

Diarrhea

Cancer and cancer treatments and medications can also cause your bowels to move much more frequently and stools to become very loose. Diarrhea is the passage of loose or watery stools three or more times a day, with or without discomfort. It occurs when the water in the intestine is not reabsorbed back into the body for some reason.

Diarrhea can sometimes be caused by an overflow of intestinal liquids around stool that is lodged (impacted) in the intestine. Other causes include bacterial and viral infections; side effects of chemotherapy, biotherapy, or radiation therapy to the abdomen and pelvis; medications; surgery; anxiety; supplemental feedings containing large amounts of vitamins, minerals, and sugar; and tumor growth. Diarrhea caused by chemotherapy or radiation therapy may continue for weeks after treatment. Talk to your doctor if you are experiencing persistent diarrhea after your treatment has ended. Ongoing diarrhea may be a sign of infection or other digestive changes, and, if left untreated, it can lead to dehydration, weight loss, and decreased strength and energy.

What to Eat to Manage Diarrhea: Low-Fiber, Low-Residue Foods

	RECOMMENDED	MAY CAUSE DISTRESS
Protein	Baked or broiled beef, pork, chicken, turkey, veal, fish, eggs, milk, cheese, yogurt	All others
Breads, cereals, rice, and pasta	Breads and rolls made from refined, white flour; pasta; converted or instant rice; refined cereals such as farina, Cream of Wheat, Cream of Rice, oatmeal, cornflakes; pancakes; waffles, cornbread; muffins; graham crackers	Whole grain breads and cereals such as whole wheat and rye bread; bran; shredded wheat; granola; wild rice
Vegetables and fruits	Soups made with allowed vegetables; cooked asparagus tips, beets, carrots, peeled zucchini, mushrooms, celery, tomato paste, tomato purée, tomato sauce; baked potato without skin; canned, frozen, or fresh fruit	Fresh, unpeeled fruit; pears, melon; all other vegetables
Beverages, desserts, and other foods	Butter, margarine; mayonnaise; salad dressing, vegetable oil; cake, cookies; flavored gelatin desserts; sherbet; fruit pie made with allowed fruit; decaffeinated beverages; salt, pepper, spices; gravy as tolerated	Desserts with nuts; coconut; dried fruit; chocolate, licorice; pickles; popcorn; foods with a lot of pepper, chili seasoning, or taco seasoning; hot sauces

Adapted from the American Dietetic Association. Grant B and Hamilton KK. *Management of Nutrition Impact Symptoms in Cancer and Educational Handouts.* (Chicago, IL: American Dietetic Association, 2004).

American Cancer Society

How to Cope with Diarrhea

If you have diarrhea, be sure to sip liquids throughout the day to prevent dehydration, which is a serious concern. When your diarrhea starts to improve, begin eating small amounts of low-fiber, easy-to-digest foods, such as rice, bananas, applesauce, low-fat yogurt, mashed potatoes, reduced-fat cottage cheese, and dry toast with jelly. Monitor the amount and frequency of your bowel movements, and try the following suggestions:

- Try a clear-liquid diet (water, weak tea, apple juice, peach nectar, clear broth, Popsicles, plain gelatin) as soon as diarrhea starts or when you feel that it is going to start. Clear liquids keep the bowels from working too hard and guard against irritation. Refer to the Clear-Liquid Diet on page 307.
- Eat frequent, small meals.
- Eat applesauce, bananas, canned peaches or pears, oatmeal, or white rice or pasta, which are easy to digest and may help thicken stool.
- Consume foods and beverages that are high in potassium, such as fruit juices and nectars, sports drinks, potatoes without the skin, and bananas. Potassium is a mineral that helps muscles function properly and is often lost during bouts of diarrhea. Do not take potassium supplements unless advised to do so by your doctor or health care team.
- Drink and eat foods that are high in sodium, such as soups, broths, sports drinks, salted crackers, and pretzels.
- Alert your doctor if your diarrhea lasts longer than two days. Stay hydrated with foods and beverages listed on the Clear-Liquid Diet. Once watery stools have stopped, slowly add low-fiber, low-residue foods as tolerated. Refer to the Low-Fiber, Low-Residue Diet on page 313.
- Drink at least a cup of liquid after each bout of diarrhea.
- Avoid caffeine-containing beverages, as caffeine can make the bowel more irritated and move faster.
- Talk to your doctor if you are taking in only clear liquids and your diarrhea lasts longer than two days in a row.

Call the doctor if you experience any of the following symptoms:

- six or more loose bowel movements per day, with no improvement in two days
- blood in or around the anal area or in the stool
- weight loss of five pounds or more after the diarrhea starts
- new abdominal cramps or pain lasting two or more days
- inability to urinate for twelve or more hours
- inability to drink any liquids for more than two days
- fever

- suddenly puffy or bloated abdomen
- constipation for several days accompanied by a small amount of diarrhea or oozing of fecal material, suggesting fecal impaction
- continuing or worsening diarrhea or stools that have an unusual odor or color (such as tan or yellow)
- undigested food particles in the stool

What to Avoid When You Have Diarrhea

Using tobacco products; drinking caffeinated, alcoholic, or carbonated beverages; and eating an excessively large meal or foods that are either very hot or very cold in temperature may irritate your digestive tract and aggravate your diarrhea.

Avoid the following foods, which can irritate your gut:

- high-fat foods such as fried, greasy, and rich foods, which can promote diarrhea
- foods that cause gas or swallowed air (such as gas-forming vegetables and chewing gum) and carbonated beverages. (You may be able to drink carbonated beverages if you leave them open for at least ten minutes before drinking.)
- sugar alcohol–containing foods such as sugar-free candies and gum. Sugar alcohols may be listed on food labels as xylitol, mannitol, or sorbitol.
- high-fiber, high-residue foods such as nuts, raw fruits or vegetables, whole grain breads, and cereals or products made with bran, which are abrasive to an irritated bowel
- strong seasonings, spices, and herbs

Lactose Intolerance

One of the symptoms of lactose intolerance is diarrhea. Milk and milk products (including creamed soups, puddings, and milk shakes) need to be used with caution if lactose intolerance is suspected. Other symptoms of lactose intolerance include abdominal gas and bloating.

Lactose intolerance means that the body is not producing enough of the enzyme lactase, which breaks down the milk sugar lactose. Lactose intolerance can result from radiation therapy or surgery to the abdomen or pelvis, chemotherapy, antibiotics, or treatments that affect the gastrointestinal tract. When lactose is not broken down, it remains in the intestine, where the body directs water to dilute it and bacteria break down the lactose and cause fermentation. The fluid retention and fermentation can cause diarrhea, gas, and cramping. These symptoms almost always disappear after treatment sessions are over or when the digestive system has healed.

How to Cope with Lactose Intolerance

You can monitor your intake of lactose to determine how much you can tolerate without having difficulty. If the lactose intolerance continues, your health care team may recommend a low-lactose or lactose-free diet. If this diet is recommended for you, keep an eye on food ingredient lists—lactose is not only found in foods containing milk products; it is also used to sweeten foods.

What to Eat When You Have Lactose Intolerance

Foods that include whey, casein, and nonfat milk solids may contribute to digestive challenges; try small portions of them to find out your level of tolerance. Gum, peppermint, butterscotch, and artificial sweeteners may also include lactose. Lactose is sometimes found as a filler in tablet medications, so check the ingredients of any medicines you take frequently and speak to your health care team about other options if problems persist.

These foods and beverages contain lactose and may need to be avoided, depending on the degree of your intolerance:

- Beverages
    - liquid or dry milk (includes skim, dried, evaporated, condensed, or acidophilus)
    - malted milk
    - hot chocolate, some cocoas and instant coffees, and other powdered drinks
    - powdered coffee creamer
    - Instant Breakfast powder
    - whey protein powder
- Other dairy, such as soft cheeses (except those naturally aged), sour cream, whipping cream, and light cream (half-and-half)
- Any kind of eggs, omelets, or soufflés made using milk, cheese, or chocolate
- Breads and dry or hot cereals
    - prepared mixes for muffins, waffles, pancakes, and biscuits
- Desserts
    - ice cream and sherbet
    - custards and puddings
    - chocolate
    - pie crust that contains margarine or butter
    - desserts with cream fillings
- Meats, fruits, and vegetables
    - creamed vegetables and meat
    - meats and vegetables to which lactose has been added during processing, such as some peas, instant potatoes, luncheon meats, or hot dogs
    - canned or frozen fruit processed with dairy products

- Sauces and sides, such as gravies, creamy sauces, dressings, and dips
- Fats, such as margarine or butter, cream, cream cheese, and peanut butter with milk solids

There are a number of alternatives to lactose-containing (dairy) products:

- Soy milk or rice milk, which come in regular, chocolate, and vanilla flavors, are alternatives to dairy milk. They often taste best when very cold. Soy and rice milk do not supply the same nutrients as cow's milk. But fortified soy or rice milk can still be good substitutes for cow's milk, especially when you are getting necessary protein and fat in other areas of your diet.
- Lactose-free products such as Lactaid and Dairy Ease dairy products (for example, milk and cottage cheese) with the enzyme lactase already added to help with digestion.
- You can often find other milk substitutes or "dairy-free" and "lactose-free" products at stores that carry health foods. Look for lactose-free soy or whey powders to boost your protein intake.
- When appropriate, choose high-calorie, full-fat substitutes over low-calorie, low-fat options to ensure your body gets all of the nutrients it needs.
- Imitation sour cream, nondairy whipped topping, and soy cheese are good lactose-free options.
- You may be able to tolerate cultured dairy products such as buttermilk, yogurt, and some aged or hard cheeses, such as aged Cheddar or Swiss; they will have less lactose, and yogurt contains active cultures that may help in digestion. Start by trying small amounts.
- Sorbet or frozen fruit juice are alternatives to ice cream or sherbet.

You may want to speak with your doctor, nurse, or registered dietitian about pills or chewable tablets that contain the lactase enzyme and can help in the digestion of milk products. An example of this lactase enzyme product is Lactaid. The product directions specify that the tablets should be taken when eating dairy foods; they must be in contact with the dairy product to break down the lactose. The tablets can make the digestion process easier without reducing the nutritional value of the dairy food. Most people who use the tablets are able to add small amounts of foods containing lactose back into their diets.

If your lactose intolerance persists, and if you are unable to eat dairy products without digestive distress, be sure to eat more of the following calcium-rich foods to get enough calcium in your diet:

- kelp
- green vegetables such as broccoli and greens
- nuts
- seeds

- beans
- tofu and soy milk fortified with calcium
- dried figs
- oysters
- canned fish that still has bones, such as sardines and salmon
- foods labeled as calcium-fortified, such as juice, crackers, and cereal

Talk with your doctor or health care team about whether you need to take calcium supplements.

Eating and Swallowing Challenges

Eating and swallowing complications are common in people with cancer, especially those with oral (mouth) cancer or cancers of the neck, esophagus, or gastroesophageal junction. This section describes eating-related complications caused by chemotherapy and radiation therapy, how to prevent them when possible, and how to cope with them.

Maintaining Good Oral Hygiene

Eating a well-balanced diet, maintaining good oral hygiene, and treating any oral problems early can help minimize oral problems and pain.

Before Treatment Begins

If your cancer treatment is likely to cause oral challenges, your doctor will have you see a dentist and dental hygienist. Your dentist and dental hygienist should be professionals who know about the complications of chemotherapy or radiation therapy to the head and neck. Before your treatment begins, you should receive a complete oral assessment, a thorough dental cleaning and fluoride treatment, and, if needed, dental work or removal of damaged or decayed teeth. If indeed dental work is needed, it should be done in a time frame that will allow your mouth sufficient time to heal before treatment begins. If you are receiving radiation therapy to the head and neck, your dentist will most likely provide you with special fluoride toothpaste and dental trays (mouth guards) to apply daily fluoride treatments at home.

Throughout Cancer Treatment

It is important to keep your mouth as clean and healthy as possible during treatment. The following daily practices can help:

- Brush your teeth after each meal or snack with a soft-bristle toothbrush. If your mouth or gums are irritated, soften your toothbrush by soaking it in warm water before using. Try a mild toothpaste or one for sensitive teeth.

- If it hurts to brush, use Toothettes (disposable oral care swabs) or cotton swabs to clean your teeth, gums, and tongue.
- Even if you do not have teeth, rinse your mouth with a homemade baking soda and salt water rinse at least three to five times a day. To make the rinse, mix together one teaspoon of baking soda and one teaspoon of salt in one quart of water.
- Avoid commercial mouthwashes that contain alcohol, which can irritate your mouth.
- If you have oral sores or if your mouth is dry, avoid lemon glycerin swabs. This type of oral swab helps to thin ropy, thick oral secretions, but it can cause significant discomfort if you have oral sores or dry mouth.
- If the type of chemotherapy you are receiving can cause inflammation or sores in the mouth or throat, ask if you might lessen this possibility by sucking on a Popsicle or an all-fruit frozen pop while the chemotherapy is being administered.
- Be on the lookout for painful, white patches in your mouth or throat. This could be thrush (also called candidiasis), a common fungal infection. If it is thrush, your doctor will prescribe an antifungal medication. In addition, rinse frequently with a baking soda and salt water solution (as described above) to help enhance healing and to keep your mouth clean.

Sore Mouth or Throat

One of the most common side effects of chemotherapy and radiation therapy to the mouth or throat area is an inflammation of the mucous membranes lining the mouth and throat, a condition known as mucositis. Mucositis can appear within seven to ten days after the start of radiation therapy to the head and neck area or after some types of chemotherapy. Mucositis can cause red, shiny, or swollen patches in the mouth and on the gums; blood in the mouth; small ulcers or sores in the mouth, on the gums, or on the tongue; white or yellow film in the mouth; pain in the mouth; mouth dryness; mild burning; increased sensitivity to hot and cold foods; soft, whitish patches or pus in the mouth; or increased mucus in the mouth. Some doctors may recommend the use of Caphosol, a supersaturated calcium phosphate rinse. This prescription medication is used to prevent and treat mucositis. Other medications prescribed to help lessen pain with eating include a topical anesthetic such as viscous lidocaine you can "swish and spit" (to numb the mouth if it is sore) or "swish and swallow" (to numb the mouth and throat if they are sore). The ingredients for these "Miracle Mouthwash" or "swish and swallow" solutions vary and often depend on the cancer center or doctor.

When treatment is over, mucositis will heal on its own in two to four weeks if there is not a viral or fungal infection. Regular rinsing throughout the day with the baking soda and salt water solution described above will help keep your mouth clean, reduce bad tastes, and help your mouth heal. In treating mucositis, your doctor will consider its severity and your white blood cell count.

How to Cope with a Sore or Irritated Mouth and Throat

Mucositis and mouth sores can make eating uncomfortable or painful. Fortunately, there are medications for treating a sensitive mouth. If mouth pain is severe or interferes with eating, ask your doctor to recommend a medicine that can either be swished and swallowed fifteen minutes before meals or dabbed on the painful areas with a cotton or oral swab before meals.

Call the doctor if you experience any of the following symptoms:
- redness or shininess in the mouth that lasts for more than forty-eight hours
- bleeding gums
- cuts or sores in the mouth
- temperature of 100.5°F or higher, when taken orally
- white patches on the tongue or on the inside of the mouth or throat

See the chart on the next page for suggestions on what to eat if your throat or mouth is sore.

Bleeding in the Mouth

Bleeding in the mouth is generally caused by mouth sores, periodontal disease (gum disease), or by a decrease in the number of blood platelets. Platelets can decrease as a side effect of radiation therapy or chemotherapy or because of the cancer itself. Platelets are responsible for blood clotting. A person with decreased platelets bleeds easily: even an everyday action such as brushing teeth can result in bleeding. Bleeding can also result from dryness of the lining of the mouth or the formation of small mouth ulcers, which can be side effects of chemotherapy or radiation therapy.

Bleeding in the mouth can take the form of blood or bruises in the mouth (or on the gums or tongue) or a rash or bright red pinpoint-sized dots on or under the tongue, on the roof of the mouth, or on the inside of the cheeks. Fortunately, bleeding in the mouth is usually a temporary problem.

How to Cope with Bleeding in the Mouth

Rinsing your mouth throughout the day with the baking soda and salt water mouth rinse (one teaspoon of baking soda and one teaspoon of salt in one quart of water) will help your mouth heal. Be sure to use a very soft toothbrush and gentle brushing when cleaning your teeth. Call the doctor if you experience any of the following symptoms:
- bleeding from the mouth for the first time
- bleeding for more than a half-hour
- vomiting blood
- feeling light headed

What to Eat When Your Throat or Mouth Is Sore

	RECOMMENDED	MAY CAUSE DISTRESS
Protein	Ground, chopped, or puréed meats, poultry, or fish; casseroles; egg, cheese, and bean dishes; cream soups; broth-based and noodle soups; puréed pea, bean or lentil soups; milk shakes, yogurt, commercial liquid nutritional supplements	Whole meats, poultry, fish dry meats
Breads, cereals, rice, and pasta	Moistened breads; cooked cereals; cold cereal soaked in milk; pasta and rice in sauce	Dry toast, hard rolls, dry crackers, English muffins, bagels
Vegetables and fruits	Frozen, cooked or puréed fruits; soft, well-cooked, or puréed vegetables	Fresh fruits and vegetables (unless very ripe, soft, and juicy, such as applesauce, bananas, and watermelon); citrus fruit, pineapple, other acidic fruit; raw and pickled fruits and vegetables
Beverages, desserts, and other foods	Fruit nectars; flavored gelatin; ice cream, sherbet, pudding; butter, margarine, vegetable oils	Carbonated beverages; cookies and cakes unless soaked in milk; crunchy snacks such as pretzels and chips; vinegar; condiments such as pepper, pepper sauces, chili powder, cloves, nutmeg, salsa

Adapted from the American Dietetic Association. Grant B and Hamilton KK. *Management of Nutrition Impact Symptoms in Cancer and Educational Handouts.* (Chicago, IL: American Dietetic Association, 2004).

Dry Mouth or Thick Oral Secretions

Radiation therapy to the head and neck can injure the glands that produce saliva, the inside of the mouth, the muscles of the jaw and neck, or the jaw bones. Dry mouth, a condition called xerostomia, occurs when there is not enough saliva in the mouth. In addition to cancer treatments, mouth breathing, dehydration, or other medications can cause dry mouth. If you have a dry mouth or thick oral secretions, you might experience dried, flaky, whitish-colored saliva in and around the mouth; thick, stringy secretions that stay attached to the lips when you open your mouth; or debris stuck to the teeth, tongue, and gums. As the mouth becomes dryer, the risk of dental decay increases. Refer to the section "Maintaining Good Oral Hygiene" on page 241 of this chapter to keep your mouth clean and healthy.

How to Cope with a Dry Mouth or Thick Oral Secretions

If you have a dry mouth or thick oral secretions, drink plenty of fluids throughout the day and incorporate moist foods into your diet as much as possible. Another way to manage dry mouth and thick secretions is to rinse your mouth regularly each day with a baking soda and salt water rinse (one teaspoon baking soda and one teaspoon salt in one quart of water) to moisten your mouth and to remove thick secretions. Try moistening your mouth with oral lubricants such as Biotene products or artificial saliva substitutes such as Salivart spray. To stimulate saliva production, swab your mouth with lemon glycerin swabs or suck on frozen grapes, sugar-free lollipops, lemon drops, or peppermints. (Avoid lemon-containing products if you have open oral sores or if your mouth is very dry.) To thin thick oral secretions, try rinsing with Alkalol (an over-the-counter product that thins secretions) or club soda.

Consider using a moist air humidifier in your home. If you sleep with your mouth open, consider placing the humidifier in an area near where you sleep. Do keep in mind that humidifiers need to be cleaned with regularity, and fresh clean bottled or distilled water must be used to keep them germ-free.

Call the doctor if you experience any of the following symptoms:
- a dry mouth for more than three days
- dry, cracked lips or mouth sores
- difficulty breathing

See the chart on the next page for suggestions on what to eat if you have a dry mouth.

What to Eat When You Have a Dry Mouth		
	RECOMMENDED	**MAY CAUSE DISTRESS**
Protein	Meats, poultry, and fish in sauces; gravies, casseroles, soups, stews	Dry meats, poultry, and fish without sauces
Breads, cereals, rice, and pasta	Bread, soft rolls; cooked and cold cereals, cereal with milk; rice soaked in gravy, sauce, broth, or milk	Dry breads, hard rolls; pasta, rice; pretzels, chips; cereal
Vegetables and fruits	Canned and fresh fruits that have a lot of moisture, such as oranges, peaches, and pineapple; vegetables in sauce or soft cooked vegetables	Bananas, dried fruit, vegetables (unless in a sauce or with a high moisture content)
Beverages, desserts, and other foods	Club soda, hot tea with lemon, fruit-ades, diluted juices, sports drinks, commercial liquid nutrition supplements, homemade milk shakes; ice cream, sherbet, pudding; butter, margarine, salad dressing; sour cream, half-and-half	Cookies, cake, pie (unless soaked in milk)

Adapted from the American Dietetic Association. Grant B and Hamilton KK. *Management of Nutrition Impact Symptoms in Cancer and Educational Handouts.* (Chicago, IL: American Dietetic Association, 2004).

Difficulty Swallowing

Difficulty swallowing and pain during swallowing can be side effects of chemotherapy or radiation therapy to the throat or chest areas. People with cancer of the head and neck, esophagus, gastroesophageal junction, or lungs are especially at risk. Difficulty swallowing can also result from a treatable fungal infection of the mouth or esophagus, such as thrush (candidiasis). Swallowing is critical to getting enough nutrition. Difficulty with swallowing can lead to dehydration and loss of appetite and weight.

Call the doctor if you experience any of the following symptoms:
- pain or discomfort with swallowing
- heartburn or esophageal reflux
- food getting stuck in your throat after swallowing
- white patches or coating on the inside of your mouth or throat
- red, shiny mouth or tongue
- ulcers in the mouth or throat or on the tongue
- severe sore throat
- temperature higher than 100.5°F, when taken orally

Cancer, surgery, and radiation therapy to the head and neck, esophagus, or chest can sometimes cause permanent changes in the ability to swallow or control food in the mouth. If foods or liquids being swallowed go into the trachea (wind pipe) instead of staying in the esophagus, aspiration can occur. Aspiration is usually signaled by coughing, but sometimes there are no symptoms. This is called "silent" aspiration. Regardless of whether there are symptoms or lack thereof, aspiration could lead to pneumonia if left untreated. For that reason, your doctor may refer you to a speech pathologist for a swallowing examination to make sure you are swallowing safely. If indicated, swallowing therapy, including exercises for strengthening the muscles involved with swallowing, may be prescribed.

Call the doctor if you experience any of the following symptoms:
- a feeling of choking when swallowing
- gagging or coughing while swallowing or drinking
- regurgitation of food
- difficulty breathing
- chest congestion
- temperature higher than 100.5°F, when taken orally

How to Cope with Difficulty Swallowing
If you have pain when swallowing, your doctor may prescribe a liquid pain reliever solution containing a local anesthetic such as viscous lidocaine to numb your throat. The ingredients for these "Miracle Mouthwash" or "swish and swallows" solutions vary and are often specific to the cancer center or doctor. Another medication to help manage difficult and painful swallowing is a

prescription medication called Carafate (a sucralfate suspension) which is used to coat your throat. Many people find that tilting the head back and forth often helps foods and liquids flow to the back of the throat for ease in swallowing.

When it is difficult to swallow, consider trying the following:

- Eat soft, moist, and easy-to-swallow foods whenever possible. Avoid dry or coarse foods when your throat is sore.
- Eat small, frequent meals and snacks. It is usually easier to eat smaller portions more frequently than larger amounts less frequently.
- Add calories to your food by using sauces, gravies, or butter whenever possible.
- Eat protein-containing foods at each meal or snack. Boost protein by adding whey, soy, or protein powders to shakes, smoothies, soups, or cereals.
- Try various temperatures for foods and liquids. Some people find icy foods more soothing, whereas others find cool or warm foods and liquids easier to swallow.
- Try different textures of foods and liquids.

What to Do if You Need to Eat Thicker Foods

Sometimes thicker fluids are more easily tolerated than thin liquids. People receiving radiation therapy to their chest for lung or esophageal cancer may find thin liquids are more painful and difficult to swallow. Choosing thicker fluids or making your favorite beverages thicker can sometimes help. You can use the following thickening products to thicken beverages or foods:

- *Gelatin.* Use unflavored gelatin to form a soft gel with cakes, cookies, crackers, sandwiches, puréed fruits, and other cold foods. Mix one tablespoon of unflavored gelatin in two cups of liquid until dissolved and pour over food. Allow food to sit until it is saturated.
- *Tapioca, flour, and cornstarch.* Use these substances to thicken liquids. Note that these products must be cooked.
- *Commercial thickeners such as Thick-It or Hydra-Aid.* Use these products to adjust a food or liquid's thickness. Follow the instructions on the package label.
- *Puréed vegetables and instant potatoes.* Use in soups. Note that these ingredients alter the food's flavor.
- *Baby rice cereal.* Use rice cereal to make very thick liquids.

You also can use a slurry as a thickener. A slurry is a thin paste of water and flour stirred into hot dishes as a thickener. When spread on top of bread or cake, it adds moisture and makes them easier to swallow.

Do not force yourself to eat if you cannot swallow. Follow your health care team's instructions for any special eating techniques.

What to Eat When You Have Trouble Swallowing

If you are having trouble swallowing, your doctor may recommend a liquid diet. If thin liquids are recommended for you, try coffee, tea, soft drinks, canned nutritional supplements, Italian ice, sherbet, broth, and thin cream soups. Once you can eat a puréed thick-liquid diet without difficulty, you may move on to what is called a "Mechanical Soft Diet," which includes thick liquids that have more substance. Refer to Appendix A for more suggestions.

	Puréed Thick-Liquid Diet (Includes foods listed on the Full-Liquid Diet [page 309] if thickened*)	Mechanical Soft Diet
Protein	Thickened milk, yogurt without fruit, cottage cheese, sour cream; casseroles; soft scrambled eggs; puréed meat, poultry, and fish	Milk, yogurt, cheeses, sour cream; all eggs; ground meats and ground meat casseroles; fish sandwiches made with ground meats or spreads
Breads, cereals, rice, and pasta	Slurry of cooked cereals such as Cream of Wheat and Cream of Rice.	Soft breads; graham crackers; cookies; soft cold cereals in milk; pancakes, waffles; pasta, rice
Vegetables and fruits	Puréed fruit and vegetables without seeds and skins; mashed potatoes	Bananas; canned fruit; soft, well-cooked, or puréed vegetables
Beverages, desserts, and other foods	Thickened juices and nectars; thick milk shakes; thickened broths and cream soups; custards, puddings; slurried cakes and cookies; syrups, honey; butter, margarine; spices as tolerated	All beverages; soft desserts that do not require much chewing, such as ice cream, sherbet, flavored gelatin, pudding, custard; soft cakes and cookies; syrups, honey; butter, margarine; spices

Adapted from the American Dietetic Association. Grant B and Hamilton KK. *Management of Nutrition Impact Symptoms in Cancer and Educational Handouts*. (Chicago, IL: American Dietetic Association, 2004).

How to Eat When You Have Difficulty Eating and Swallowing

Avoid tart, acidic, or salty foods, such as pickled and vinegary foods, citrus fruits, tomato-based foods, some canned broths.

Avoid citrus fruit juices and carbonated beverages.

Avoid rough-textured foods, such as dry toast, pretzels, granola, and raw fruits and vegetables.

Avoid foods that need a lot of chewing, such as meats, chewy candy, or raw, whole vegetables.

Try eating foods at different temperatures to find which temperature is most soothing to your mouth or throat, unless your treatment does not allow cold foods or beverages.

Stay away from alcohol, caffeine, and tobacco.

Avoid irritating spices such as chili powder, cloves, curry, hot sauces, nutmeg, horseradish, and pepper.

Eat soft, bland, creamy foods high in calories and protein, such as cream soups, cheeses, mashed potatoes, yogurt, eggs, custards, puddings, cooked cereals, ice cream, casseroles, gravies, syrups, milk shakes, and canned nutritional supplements.

Blend and moisten dry or solid foods with gravies, yogurt, milk, broth, creams, butter, or margarine.

Drink through a straw.

Avoid hot drinks (Heat dilates blood vessels and increases bleeding.)

Try chilled foods and fluids, such as Popsicles, applesauce, yogurt, frozen yogurt, sherbet, and ice cream, unless your treatment does not allow cold foods or beverages.

Eat six to eight small meals a day.

	Irritated or Sore Mouth	Mouth Sores or Oral Bleeding	Thick Oral Mucous Secretions	Dry Mouth	Sore and Irritated Throat	Difficulty Swallowing
	X	X	X	X	X	
	X	X	X		X	X
	X	X	X	X	X	X
	X	X	X	X	X	X
	X	X	X	X	X	X
	X	X	X	X	X	X
	X	X	X	X	X	X
	X	X	X	X	X	X
	X	X	X	X	X	X
	X	X				
	X	X	X			
	X	X	X	X	X	X
	X	X	X	X	X	X

Caring for Your Mouth When You Have Swallowing Problems

Clean and rinse your teeth (including dentures) with a salt and baking soda solution after eating and every two hours (recipe on page 242).

Brush your teeth using a very soft or soft nylon-bristle toothbrush or a Toothette (a foam swab on a stick) and use a nonabrasive (sensitive), fluoride-containing toothpaste. Rinse toothbrush well after each use and store in a cool, dry place.

Ask your doctor or nurse about an oral lubricant or gel to moisten your mouth.

Ask your doctor or nurse about an artificial saliva substitute.

Use petroleum jelly or lip balm to moisten lips.

Look for oral sores and white patches by checking your mouth twice a day using a small flashlight and a padded tongue blade; if you wear dentures, remove them first.

Remove thick oral secretions by using a soft toothbrush or Toothette or gauze dipped in saltwater. Rinse and clean your mouth regularly throughout the day with a salt and baking soda rinse.

Report any change in appearance, taste, or feeling in your mouth or throat to your doctor or nurse.

Use a cool mist humidifier to moisten room air, especially at night. Be sure to use distilled water and keep the humidifier clean to avoid spreading mold in the air.

To stay hydrated, drink at least forty-eight to sixty-four ounces of healthy fluid daily. If you are at risk for aspiration or if you are receiving nutrition support, check with your doctor about your fluid needs.

Try sipping warm (not hot) beverages to soothe your mouth and throat.

Ask your doctor about a prescription for "Miracle Mouthwash",* a solution that can soothe and numb the mouth and throat.

* Most cancer centers or doctors have their own name and recipe for this type of solution.

Irritated or Sore Mouth	Mouth Sores or Oral Bleeding	Thick Oral Mucous Secretions	Dry Mouth	Sore and Irritated Throat	Difficulty Swallowing
X	X	X	X		
X	X	X	X		
X	X		X		
X			X		
X	X		X		
X	X	X	X		
		X	X		
X	X	X	X	X	X
X		X	X	X	X
			X		X
X	X			X	X
X	X			X	X

Appetite Challenges

Things like the feeling of fullness or changes in taste and smell can cause changes in appetite. Having a decreased appetite can make getting the calories and nutrients you need a challenge. Do not be afraid to break the rules, try new things, and eat what you want when you want to eat it. Try eating smaller meals and snacks more often. If breakfast foods taste best to you at night, or if you crave a hearty dinner at lunchtime, feel free to depart from tradition.

Changes in Taste and Smell

Common problems that can occur during and after your chemotherapy or radiation therapy are changes in your senses of smell and taste. Food may taste bitter, metallic, or even too salty, sweet, or sour. Some people may even experience a complete loss of taste. Aversions to the odor of food and the aroma of nonfood items such as perfumes and soap also can happen. These changes are usually temporary and go away after your treatment is over, but they can affect your appetite and what you eat.

Changes in your sense of taste and smell can mean that your favorite foods do not taste the same to you anymore. If you are having a problem with food aversions, try foods or beverages that are different from ones you usually eat. To keep from developing additional food aversions, try new foods and nutritional drinks when you're feeling well. Eat lightly (small portions of lower-fat, bland foods) on the morning of or several hours before receiving chemotherapy.

Do not taste new foods when you are around unpleasant odors. Also, keep your mouth clean by rinsing and brushing, which may help foods taste better to you.

Thrush (also called candidiasis), a common fungal infection in the mouth and throat, can also cause taste alterations. Fortunately, once identified, thrush is easily treated. Refer to page 241 in this chapter for information about maintaining good oral hygiene.

How to Cope When You Cannot Tolerate the Smell of Food

Try the following when food odors make you feel ill or nauseated:

- Ask another person to cook for you. Ask them to take off any food covers to release food odors before entering your room or eating area.
- Consider using prepared foods from a reliable, clean deli. This is not recommended if your white blood cell counts are low.
- Avoid eating in a room that has cooking odors or other smells. To reduce cooking odors, cook outside on the grill, use boiling bags, or use a slow-cooker on the back porch or in the garage. Kitchen fans and small portable fans can be used to direct food odors away from you.

- Avoid cooking foods with strong odors, such as onions, cruciferous vegetables (cabbage, broccoli, Brussels sprouts), heavy meats, or fish.
- Get creative; if smells from cooking appliances such as coffeemakers or toasters make you queasy, consider placing them in another part of the house or in the garage.
- Order take-out food from restaurants you know to be clean to avoid preparing food and creating strong smells at home. However, avoid buffet-style restaurants or take-out foods from buffets.
- Prepare cold foods such as sandwiches, pasta salads, cottage cheese, or yogurt instead of hot foods, which release odors in the rising steam.

How to Cope When Food Does Not Taste the Same

Chemotherapy, biotherapy, radiation therapy, oral surgery, or cancer itself can alter your sense of taste. You may find that food has a bitter or metallic taste or not much taste at all. You may start to dislike sweet foods, or meat and poultry may taste very different. As your tastes evolve, try these ways of coping:

- Try using plastic utensils if you have a metallic taste in your mouth.
- Serve foods cold or at room temperature. This can decrease the potency of flavors and smells, making foods easier to tolerate.
- Rinse your mouth with tea, ginger ale, or a baking soda and salt rinse before eating to help cleanse your palate.
- Add tart flavors by seasoning foods with lemon juice, lemonade, other citrus fruits, or vinegar, or eat pickled foods. (Avoid these foods if you have a sore mouth or throat or open oral sores.)
- Increase the sugar in foods to enhance pleasant tastes and decrease salty, bitter, or acidic ones.
- Flavor foods with onion, garlic, chili powder, basil, oregano, rosemary, tarragon, barbecue sauce, mustard, ketchup, or mint.
- Marinate meat or poultry in sauces such as barbecue, soy, or teriyaki or in oil and vinegar salad dressing to improve flavors and eliminate possible bitter tastes.
- Suck on lemon drops, mints, or other tart hard candies or chew gum to get rid of unpleasant tastes in your mouth after eating. (If you have diarrhea, avoid sugarless candies and gums.)
- Freeze fruits such as grapes and cut-up pieces of cantaloupe, oranges, and watermelon. Fruit smoothies and frozen fruit desserts such as sorbet or sherbet may be appealing.
- Rather than force yourself to eat foods that taste bad to you, find substitutes. If red meat tastes different or strange, try other protein sources, such as chicken, turkey, fish, eggs, cottage cheese, cheese, yogurt, or tofu.
- Eat clean, fresh vegetables, as they are often more appealing than canned or frozen ones.

FAT, ACID, SALT, AND SWEET

Chef Rebecca Katz of the Commonweal Cancer Help Program encourages people experiencing changes in taste to experiment with "FASS." FASS stands for fat, acid, salt, and sweet. Using FASS when preparing and cooking food helps to add simple, healthy ingredients to balance out flavors in dishes and make them taste their best.

FAT: Fats coat the tongue and allow flavors to spread around the tongue and mouth. Fats also add heft to a dish and help you feel full.
> **What works well:** Cold-pressed extra virgin olive oil has a nice, clean taste. Naturally occurring, un-hydrogenated vegetable oils, such as canola, safflower, sunflower, or other olive oils, will also work.

ACID: Acids—especially citric acid—counterbalance the sweet flavor in a dish.
> **What works well:** Fresh lemon and lime. Many types of vinegar, including brown rice, red wine, and balsamic, also work nicely.

SALT: Salt "unlocks" the flavor in every food it comes in contact with.
> **What works well:** Sea salt. Sea salt has more flavor than regular table salt, but table salt can be used, too.

SWEET: Adding a sweet ingredient can cut an acid or bitter taste in a dish.
> **What works well:** If you can find it, Grade B organic maple syrup works particularly well. It has a more complex, satisfying flavor than refined sugar, and you need much less of it. Honey, brown rice syrup, and agave nectar will also work in a pinch.

Reprinted, with permission, from Rebecca Katz. "One Bite at a Time: Nourishing Recipes for Cancer Survivors and their Friends" (Berkeley, CA; Celestial Arts Press: 2008).

- No-salt-added or low-salt canned soups or vegetables can have a metallic taste. You may want to avoid them unless you have high blood pressure and have been advised to eat a low-salt diet.
- You might be able to eat mild pasta dishes and milk products.
- Carrot peel often tastes extremely bitter to people having cancer treatment. Peeled sweet baby carrots or peeled large carrots will not have this bitter flavor. Try dipping carrots in salad dressing or hummus for extra flavor and nutrition.
- Get a dental checkup to rule out dental problems that could be causing a bad taste in the mouth.
- Clean your mouth, including your teeth, gums, and tongue, regularly.

Loss of Appetite

A person with a poor or no appetite (also called anorexia—not to be confused with anorexia nervosa, an eating disorder) eats much less than he or she normally would or does not eat at all. Loss of appetite or poor appetite is one of the most common problems that occur with cancer and its treatment. Sometimes loss of appetite results from treatment side effects, such as nausea, vomiting, difficulty swallowing, feeling full, or changes in senses of taste or smell. Tumor growth, depression, or pain can also make you uninterested in food. Speak to your health care team about how best to address these causes of poor appetite.

Many people find that their appetite is greatest in the morning. If this is true for you, take advantage of it. Consider having your main meal of the day early. Then have commercial nutritional supplements or liquid meal replacements such as Ensure, Boost, or Instant Breakfast later on if you do not feel like eating.

How to Cope with Appetite Challenges

Most people lose their appetite for just a day or two; for others, it is an ongoing concern. There are a number of ways to cope with treatment side effects and increase appetite:

- Ask your doctor about medications to help relieve constipation, nausea, pain, or other side effects that interfere with appetite.
- Eat food cold or at room temperature to decrease its smell and taste.
- Drink beverages between meals instead of with meals; drinking liquids at mealtime can lead to early fullness. Do take sips of fluids with meals to aid swallowing.

How to Eat When You Have Appetite Challenges

Whatever the reason for your loss in appetite, the following suggestions may help you cope:

- Try to eat small meals or snacks of favorite foods throughout the day. It may be easier to eat more that way, and you won't get so full.
  - Keep snacks within easy reach so you can have something easy to eat whenever you feel like it. Cheese and crackers, muffins, nut butters, and fruit are good possibilities.
  - Take portable snacks such as granola or energy bars, peanut butter crackers, or small boxes of raisins with you when you go out.
  - Eat only as much as you want, but try to eat at least a little bit of food every two to three hours while you are awake. This means you may be eating four to six (or more) small meals or snacks a day.
  - Start the day with breakfast. Use a timer or an alarm clock to help remind you to eat. Try to eat frequently at set times each day rather than waiting until you get hungry.

- Build up your appetite and motivate yourself to eat.
  - Make eating more enjoyable by eating with friends, setting the table with pretty dishes and flowers, playing your favorite music, or watching a television show.
  - Think of food as a necessary part of treatment.
  - With your doctor's approval, try light exercise an hour before meals.
  - If it is all right with your doctor, try having a small glass of beer or wine before eating.
- Increase calories and protein.
  - Try liquid or powdered meal replacements such as Instant Breakfast drinks when it is hard for you to eat food.
  - Try to keep easy-to-eat foods that are high in calories on hand. These could include pudding, chocolate pieces, ice cream, or yogurt. Meal replacement bars such as Power Bars, Clif bars and Odawalla bars are also good choices for high-calorie, high-protein, easy-to-eat meals.
  - Avoid low-calorie foods that fill you up, such as lettuce, broth, and diet soda.
  - Keep high-calorie, high-protein snacks on hand, such as hard-boiled eggs, peanut butter, cheese, granola bars, and canned nutritional supplements.

Eating well and eating enough are important to your recovery from treatment. But on those days when you cannot eat at all, don't worry. Do what you can to make yourself feel better. Come back to eating as soon as you can, and let your doctor know if your appetite does not improve within a couple of days.

Nutrition Support

If you are losing weight and are unable to eat because of cancer or cancer treatment, your doctor may suggest nutrition support measures. Nutrition support involves providing calories (from protein, fat, and carbohydrates) and vitamins and minerals—either intravenously or directly into your gastrointestinal tract—to prevent weight loss and malnutrition. Other reasons your doctor may prescribe nutrition support include severe nausea and vomiting that cannot be controlled or an obstruction that prevents food from passing through your gastrointestinal tract. If you are having difficulty eating and maintaining your weight because of your cancer or treatment-related side effects, talk to your doctor about whether nutrition support may be needed.

The two main types of nutrition support are enteral and parenteral nutrition:
1. *Enteral nutrition*, or tube feeding, provides nutrition directly to the gastrointestinal tract, where it is digested and absorbed. Nutritional formula is given through a tube placed in the nose, stomach, or intestine.

2. *Parenteral nutrition* provides specialized intravenous (IV) nutrition. Veins are accessed by a catheter placed in the chest or arm, and IV nutrition is given into the vein. This type of therapy is also called hyperalimentation or total parenteral nutrition (TPN).

An important safety concern when receiving nutrition support is that anything that goes into the intravenous line must be sterile (completely germ free) to avoid putting germs into the bloodstream and causing infections. Parenteral nutrition and equipment must be handled carefully to keep germs out of the body. Enteral nutrition formula and equipment also require special handling and care. Your doctor will refer you to nutrition support professionals (registered dietitians or nurses) to teach you how to give yourself the specialized nutrition and how to care for your intravenous line or feeding tube. It is always helpful to have a family member or caregiver present when receiving this special training and instruction.

The nutrition support professionals and your doctor will determine how much nutrition support you need. They will also help you decide on the best method and schedule (time of day) of feeding for you.

For most people, nutrition support is only needed temporarily. Once cancer treatment has ended and you have recovered from your treatment, you will be able to eat again. A registered dietitian can help you with the transition from nutrition support back to eating regularly.

Be sure to ask your doctor or nutrition support professional whether your tube feeding formula, supplies, and equipment (such as syringes, feeding bags, and feeding pump) are covered by your health insurance. If they are not covered or if you do not have health insurance, ask about patient assistance programs available through your hospital, clinic, or from the manufacturers of the formula, such as Nestle Nutrition and Abbott Nutrition.

Methods of Enteral Feeding (Tube Feeding)

- *Nasogastric feeding tube.* A nasogastric feeding tube (or NG tube) is placed in the nose, down the esophagus, and into the stomach. This method of feeding is often used for people needing nutrition support for a short period (up to two weeks). Special tube feeding formula can be given three different ways: by using a syringe (bolus feeding), a bag (gravity feeding), or a pump, all specially designed to facilitate tube feeding. Your doctor or registered dietitian will determine which feeding method is right for you.
- *Gastrostomy feeding tube.* A gastrostomy tube (G tube) is placed by a doctor directly into the stomach through a small opening on the outside of the abdomen. Another term for this type of feeding tube is percutaneous endoscopic gastrostomy, or "PEG." This method is used for people needing nutrition support for longer than two weeks. Tube feeding formula is given through a syringe by a bolus method, by a gravity tube feeding

bag, or by using a pump. Your doctor or registered dietitian will determine which feeding method is right for you.

- *Jejunostomy feeding tube.* A jejunostomy tube (J tube) is placed by a surgeon into the upper part of the small intestine (jejunum) through a small opening on the outside of the abdomen. This type of feeding is also called a percutaneous endoscopic jejunostomy, or "PEJ." This method is used for people needing nutrition support for longer than two weeks. Jejunostomy feedings can only be given using a pump to deliver the nutrition formula. Bolus or gravity methods of feeding into the jejunum can cause severe intestinal bloating, cramping, and diarrhea. Jejunostomy feeding tubes are used for people who cannot tolerate a tube feeding into the stomach. Portable pumps and easy-to-carry backpacks allow people who need this kind of nutrition support to get around easily.

The formula used in tube feedings usually consists of products such as Jevity and Osmolite (made by Abbott Nutrition) or Isosource and Fibersource (made by Nestle Nutrition). People with diabetes may use products called Glucerna (Abbott Nutrition) or Glytrol (Nestle Nutrition) These products are nutritionally complete and will provide you with needed protein, calories, vitamins, and minerals.

Tube feedings are given at room temperature. Refrigerate any unused product. Bring any leftover product back to room temperature before infusing. Unused product should be thrown out after twenty-four hours. Be sure you are comfortable with the method of feeding you are using. Follow your nutrition support professional's instructions for feeding, and be sure to check the skin around your tube each day for redness, drainage, skin problems, or signs of infection.

Methods of Parenteral Feeding (Intravenous Feeding)

- *Intravenous hydration.* While undergoing intensive chemotherapy or radiation therapy, some people may need infusions of intravenous fluid and electrolytes to help them avoid dehydration because of side effects such as severe nausea and vomiting. Intravenous hydration is most often given in the outpatient clinic or chemotherapy infusion area. If you have health insurance, some policies cover the cost for these services to be provided in your home.
- *Peripheral parenteral nutrition.* Some people may not be able to take in enough calories, protein, and fluid while undergoing or recovering from cancer treatment. Their doctor may prescribe supplemental intravenous nutrition for maintaining weight and avoiding dehydration. This type of parenteral nutrition can be given in the outpatient clinic or chemotherapy infusion area. If you have health insurance, your policy may cover the cost for this type of nutrition to be given in your home.

- *Total parenteral nutrition (TPN).* Some people who receive aggressive cancer treatment may experience serious side effects that keep their gastrointestinal tracts from functioning normally. Some people may have a cancer that has caused an obstruction in the gut, meaning food cannot pass. TPN may be prescribed by your doctor to provide for all of your nutrition needs while you undergo and recover from cancer treatment. If medically indicated, many health insurance policies will cover the cost for this type of nutrition to be given in your home if you are an outpatient. Portable pumps and easy-to-carry backpacks allow people needing this type of support to easily carry their nutrition wherever they go.

Your nutrition support professional will teach you exactly how to begin and end each infusion. Depending upon the amount of calories, protein, and fluid that you need, your parenteral nutrition infusion may run for several hours or up to twenty-four hours a day.

A parenteral nutrition pump can be plugged into the wall when you are home. This type of pump is also battery powered, so you can take it with you wherever you go. Check with your nutrition support professional about how often the pump will need to be recharged or when batteries will need to be changed. Be sure you have enough batteries for your pump and that you know how and when to replace or recharge them.

Keep a clean work area for supplies. If possible, use a separate place in the refrigerator (or a separate refrigerator if you have an extra one) for parenteral nutrition solutions. Throw away all needles and syringes in a metal coffee can with a lid, a bleach bottle, or in a container provided by your nutrition support professional. Keep the container out of the reach of children, pets, and others.

References

Acupuncture reduces side effects of chemotherapy: electroacupuncture treatments help control chemotherapy-related vomiting. American Cancer Society Web site. http://www.cancer.org/docroot/NWS/content/NWS_1_1x_Acupuncture_Reduces_Side_Effects_of_Chemotherapy.asp. Published December 27, 2000. Accessed December 13, 2009.

American Cancer Society. *Cancer Caregiving A to Z: An At-Home Guide for Patients and Families*. Atlanta, GA: American Cancer Society; 2008.

Besser J, Ratley K, Knecht S, Szafranski M. *What to Eat During Cancer Treatment: 100 Great-Tasting, Family-Friendly Recipes to Help You Cope*. Atlanta, GA: American Cancer Society; 2009.

Calhoun S, Bradley J. *Nutrition, Cancer and You: What You Need to Know and Where to Start*. Lexena, KS: Addax Publishing Group; 2002.

Elliott L, Molseed LL, McCallum PD, Grant B. *The Clinical Guide to Oncology Nutrition*. 2nd ed. Chicago, IL: American Dietetic Association; 2006.

FASS tip sheet. Caring 4 Cancer Web site. http://www.caring4cancer.com/go/cancer/nutrition/chef-rebecca-katz/fass-tip-sheet.htm. Accessed November 20, 2009.

Food just doesn't taste the same. University of Michigan Comprehensive Cancer Center Web site. http://www.cancer.med.umich.edu/support/food_taste.shtml. Accessed December 13, 2009.

Goldwein JW, Vachani C. Chemotherapy: the basics. Oncolink Web site. http://www.oncolink.com/treatment/article.cfm?c=2&s=9&id=319. Updated December 8, 2006. Accessed December 13, 2009.

Grant B, Hamilton KK. *Management of Nutrition Impact Symptoms in Cancer and Educational Handouts*. Chicago, IL: American Dietetic Association; 2004.

Katz R, Edelson M. *The Cancer-Fighting Kitchen*. Berkley, CA: Celestial Arts; 2009.

Margie JD, Bloch AS. *Nutrition and the Cancer Patient*. Radnor, PA: Chilton Publishing; 1984.

National Cancer Institute. Eating hints: before, during, and after cancer treatment. National Cancer Institute Web site. http://www.cancer.gov/cancerinfo/eatinghints. Published September 2009. Accessed November 20, 2009.

National Cancer Institute. Gastrointestinal complications (PDQ®). National Cancer Institute Web site. http://www.cancer.gov/cancertopics/pdq/supportivecare/gastrointestinalcomplications/Patient. Updated October 8, 2009. Accessed December 13, 2009.

National Cancer Institute. Nausea and vomiting (PDQ®). National Cancer Institute Web site. http://www.nci.nih.gov/cancertopics/pdq/supportivecare/nausea. Updated October 2, 2009. Accessed December 13, 2009.

National Cancer Institute. Nutrition in cancer care (PDQ®). National Cancer Institute Web site. http://www.nci.nih.gov/cancertopics/pdq/supportivecare/nutrition/patient. Updated April 29, 2009. Accessed December 13, 2009.

National Cancer Institute. Oral complications of chemotherapy and head/neck radiation (PDQ®). Physician data query. National Cancer Institute Web site. http://www.nci.nih.gov/cancertopics/pdq/supportivecare/oralcomplications. Updated November 6, 2008. Accessed December 13, 2009.

National Comprehensive Cancer Network and the American Cancer Society. *Nausea and Vomiting: Treatment Guidelines for Patients with Cancer*. Version 1 [patient education material]. Publication number 01-50M-No.9418-HCP. Atlanta, GA: National Comprehensive Cancer Network and the American Cancer Society; January 2001.

National Library of Medicine, National Institutes of Health. Lactose intolerance. Medline Plus Web site. http://www.nlm.nih.gov/medlineplus/lactoseintolerance.html. Updated December 8, 2009. Accessed December 13, 2009.

Poor appetite. University of Michigan Comprehensive Cancer Center Web site. http://www.cancer.med.umich.edu/support/nutrappetite.shtml. Accessed December 13, 2009.

US Department of Health and Human Services and United States Department of Agriculture. Dietary Guidelines for Americans, 2005. US Department of Health and Human Services Web site. http://www.health.gov/dietaryguidelines/dga2005/document/default.htm. Published January 2005. Accessed December 13, 2009.

Yarbo CH, Goodman M, Frogge MH. *Cancer Symptom Management*. 3rd ed. Sudbury, MA: Jones and Bartlett Publishers; 2003.

Zick SM, Ruffin MT, Lee J, Normolle DP, Siden R, Alrawi S, Brenner DE. Phase II trial of encapsulated ginger as a treatment for chemotherapy-induced nausea and vomiting. *Support Cancer Care*. 2009;17(5):563-572.

American Cancer Society

Chapter Thirteen

Lifestyle Choices to Enhance Health for Cancer Survivorship

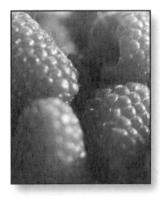

MORE AND MORE PEOPLE LIVE LONG, HEALTHY LIVES after cancer treatment. Living a healthy lifestyle after treatment includes eating a balanced diet and being physically active. Eating well is important during treatment and remains so after treatment, as you look toward a future beyond cancer.

After cancer treatment, some cancer survivors continue to have eating-related side effects and concerns, such as fatigue, weight loss or weight gain, or bowel irregularities. Many of these conditions are a result of necessary treatments for their cancer. The good news is that all or most of these issues will improve with time and the adoption of a healthy diet and regular physical activity—a goal we should strive for regardless of whether we have had a cancer diagnosis.

Some people treated for cancer report that they believe their precancer diet and physical activity choices were contributing factors to their initial cancer diagnosis. For many people, adopting healthier habits is a priority for reducing the risk of cancer recurrence. While it is not always easy to adopt new lifestyle habits, resources do exist to help survivors make healthy eating and physical activity priorities.

Healthy Eating After Treatment

After reading this book, you are aware of the benefits of eating well throughout treatment. Now that treatment is over, you may wonder how nutrition and exercise can affect your quality of life as well as your risk for cancer recurrence, the development of another cancer, or lingering or late-occurring side effects of your cancer treatment, such as weight gain, heart disease, or osteoporosis.

Although a lot is known from research about how nutrition and physical activity influence the incidence of cancer, less is known about how these factors affect cancer recurrence. Most research has focused on which foods and dietary patterns prevent cancer in the first place. The American Cancer Society regularly publishes a document compiling the views of many experts in the field outlining the current nutrition and physical activity recommendations to promote health during and after cancer treatment. These recommendations are consistent with what is recommended for the prevention of cancer:

- Maintain a healthy body weight.
  - Balance caloric intake with physical activity. Achieving and maintaining a healthy body weight is particularly important for obesity-related cancers such as breast, prostate, endometrial, colorectal, gallbladder cancer, and others.
  - Avoid excess weight gain. While some people lose weight with treatment, many people actually gain weight (see chapter 8), a problem that may contribute to cancer recurrence or other conditions such as early-onset heart disease, hypertension, or diabetes.

- Adopt a physically active lifestyle.
  - Try to do moderate activity, such as walking, for at least thirty minutes five or more days per week. You may be tired after treatment, but becoming more physically active is important. Start small and work your way toward an increasingly active lifestyle.
- Consume a healthy diet with an emphasis on plant sources.
- If you drink alcohol, limit consumption.
  - Drink no more than one alcoholic beverage per day for women and two beverages per day for men.

Make sure to work with your health care team to develop a follow-up care plan that includes guidelines for increased cancer screening.

Because people who have had cancer may also be at risk for other cancers, heart disease, diabetes, or osteoporosis, the health guidelines established to prevent those diseases should be considered as well.

Ongoing Eating Concerns for People Finished with Treatment

You may have coped with treatment side effects for some time. Now that your treatment has ended, so will most of its eating-related effects. However, sometimes you may continue to experience treatment-related side effects such as poor appetite, dry mouth, changes in senses of taste or smell, difficulty swallowing, or significant weight loss. You may have had surgery to remove part of your stomach or intestines or had radiation therapy to the abdomen, all of which can cause longer-lasting or permanent effects on eating and digestion. If you continue to have eating concerns, talk to your health care team so you can work together on a plan to address any remaining problems.

Depending upon your specific cancer treatment, your doctor will also monitor you for late-occurring side effects. For example, people who have received head and neck radiation therapy are at greater risk for dental decay because of treatment-related dry mouth, and people who have received chest irradiation may experience difficulty with swallowing some foods because of treatment-related changes to their esophagus.

The Role of Dietary Supplements After Cancer Treatment

If you have been unable to eat a nutritious diet or are eating less than normal because of your cancer and cancer treatment, your health care team may recommend that you continue taking a daily multivitamin/mineral supplement after treatment. In special instances, if you have a specific nutrient deficiency, such as iron-deficiency anemia, because of your cancer or cancer treatment, you may be asked to take an additional dietary supplement. If you are considering taking any dietary supplements now that your cancer treatment is over, be sure to check with your doctor before doing so. At this time, there is little research on whether dietary supplements, certain foods, or specific dietary regimens improve the health of people who have had cancer and have undergone cancer treatment. Despite the lack of scientific evidence of benefit, it is estimated that more than 60 percent of all American adults have used complementary and alternative medicine practices, including dietary supplements, special diets, prayer, meditation, and yoga along with their conventional treatment because they believed it would be helpful.

You are likely eager to preserve your health, so do your research before embarking on a nutritional plan that includes various controversial dietary supplements or suggests making drastic dietary changes. While you no longer need to be concerned about interactions with your cancer treatment, the safety and efficacy of these products and regimens should be evaluated by your doctor or a member of your health care team. Do not invest time or money in something that will not benefit you or your health.

Although many commercial dietary supplements claim to boost the immune system, some can actually inhibit the immune system. Some people's immune systems may be compromised for months after treatment. Eating a well-balanced diet with adequate protein and nutrients is important for improving and regaining your health. Be wary of taking high doses of any dietary supplement or making dramatic dietary changes—a deficiency of any essential vitamin or mineral during recovery from treatment can further weaken your immune system.

At the time of diagnosis, many people with cancer have lower levels of antioxidants in their blood than people without cancer, but it is unclear whether this difference contributes to risk or is caused by cancer itself. Because of this possible correlation, many cancer patients and survivors begin taking antioxidant dietary supplements. Rather, eating a varied diet with adequate sources of diverse antioxidants and phytonutrients is the best approach.

A New Eating Plan: Healthy Eating for Life

Your ideal nutrition and wellness plan after treatment will be designed to replenish nutrient stores in your body, rebuild muscle strength, and help correct problems like anemia or organ dysfunction. Eating enough to maintain a healthy weight and being physically active are crucial for a speedy recovery. Your registered dietitian and other members of your health care team can set up a plan tailored to your needs. A diet containing a variety of low-fat protein (such as lean meats, fish, and poultry), vegetables, fruits, whole grains, and legumes reduces cancer risk in people who have never had cancer. These foods contain vitamins, minerals, and phytochemicals that help the body fight cancer. This diet may also reduce the risk of cancer recurrence and secondary cancers.

Good nutrition can help improve strength, rebuild tissue, and increase feelings of wellness.

Making positive changes to your diet will help you feel empowered in the process of staying well and feeling good. Take advantage of your motivation to change your lifestyle now that your cancer treatment is over. A cancer diagnosis can be extremely motivating and can help set you on a path to better health.

Research suggests the following diet modifications and lifestyle habits have the potential to improve and promote your health:

- achieving and maintaining a healthy body weight
- achieving and maintaining a physically active lifestyle
- eating at least five servings of colorful vegetables and fruits daily
- eating more whole grains and whole grain products
- reducing red and processed meat intake
- increasing fish intake (both flaky fish and firmer fish)
- eating nuts and seeds
- choosing monounsaturated fats such as olive oil and canola oil over trans fats
- choosing foods and beverages low in fat and added sugars to help maintain a healthy weight
- limiting alcoholic beverages—if you choose to drink—to no more than one beverage daily for women and no more than two beverages daily for men

Strive to Achieve a Healthy Body Weight

Cancer treatments may have caused you to gain or lose weight. Talk to your doctor or a registered dietitian about what you should weigh and how to achieve a healthy body weight. Get their support as you work toward your goal.

If you need to gain weight, your doctor, nurse, or registered dietitian may suggest frequent meals that incorporate high-calorie, high-protein snacks, such as canned nutritional supplements, homemade or commercially prepared milk shakes and smoothies, peanut butter, hummus and vegetables, whole grain bread, and cheese. These foods can help you increase your weight slowly. Gaining weight is not easy for everyone. Do not be discouraged if you do not gain your weight back quickly. A gain of a pound or two of body weight each week is excellent progress.

If you gained weight during treatment and would like to return to a healthy weight, talk to your doctor or registered dietitian. Losing extra pounds should occur slowly and should only happen after all side effects of your cancer treatment have resolved. (One exception may be women with breast cancer, who may benefit from slow, healthful weight loss during treatment. Generally, the recommended amount of weight loss is defined as one to two pounds per week.) Pay attention to portion sizes and include more vegetables, fruits, and other plant-based foods that are high in nutrients and low in calories and saturated fat. See the portion sizes table on page 174 for a reminder.

Ease into Healthy Eating and Cooking

Even if your treatment is over and you are feeling much better, you still may not feel completely like your old self. Your usual appetite may not return immediately. You may also continue to experience taste changes, changes in bowel and urinary function, and struggle with pain or queasiness. All of these treatment-related side effects can affect your appetite and ability to eat. It is also sometimes difficult to muster the strength and energy to plan, shop, and cook your meals. Here are some other ways to help you ease into preparing meals and eating well:

- Take it easy. Do not get overly ambitious and plan large labor-intensive meals; enjoy simple dinners at home when you first get back into cooking and eating.
- Think about ways you used to make mealtime special and try them again. These could be eating by candlelight, setting the table with cloth napkins, having a picnic in front of the TV, or inviting a friend over to share a leisurely conversation-filled meal.
- Do not be afraid to ask a friend or family member for help with shopping or cooking. Your support system is still important during your recovery from cancer treatment. People are often willing to help; they may just need to be asked and given instruction and ideas of how to help.
- Try buying the supermarket's washed and cut produce, seasoned meat or fish, or prepared foods (such as a rotisserie chicken) to make mealtimes easier. Remember to wash produce again before eating.
- Refer to the food safety guidelines on pages 197–204 in chapter 10 if you need a refresher on keeping your kitchen and food free of bacteria, as well as tips on eating out safely.

Shop for Health

Once you are on the road to recovery and striving to achieve or maintain a healthy body weight, here are some easy ways to bring lower-calorie, healthier choices into your home for you and your family:

- Try a new healthy food—whether a fruit, vegetable, or whole grain product (bread, pasta, rice, cereal, or other grain)—each time you shop for groceries.
- Choose low-fat or nonfat milk and dairy products.
- Choose healthy fats, lean meats, poultry, fish, and eggs enriched with omega-3 fatty acids. Olive oil, canola oil, walnuts, almonds, and fish such as salmon, halibut, and cod are sources of "good" fats.
- Minimize your intake of saturated fat, salt, sugar, smoked or pickled foods, and alcohol.
- Reduce or avoid intake of sugar-sweetened beverages such as soda, fruit punch, or other fruit-flavored beverages.
- Choose small portions (totaling no more than six to seven ounces a day) of poultry without skin or lean meat.

ON THE HORIZON: EARLY RESEARCH STUDIES OF INTEREST

Update: Diet and Cancer

People who have had cancer (compared with those who have not) are at equal or greater risk for many diseases, such as other cancers, heart disease, and diabetes. Although there are only a few studies addressing the issue of diet and cancer recurrence, findings continue to suggest that a balance of physical activity, a healthy diet, and a healthy weight is helpful in preventing cancer recurrence. The evidence of benefit is even stronger when considering the risk of developing a new cancer and several other noncancerous diseases.

Body mass index, or BMI, is a way to evaluate whether a person is at a healthy weight. However, your BMI should be used only as a general guide, and it is not the only factor one should consider when determining a healthy weight. (You can calculate your BMI by using the formula on page 164 or by visiting the Web site mentioned there.) Another important measure is your waist circumference. Pay attention to changes in the size of your pants and even ask your health care provider to measure your waist with a tape measure at each visit to monitor changes over time. Higher waist circumference may increase your risk of metabolic syndrome, diabetes, hypertension, stroke, heart disease, high insulin and glucose levels, and maybe even cancer.

Based on 2005–2006 data from the Centers for Disease Control and Prevention, almost 65 percent of adults in the United States are overweight or obese (with a BMI greater than twenty-five), and 33 percent of men and 35 percent of women are obese (with a BMI greater than thirty). In the United States, more than one hundred thousand deaths each year are associated with obesity. The World Health Organization has called obesity a global epidemic.

Being overweight may be related to increased risk for cancer recurrence and a decrease in life expectancy. Evidence continues to associate obesity with breast cancer recurrence, and the body of data is growing on the effects of obesity on prognosis for people with other types of cancer. Those who have or have had cancer and are overweight or obese are at greater risk for other obesity-associated diseases such as hypertension, diabetes, cardiovascular disease, and other types of cancer. There is some concern that overweight cancer survivors may face a diagnosis of these diseases at an earlier age than others who have not had a cancer diagnosis and treatment. Cancer survivors can take control of their health by incorporating physical activity into their lives, eating a variety of fresh vegetables and fruits, selecting healthier fat sources and whole grains, and maintaining a healthy weight throughout life.

Now You're Cooking

Cooking lower-calorie, healthier meals is not difficult. Here are some suggestions to modify your cooking for better health:

- Start with familiar, easy-to-prepare recipes and lighten them up. Having a hard time with making a family favorite meal or recipe healthier? Ask a registered dietitian for help or try looking at healthy cooking magazines and cookbooks.
- Use a slow cooker. Slow-cookers are an easy way to provide you and your family with delicious and nutritious meals.
- Try out some new dishes or recipes with your favorite spices and seasonings in them. Wake up your tastebuds!
- Cook enough for two or three meals and freeze portions for later. (This works especially well with casseroles and many soups.)
- Remember to try healthy cooking methods like baking and broiling instead of frying.

Get Even More Than "Five a Day"

Trying to think of ways to get vegetables and fruits in your diet each day, let alone more than five servings a day? Here is one way to start: visualize your plate and imagine this—two-thirds of your meal should be vegetables, fruits, whole grains, or beans, and *one-third (or less)* should be meat or dairy products.

The following are simple ways to increase your intake of plant-based foods:

- Try hearty meatless meals, such as spinach lasagna, vegetarian chili, or vegetarian pizza, a couple of times a week.
- Try plant-based foods that can take the place of meat, such as tofu, tempeh, and beans, or try portobello mushrooms or eggplant for a firm, meaty texture. These foods help satisfy your hunger, too. Some easy choices are marinated, roasted portobello mushrooms, baked eggplant with tomatoes and onion, or firm tofu mixed into a stir fry with whole grain rice and vegetables.
- Experiment with one new produce item each time you shop for groceries. Try making a mango salsa with onion, cilantro, and red bell pepper; add some julienned jicama to your salad; or bake a spaghetti squash and serve as a side dish.
- Choose fresh fruit or 100 percent fruit juice and only whole wheat breads or high-fiber (more than six grams per serving) cereals at breakfast. Add raisins, dried cranberries, or apple slices to your oatmeal. Add berries or other fruit to your cereal.
- Snack on bell pepper strips, baby carrots, or other favorite vegetables dipped in hummus, or sliced, fresh fruit and low-fat or nonfat cottage cheese or yogurt.

Each vegetable and fruit contains its own special combination of vitamins, minerals, and antioxidants and phytochemicals. Buy a variety of produce so your body gets lots of combinations of healthy nutrients.

Eat Wisely When Eating Out

Eating fewer calories and understanding simple ways to control your portions will help you eat out without overdoing it and eating too much. As you consider strategies for eating restaurant food without blowing your diet, remember the following:

- If you know you are going to eat out, eat smaller portions throughout the day so as to stay within your "calorie budget."
- Restaurants are in the business of serving customers. Do not be afraid to ask for items specially prepared the way you want them.

Try not to skip meals, which may make you overindulge later. And most important, try not to show up at the restaurant famished. Commit to sticking to your plan once in the restaurant. If you would like to splurge on a high-calorie entrée, skip dessert. Eating out does not have to wreak havoc with your diet. Try some of the following tactics to help make restaurant foods fit into your own eating plan:

- Get exactly what you want by ordering each item separately (à la carte). For example, order one chicken enchilada (easy on the sauce), side salad, and fruit dessert instead of the enchilada plate with rice, refried beans, sour cream, and guacamole.
- Ask how dishes are prepared and request that the cook grill the chicken, steam the vegetables, put sauces and salad dressings on the side, or use just a dollop of cream sauce on the pasta primavera and add extra grilled vegetables.
- Don't tempt yourself! Have the waiter remove the bowl of chips or peanuts or the basket of bread after you've had a small portion. Calories from mindless nibbling can add up quickly.
- Limit alcohol. It is high in calories, has few nutrients, and can weaken your willpower.

The following foods and methods of preparation are good choices to help you stay within a healthy eating plan:

- soups with a clear-broth base, such as Chinese wonton or hot and sour soup, consommé, tortilla soup, or minestrone
- raw vegetables (crudités) with a small amount of low-calorie dip
- lettuce or spinach salads with vegetables and with dressing on the side (Go easy on the bacon bits, croutons, cheese, and mayonnaise-based items like macaroni salad or tuna salad. One-quarter cup of tuna salad has 190 calories.)

- steamed vegetables with a slice of lemon; grilled veggies if not drenched in oil
- meats that are grilled (but not charred), broiled, roasted, or baked without added fat
- seafood that is broiled, baked, steamed, blackened, or poached—think tender sole poached in parchment with broth, savory vegetables, and herbs
- three to six ounces of steak
- lean meat cuts served au jus, with a piquant fruit sauce, or stir-fried with vegetables (Go easy on rich sauces.)
- a baked potato with a pat of butter or small amount of sour cream (Top with broccoli, lean chili, or salsa.)
- sandwiches on whole wheat or multigrain breads or pita; with lean meats and reduced-fat cheeses; and with mustard, relish, ketchup, or light mayonnaise (Add flavor and vitamins with roasted sweet peppers, lettuce, tomato slices, jalapenos, or chopped olives in small amounts.)
- fresh fruit, sherbet, or angel food cake for dessert

GOOD GRILLING

Cooking meats at high temperatures creates carcinogens, which are chemicals that may increase the risk of cancer. To enjoy grilling and prevent formation of carcinogens, remember the following:

- Choose lean cuts of meat and trim excess fat from meat and poultry.
- Line the grill with foil and poke small holes in the foil so some fat can drain down but not all the smoke can come back onto the food.
- Avoid charring food and do not eat any part that is especially burned and black.
- Marinate meat and poultry with a vinegar- or lemon juice–based marinade and a little oil before grilling.
- Precook meat a bit inside the house (such as in the microwave) then drain away the juices before putting the meat on the grill.
- Watch portion size; aim for a three-ounce meat portion (about the size of a bar of soap). You might want to start by halving your usual portion if this is a drastic change in portion size. Consider supplementing with grilled vegetables—see below.
- Grill marinated vegetables, veggie burgers, or veggie hot dogs. Plant-based foods do not form cancer-promoting substances when cooked on the grill.

The following descriptions mean higher-calorie choices: pan-fried, sautéed, battered, breaded, au gratin, cheesy, creamy, buttered, deep-fried, béarnaise, or crispy—as in the "crispy," deep-fried tortilla bowl holding the salad.

Pay Attention to Portions

Eating smaller portions of food is one of the most obvious ways to cut back on calories. But it can also be one of the most challenging, especially with the current trend of super-sizing. Huge portions, all-you-can-eat buffets, and extra-large "single servings" of chips, candy bars, and other snack foods can all contribute to overeating.

Even bagels have become super-sized, which gives this reasonably healthful breakfast item a high calorie count. Bakeries and grocery stores often carry jumbo bagels that measure four and a quarter inches across and contain three hundred to four hundred calories each. A regular, three-inch bagel has about one hundred fifty calories and counts as two servings of bread in the grain group.

There are a number of ways to eat smaller portions when eating out:

- Order regular portion sizes instead of jumbo sizes. Choosing a regular hamburger instead of a larger one at your favorite fast food stop can save about one hundred fifty calories. Have the small fries instead of the super-sized and save about three hundred calories. Order the small soda. It has about one hundred fifty fewer calories than the large one. (Diet sodas have few or no calories.)
- Try an appetizer, half an entrée, or share a meal with a friend and order an extra side salad.
- Ask for half the entrée to be wrapped up to go before the food is brought to the table. Eat it for lunch the next day.

Similarly, try some of these tips at home:

- Don't eat from the bag. When snacking, place a few chips, crackers, or cookies in a bowl to help prevent overeating.
- Buy single portions of snack foods so you're not tempted to eat a whole bag or box.
- Dress your foods with half the amount of butter, sour cream, cream cheese, cheese, or mayonnaise as you would normally.

Health Risks Associated with Being Overweight or Obese

It is estimated that one-third of all cancer deaths in the United States are related to nutrition and physical activity factors, including excess weight. Overweight and obesity will soon surpass smoking as the leading cause of preventable deaths, and many of those deaths will be from cancer. Despite this fact, many people do not fully understand the risks of being overweight or obese, and many people do not realize the impact that excess weight can have on cancer risk (and the risk of other chronic diseases). Being overweight or obese is a risk factor for many types of cancers but, in particular, for hormone-related cancers (such as breast and prostate cancer), possibly because of a change in the metabolism of estrogen and other hormones.

Physical Activity and Cancer Survivorship

A growing number of studies have examined the effects of exercise and physical activity during recovery and long-term survival after cancer treatment. The studies have mainly been done with women who have had breast cancer, men who have had prostate cancer, people who have had colorectal cancer, and people who have received a bone marrow transplant. The results suggest that exercise has important benefits in physical fitness and overall quality of life. In one study of men, each hour of moderate daily physical activity was shown to reduce the risk of death related to cancer by 12 percent.

Studies also suggest that exercise is related to the prevention of some cancers and other chronic diseases like heart disease and diabetes. The preventive benefits will also likely be found to apply to people who have had cancer. Physical activity is therefore probably helpful in preventing second cancers and other chronic diseases in people who have had cancer. The American Cancer Society and other health organizations recommend at least thirty minutes of moderate physical activity at least five days per week for members of the general population. These levels of activity have not been studied or tested specifically in people who have had cancer, but the health benefits of exercise are in general greater with increased intensity of activity and time spent exercising. (However, excessive overtraining can result in an increased risk for lower immune system functioning.) Please see a list of light, moderate, and vigorous activities on page 188 of chapter 9.

Staying Active

After cancer treatment, it is important to increase body strength and regain your pretreatment fitness level (or improve it). The benefits of exercise in improving overall quality of life are well known. Increased physical activity can positively influence heart rate, lung capacity, and lean body mass in people who have had cancer (these effects are similar to those in people who have not had cancer). If you had or have physical limitations, or if you have not been physically active in the past, develop a physical activity plan with your health care team before jumping into an exercise regimen.

Exercise can help you regain strength and flexibility, reduce stress, maintain an optimal weight, and even relieve symptoms such as depression, anxiety, or irregular bowel movements. Physical activity may strengthen the immune system. Regular exercise can also reintroduce a sense of autonomy that is sometimes lost during treatment.

A well-rounded activity plan includes aerobic exercise (which increases the heart rate and the amount of oxygen your body uses), strength training with weights, and flexibility exercises. Even when performed in small but regular increments, this balanced approach to physical activity provides real benefits for the body.

Performing moderately intense aerobic exercise frequently—three to five times per week for thirty to sixty minutes—is a good goal. This exercise can be accomplished in ten-minute increments throughout the day. Walking, running, cycling, swimming, and stair-climbing are examples of activities that exercise the major muscle groups. Vigorous housework and yardwork count, too—as does any activity that makes you breathe as intensely as you do when walking quickly.

A well-rounded program of resistance or strength training will help improve muscular strength and endurance, body composition, and flexibility. General stretching exercises involving the major muscle and tendon groups can help maintain range of motion in joints and overall flexibility throughout the life cycle.

Despite the known benefits of physical activity, it can sometimes be difficult for cancer survivors to get moving. Fatigue, lack of interest, sedentary lifestyle prior to the cancer diagnosis, and even body image issues are all possible barriers to increasing activity.

However, much like healthy eating, increasing physical activity can be achieved by making a few simple changes. Here are some helpful ways to be more active:

- Use stairs rather than an elevator or escalator.
- If you can, walk or bike to your destination.
- Exercise at lunch with your workmates, family, or friends.
- Take a ten-minute exercise break at work to stretch or to take a quick walk.
- Walk to visit coworkers rather than sending e-mails or calling.
- Go dancing with your spouse or friends.
- Plan active vacations rather than driving-only trips.
- Wear a pedometer every day and watch your daily steps increase. (Try to work up to ten thousand steps per day.)
- Park far from a store and walk through the parking lot.
- Stroll through the neighborhood.
- Join a sports team.
- Pedal a stationary bicycle while watching TV.
- Plan your exercise routine for gradual increases in the days per week and minutes per session.

If it helps, involve friends, family members, or even coworkers to help keep you motivated! Also keep in mind that many people may feel more tired when they first start to push physical activity especially if they try to do too much too soon. Start slowly, and, if necessary, make time for naps.

If you are fatigued and unable to be physically active just after you finish treatment, consult your doctor and ask for advice on creating an individualized exercise program. Then start slowly and work up to a moderate level of exercise as you are able. The ultimate goal is to incorporate exercise as a permanent lifestyle change.

Physical Activity and Older-Aged People

If you are sixty-five or older, a balanced exercise program can help restore joint and muscle flexibility. By including flexibility training—such as stretching exercises —in your exercise programs, you can help offset naturally occurring muscular and skeletal changes that can have an impact on daily life. Flexibility exercises can improve the function and range of motion of your joints and can also be important in preventing musculoskeletal injuries. In addition, exercise helps relieve depression and keeps your mind sharp.

People aged sixty-five or older also may need longer periods to adapt to an exercise program. Whether you are in good health or you have health challenges, you can make significant increases in your strength and muscle mass through resistance and strength training. You should strive to be up and moving seven days a week, and aim to spend time doing extra flexibility exercises or walking on five of those days. Start with five minutes of stretching, then add a few minutes of walking. Build up the amount of time spent exercising as you can.

Special Concerns with Physical Activity After Treatment

If you are confined to bed because of cancer, cancer treatment, or other reasons, talk to your health care team about physical therapy to help you stay strong and keep your joints moving. If you have been in bed a long time, your endurance, muscle strength, and fitness level will have decreased. This can make everyday tasks more tiring. If you are confined to bed, light physical activity can actually help you cope with fatigue, stress, and emotional lows.

If you have been dehydrated and have had an imbalance of electrolytes, your energy level may be low. Even with limited activity, make sure to drink plenty of liquids. If you have had cancer in your bones or treatment that affected your bone strength, abrupt jumping or vigorous twisting might fracture the bone; talk to your health care team about appropriate activities. Remember, physical activity that includes weight-bearing exercise will increase bone health.

If you have lymphedema following surgery or radiation to the lymph nodes under the arm, begin to use your affected arm for everyday activities about four to six weeks after treatment, but be careful not to overdo activity. Talk to your health care team before beginning tennis or weightlifting, which could tire out your arm. Recent evidence suggests that using the arm to perform daily activities can be done safely and may even protect against lymphedema. Ask your doctor about working with a lymphedema therapist.

Community and gym programs often offer options for people beginning physical activity for the first time or taking it up after a time of inactivity. Some classes focus on people with special needs regarding physical activity. If you were extremely active before treatment, take it slow when you first get back into exercise. Your health care team and an exercise specialist can help you develop activities appropriate for the time immediately after treatment and beyond. Look for a LIVESTRONG at the YMCA cancer survivor program in your community. The purpose of this program is to support cancer survivors and their caregivers in reaching their health goals. Physical activity and health information is provided by specially trained YMCA staff. By 2011, more than 150 LIVESTRONG at the YMCA programs should be available across the United States. For more information, go to www.LIVESTRONG.org/YMCA.

The effects of physical activity on heart disease and diabetes have not been studied in people with cancer, but they would be expected to be as favorable as outcomes seen in the general population. Resistance exercise (resistance training and weightlifting) has been reported to improve bone strength in persons without cancer, but the effectiveness of resistance exercise in people with cancer is not yet known.

Women who go through menopause during or after treatment and men who are treated with long-term hormonal therapy (antiandrogenic medications) are at greater risk for osteoporosis. Studies of the general population indicate that people at risk for osteoporosis after treatment might benefit from resistance training. Physical activity can also lead to improved lean body mass and balance, which might also reduce the risk of falls and fractures. Clinical trials are under way, testing the effects of aerobic and resistance exercise on bone density in women who have postmenopausal breast cancer.

The following other situations should be discussed with your health care team before starting physical activity:

- If you have severe anemia, wait to exercise until you have recovered from treatment.
- If you have compromised immune function, avoid public gyms and other public places until your white blood cell counts are back to normal. Instead, exercise at home or outdoors for a time. (If you have had a bone marrow transplant, your health care team may advise you to avoid public places with risk of microbial contamination, such as gyms, for a year after the transplant.)
- If you have severe fatigue and do not feel up to an exercise program, your health care team might encourage you to instead do ten minutes of stretching exercises each day.
- If you have significant peripheral neuropathies (tingling and burning sensations or weakness or numbness in your hands and feet), you may not be able to exercise your affected limbs. You may also feel off balance and may prefer pedaling a reclining bicycle, for example, rather than walking on a treadmill.

Cancer treatment is challenging. After treatment, many people are ready to live life to its fullest—and are willing to take extra steps to make sure they are around to enjoy more of it. Making simple changes in your daily life, like eating well, being active, and keeping a healthy weight, can help you reach those goals.

Long-term Health of Cancer Survivors

As the population of cancer survivors continues to increase, there is more and more interest on the potential health consequences of cancer treatments. For example, do cancer survivors have higher rates of obesity, diabetes, hypertension, or osteoporosis than others of their same age? Much research needs to be done to answer these questions. But this is what current evidence suggests:

- Cancer treatments can affect bone health, particularly if the bone is irradiated or if people are placed on medications that reduce hormone levels that are important to bone health. And some reports suggest some cancer survivors have higher risk of osteoporosis. But, it seems that with proper intervention, improvements in bone health can be made. The following are suggested recommendations to improve bone health:
  - Select low-fat or nonfat dairy products to increase calcium, vitamin D, and phosphorus intake. Green vegetables are another food source of calcium.
  - If your doctor has not checked your vitamin D blood level, ask your doctor to check it during a routine blood evaluation to make sure it is in the normal range.
  - Try to consume the recommended amounts of calcium and vitamin D each day from food and/or dietary supplements. If you have osteopenia, osteoporosis, or if your vitamin D level is low, your doctor will provide you with specific information regarding what amounts are right for you.
    - For postmenopausal women, the recommended daily intake is fifteen milligrams of calcium and eight hundred to one thousand milligrams of vitamin D.
    - For younger women, the recommended daily intake is one thousand to twelve hundred milligrams of calcium and four hundred to eight hundred milligrams of vitamin D.
  - Try to get fifteen to twenty minutes of sunshine a day to promote vitamin D health. Five to ten minutes is enough in sunny areas or in mid-summer.
  - Engage in weight-bearing exercises daily (for example, walking, jogging, or tennis).
  - Take bone-promoting medications as prescribed by your health care provider.
  - Ask your doctor for a bone mineral density test to evaluate the density of your bones.

- Some chemotherapy drugs may affect cardiovascular health. Cancer survivors should have their serum cholesterol, HDL, LDL, C-reactive protein, and homocysteine tested annually. Depending on your levels, you may require dietary and lifestyle changes or even medications. The following can help reduce your risk for heart disease:
  - Achieve and maintain a healthy weight.
  - Be active daily for at least thirty minutes.
  - Eat fish, lean meats, and poultry, and avoid processed meats.
  - Eat soluble fiber such as in oats, oatmeal, and corn bran.
- Up to 80 percent of cancer survivors experience fatigue. This side effect is thought to be more common after radiation therapy, but surgery and chemotherapy can also cause fatigue, as can the stress of a cancer diagnosis. The following can help reduce fatigue:
  - Eat small, frequent meals.
  - Reduce your intake of sweets and sugars.
  - Achieve and maintain a healthy body weight.
  - Be active—small spurts of activity several times a day may work best.
  - Get adequate rest—eight hours of sleep a night is recommended; consider napping as well
- There is not strong evidence that cancer survivors are at greater risk for diabetes, but some types of cancer are more common in overweight people. And if weight gain continues after treatment, the risk for diabetes does rise. Many overweight cancer patients develop what is called metabolic syndrome, or prediabetes. The signs of this syndrome are high blood cholesterol with low HDL cholesterol or triglycerides, high blood pressure, and larger waist measurements. The following can help reduce your risk of prediabetes:
  - Achieve and maintain a healthy body weight.
  - Stay active.
  - Eat a diet low in sugar-containing foods.
  - Restrict intake of sweetened beverages.
  - Select low- or nonfat dairy products.
  - Select fish and lean meats and poultry.
  - Add nuts or seeds to your daily diet (for example, eight to ten walnuts, pistachios, or almonds).

It is not known whether cancer treatment changes your risk for the illnesses we have just described. There is some evidence that people who have completed treatment may have a slightly increased risk for some of these problems or may show evidence of them at a slightly earlier age than most people. But more research is needed before we can say this with certainty. What seems most important is that cancer survivors first understand that these potential risks exist and then make lifestyle choices to reduce the risks and promote a long, healthful life.

Living with Advanced Cancer

Some individuals are cured of cancer or experience it as a controllable chronic disease, whereas others live with advanced cancer (cancer that cannot be cured or controlled) for years. For these people, good nutrition can be an important part of creating and maintaining a sense of well-being. Eating well, maintaining a healthy weight, and being physically active may even improve quality of life. If you have advanced cancer, focus on eating healthy, nutritious foods that are easy to tolerate.

Weight loss is a common problem for people living with advanced cancer. Healthy food choices and changes in your diet can help in preventing further weight loss, meeting nutritional needs, and managing symptoms and side effects such as pain, constipation, and loss of appetite. Medications can help minimize symptoms that interfere with eating, such as pain or constipation. Other medications (such as Megace, Megace ES, or Marinol) may be prescribed to help increase your appetite. Some evidence indicates that omega-3 supplements may help to stabilize or improve your nutritional status, body weight, and overall functioning. Other types of nutritional support can help if you cannot eat enough. Talk to your health care team about ways to improve your feeling of well-being.

Some level of doctor-approved physical activity is helpful for people with advanced cancer, since physical activity—even if you are confined to bed—may help increase appetite, reduce constipation, and counteract fatigue. But there is very limited research on exercise in people with advanced disease. Therefore, talk to your health care team about exercise recommendations based on your needs and situation.

People living with advanced cancer can be particularly susceptible to information and products promoted as cancer cures or treatments. The old adage "if it sounds too good to be true, it probably is" should be applied to nutrition regimens and diets promoted as cancer cures when scientifically sound treatments have not produced the same effect. Talk to your health care team before you forgo conventional (traditional) medical care and embark on an alternative treatment. Ask your doctor to help you evaluate these claims.

See the "How to Eat When You Have Appetite Challenges" section on pages 256–257 for additional information about nutrition options for people with special concerns.

Sometimes people are in treatment for long periods or they may be prescribed different types of therapies to treat their cancer. If your side effects become worse or if they are hard to manage, ask your doctor and registered dietitian for information about how to cope with your specific eating-related concerns. They can help in developing a plan that meets your individual nutritional needs.

Nutrition Studies with Cancer Survivors

Recently, the results of two large dietary intervention trials, which together included more than 5,000 breast cancer survivors, showed that diet can make a difference in the risk of cancer recurrence. The Women's Intervention Nutrition Study (WINS) was conducted at thirty-nine sites across the United States and included postmenopausal women previously treated for early-stage breast cancer. Women either followed their usual diet or were asked to follow a diet that was very low in fat. Registered dietitians helped the women achieve and maintain their low-fat diet for an average of just over eight years.

Among women with breast tumors that were estrogen receptor–negative, those who followed the low-fat diet had a 42 percent reduction in risk for recurrence relative to women who ate their usual diet. However, the low-fat diet did not significantly reduce risk in women with estrogen receptor–positive disease. For these women, the current estrogen-modulating drugs (tamoxifen, aromatase inhibitors) are significantly improving survival. Of importance, the women on the low-fat diet were able to drop their weight slightly (about six pounds on average). This could mean that even a small weight loss may contribute to reducing risk for recurrent breast cancer. The conclusion seems to be that women treated for early-stage postmenopausal breast cancer that is estrogen receptor–negative should adopt a lower-fat diet. It may reduce their risk for recurrent disease.

In this study, registered dietitians set goals for women's daily intake of fat grams. By dividing each woman's body weight in pounds by six, the dietitians arrived at the maximum number of grams of fat each woman was to consume daily. For example, a 188-pound woman would divide 188 by six with a result of 31, meaning she should limit herself to 31 grams of fat per day. If you are trying to pursue a lower-fat diet, consider meeting with a registered dietitian to help identify and reduce fat sources in your diet. Keep a daily log of intake of fat grams—it will help keep you on track for the short and the long run.

Results from the Women's Healthy Eating and Living (WHEL) Study of 3,088 pre-menopausal and postmenopausal breast cancer survivors were published in 2007. In this study, women either followed the National Cancer Institute's 5-A-Day eating plan or adopted a diet very high in plant foods. The diet high in plant foods consisted of the following:

- five servings of vegetables daily
- three servings of fruit daily
- more than thirty grams of fiber daily
- fat calories consisting of no more than 20 percent of total calories

The diet high in plant foods was no better than the 5-A-Day diet in terms of lowering breast cancer recurrence. However, the women in the 5-A-Day group actually averaged more than seven servings of vegetables and fruit daily, while the women who ate the diet high in plant foods averaged twelve servings daily. This means that there was little difference between eating seven servings versus twelve for lowering breast cancer recurrence.

Of importance here is that eating seven servings of vegetables and fruits is a good idea. Further, when the women's dietary patterns prior to the study were analyzed, the following became clear:

1. Among women who ate more than five vegetables and fruits daily and participated in regular physical activity (thirty minutes walking, six times a week), there was a 44 percent reduction in risk for recurrent breast cancer.
2. High blood levels of carotenoids—phytochemicals from vegetables and fruits—also reduced breast cancer recurrence by an estimated 43 percent.
3. Recent unpublished data from the WHEL study shows that eating high amounts of vegetables, particularly cruciferous vegetables, may also protect against recurrence in women taking tamoxifen. More research is needed.
4. Higher fiber intake was associated with lower estrogen/estradiol levels, which in turn was associated with lower cancer recurrence rates.

Several large-scale, long-term studies are evaluating the effects of various dietary factors on cancer recurrence or secondary cancers. Here is a look at some promising studies that are currently under way:

The FRESH START Study. A mailed, tailored nutrition and physical activity intervention program developed to increase healthy behaviors among more than five hundred males with prostate cancer and females with breast cancer resulted in improved food and activity choices during a ten-month period. These results suggest that when information is provided in a tailored fashion and provides people with specific recommendations to improve their own individual health, behavioral change can occur even in the absence of face-to-face counseling.

Nurses' Health Study. This twenty-seven–year-old, ongoing study looks at women's use of hormones, diet, and lifestyle factors to determine the effects on health. Researchers primarily use questionnaires to assess these lifestyle factors. These phase I and II studies are among the largest investigations for major chronic diseases in women and have resulted in many research findings about women and their health. A phase III study was launched in the fall of 2008.

In recent years, researchers have become interested in the increasing number of people in this study who have had cancer. They have published preliminary results from one study in which women with breast cancer who ate a diet rich in poultry, fish, and vegetables lived longer than those who didn't. Researchers involved with this study continue to investigate lifestyle factors that may help women with cancer live longer and healthier lives.

Other studies have looked at people's lifestyles after cancer. In one study of cancer survivors, two-thirds of those interviewed said they made at least one change in their behavior after the cancer diagnosis. Approximately 40 percent improved their diet; 20 percent became physically active; and others began taking multivitamins. Those interviewed reported that their efforts improved their quality of life.

In another study, many women reported making positive dietary changes in the year after their breast cancer diagnosis. The changes typically included following nutritional guidelines recommended for overall health and cancer prevention. The women who made changes in their diet were concerned about reducing the risk of recurrence, coping with and establishing a sense of control over cancer, and improving their prognoses.

In contrast, results from a recent study in Australia suggested that overall, people previously treated for cancer have similar lifestyle habits to the remainder of the population, with similar—and possibly even higher—rates of smoking, alcohol intake, inactivity, and obesity. This points to the importance of supporting positive health choices among cancer survivors as well as for survivors to be assertive in locating the people, tools, and resources needed to help promote healthful choices each and every day.

More and more studies are being conducted to determine whether dietary and lifestyle changes affect the likelihood of cancer recurrence and co-occurring conditions such as diabetes and obesity. In the meantime, living according to the American Cancer Society's cancer prevention guidelines will benefit your overall health. In fact, a recent review of studies of diet and prostate cancer concluded that following those guidelines and emphasizing intake of plant foods can improve prognosis.

We do not really know much yet about how diet may change cancer risk among survivors of cancers other than breast cancer. One study tested the difference in overall survival among cancer survivors eating a prudent diet that included five vegetables and fruits, less fat, and more fiber versus a typical Western diet, which contains few fruits and vegetables, high fat intake, and frequent intake of fast-foods. The prudent diet reduced risk of death from causes other than breast cancer and therefore seems to generally improve health. In addition, the study showed an increased risk of recurrence for colon cancer survivors who ate the typical Western diet.

Although more research is needed, current evidence suggests the best advice for cancer survivors to decrease risk of recurrence, additional cancers, or other chronic diseases is to eat well, live a physically active lifestyle, and maintain a healthy weight.

References

Ahmed RL, Thomas W, Yee D, Schmitz KH. Randomized controlled trial of weight training and lymphedema in breast cancer survivors. *J Clin Oncol.* 2006;24(18):2765-2772.
> Erratum in:
> *J Clin Oncol.* 2006;24(22):3716.

American Cancer Society. *A Breast Cancer Journey: Your Personal Guidebook from the Experts at the American Cancer Society.* 2nd ed. Atlanta, GA: American Cancer Society; 2004.

The American Cancer Society's skinny on trimming the fat. American Cancer Society Web site. http://www.cancer.org/docroot/MED/content/MED_2_1X_The_American_Cancer_Society_s_Skinny_on_Trimming_the_Fat.asp. Published February 24, 1998. Accessed May 20, 2009. Content no longer available.

At first-ever conference on nutrition for cancer survivors, researchers vow to find needed answers. Article 00244. Charity Wire Web site. http://www.charitywire.com/charity10/00244.html. Published May 8, 2001. Accessed December 14, 2009.

Barnes P, Powell-Griner E, McFann K, Nahin R. Complementary and alternative medicine use among adults: United States, 2002. *CDC Advanced Data Report.* 2004;(343):1-19.

Berkow SE, Barnard ND, Saxe GA, Ankerberg-Nobis T. Diet and survival after prostate cancer diagnosis. *Nutr Rev.* 2007;65(9):391-403.

Chlebowski RT, Blackburn GL, Thomson CA, Nixon DW, Shapiro A, Hoy MK, Goodman MT, Giuliano AE, Karanja N, McAndrew P, Hudis C, Butler J, Merkel D, Kristal A, Caan B, Michaelson R, Vinciguerra V, Del Prete S, Winkler M, Hall R, Simon M, Winters BL, Elashoff RM. Dietary fat reduction and breast cancer outcome: interim efficacy results from the Women's Intervention Nutrition Study. *J Natl Cancer Inst.* 2006;98(24):1767-1776.

Controlling portion sizes. American Cancer Society Web site. http://www.cancer.org/docroot/PED/content/PED_3_2x_Portion_Control.asp. Updated November 2, 2009. Accessed December 13, 2009.

Doyle C, Kushi LH, Byers T, Courneya KS, Demark-Wahnefried W, Grant B, McTiernan A, Rock CL, Thompson C, Gansler T, Andrews KS; 2006 Nutrition, Physical Activity and Cancer Survivorship Advisory Committee; American Cancer Society. Nutrition and physical activity during and after cancer treatment: a guide for informed choices by cancer survivors. *CA Cancer J Clin.* 2006;56(6):323-353.

Eakin EG, Youlden DR, Baade PD, Lawler SP, Reeves MM, Heyworth JS, Fritschi L. Health behaviors of cancer survivors: data from an Australian population-based survey. *Cancer Causes Control.* 2007;18(8):881-894.

Haydon AM, Macinnis RJ, English DR, Giles GG. Effect of physical activity and body size on survival after diagnosis with colorectal cancer. *Gut.* 2006;55(1):62-67.

Holmes MD, Stampfer MJ, Colditz GA, Rosner B, Hunter DJ, Willett WC. Dietary factors and the survival of women with breast carcinoma. *Cancer.* 1999;86(5):826-835.
> Erratum in:
> *Cancer.* 1999;86(12):2707-2708.

Kellen E, Vansant G, Christiaens MR, Neven P, Van Limbergen E. Lifestyle changes and breast cancer prognosis: a review. *Breast Cancer Res Treat.* 2009;114(1):13-22.

Kroenke CH, Fung TT, Hu FB, Holmes MD. Dietary patterns and survival after breast cancer diagnosis. *J Clin Oncol.* 2005;23(36):9295-9303.

LiveStrong at the YMCA. LiveStrong Web site. http://www.livestrong.org/site/c.khLXK1PxHmF/b.5119497/k.5FD9/LIVESTRONG_at_the_YMCA.htm. Accessed November 20, 2009.

Maunsell E, Drolet M, Brisson J, Robert J, Deschênes L. Dietary change after breast cancer: extent, predictors, and relation with psychological distress. *J Clin Oncol.* 2002;15;20(4):1017-1025.

Meyerhardt JA, Giovannucci EL, Holmes MD, Chan AT, Chan JA, Colditz GA, Fuchs CS. Physical activity and survival after colorectal cancer diagnosis. *J Clin Oncol.* 2006;24(22):3527-3534.

Miller MF, Bellizzi KM, Sufian M, Ambs AH, Goldstein MS, Ballard-Barbash R. Dietary supplement use in individuals living with cancer and other chronic conditions: a population-based study. *J Am Diet Assoc.* 2008;108(3):483-494.

National Cancer Institute. Eating hints: before, during, and after cancer treatment. National Cancer Institute Web site. http://www.cancer.gov/cancerinfo/eatinghints. Published September 2009. Accessed November 20, 2009.

Nutrition and exercise important after treatment. American Cancer Society Web site. http://www.cancer.org/docroot/NWS/content/update/NWS_2_1xU_Nutrition_and_Exercise_Important_After_Treatment_.asp. Published July 18, 2001. Accessed December 13, 2009.

Nutrition and physical activity guidelines: points to remember. American Cancer Society Web site. http://www.cancer.org/docroot/SPC/content/SPC_1_Nutrition_and_Physical_Activity_Guidelines_Points_To_Remember.asp. Accessed December 13, 2009.

Nutrition and the cancer survivor [patient brochure]. American Institute for Cancer Research Web site. http://www.aicr.org/site/DocServer/Nov2007_Nutrition_and_Cancer_Survivor_FINAL.pdf?docID=1566. Published 2001. Updated November 2007. Accessed December 14, 2009.

Orsini N, Mantzoros CS, Wolk A. Association of physical activity with cancer incidence, mortality, and survival: a population-based study of men. *Br J Cancer.* 2008;98(11):1864-1869.

Patterson RE, Neuhouser ML, Hedderson MM, Schwartz SM, Standish LJ, Bowen DJ. Changes in diet, physical activity, and supplement use among adults diagnosed with cancer. *J Am Diet Assoc.* 2003;103(3):323-328.

Peters U, Littman AJ, Kristal AR, Patterson RE, Potter JD, White E. Vitamin E and selenium supplementation and risk of prostate cancer in the Vitamins and lifestyle (VITAL) study cohort. *Cancer Causes Control.* 2008;19(1):75-87.

Pierce JP, Natarajan L, Caan BJ, Parker BA, Greenberg ER, Flatt SW, Rock CL, Kealey S, Al-Delaimy WK, Bardwell WA, Carlson RW, Emond JA, Faerber S, Gold EB, Hajek RA, Hollenbach K, Jones LA, Karanja N, Madlensky L, Marshall J, Newman VA, Ritenbaugh C, Thomson CA, Wasserman L, Stefanick ML. Influence of a diet very high in vegetables, fruit, and fiber and low in fat on prognosis following treatment for breast cancer: the Women's Healthy Eating and Living (WHEL) randomized trial. *JAMA.* 2007;298(3):289-298.

Pierce JP, Stefanick ML, Flatt SW, Natarajan L, Sternfeld B, Madlensky L, Al-Delaimy WK, Thomson CA, Kealey S, Hajek R, Parker BA, Newman VA, Caan B, Rock CL. Greater survival after breast cancer in physically active women with high vegetable-fruit intake regardless of obesity. *J Clin Oncol.* 2007;25(17):2345-2351.

Reid ME, Duffield-Lillico AJ, Slate E, Natarajan N, Turnbull B, Jacobs E, Combs GF Jr, Alberts DS, Clark LC, Marshall JR. The nutritional prevention of cancer: 400 mcg per day selenium treatment. *Nutr Cancer.* 2008;60(2):155-163.

Restaurant eating tips. American Cancer Society Web site. http://www.cancer.org/docroot/PED/content/PED_3_2x_Restaurant_Eating_Tips_Mar_03.asp?sitearea=&level=. Updated October 2, 2006. Accessed December 13, 2009.

Rock CL, Flatt SW, Natarajan L, Thomson CA, Bardwell WA, Newman VA, Hollenbach KA, Jones L, Caan BJ, Pierce JP. Plasma carotenoids and recurrence-free survival in women with a history of breast cancer. *J Clin Oncol.* 2005;23(27):6631-6638.

Thomas R, Davies N. Lifestyle during and after cancer treatment. *Clin Oncol (R Coll Radiol).* 2007;19(8):616-627.

UC Davis researchers need volunteers to study diet's effects on breast cancer recurrence [press release]. Sacramento, CA: UC Davis Health System; October 7, 1998. UC Davis Health SystemWeb site. http://www.ucdmc.ucdavis.edu/news/whelstudy.html. Accessed December 13, 2009.

World Cancer Research Fund. American Institute for Cancer Research (AICR). Food, nutrition, physical activity, and the prevention of cancer: a global perspective. Washington, DC: AICR; 2007.

Young LR, Nestle M. Expanding portion sizes in the U.S. marketplace: implications for nutrition counseling. *J Am Diet Assoc.* 2003;103(2):231-234.

Chapter Fourteen

Resource Guide

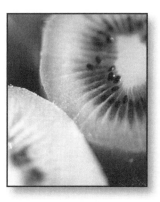

American Cancer Society

250 Williams Street, NW
Atlanta, GA 30303
Toll-free: 800-227-2345
Web site: http://www.cancer.org

The American Cancer Society is the nationwide community-based volunteer health organization dedicated to eliminating cancer as a major health problem by preventing cancer, saving lives, and diminishing suffering from cancer, through research, education, advocacy, and service. For comprehensive, up-to-date cancer information, visit the Web site or call the National Cancer Information Center, toll-free, 24 hours a day, 7 days a week. The American Cancer Society offers a wide variety of education programs, services, and referrals, as well as information related to nutrition during cancer treatment.

About the Resources

Listings in this section represent organizations that operate on a national level and provide some type of service or resource to consumers related to cancer, cancer research, or public health. This list is designed to offer a starting point for seeking information, support, and needed resources. Most of the organizations listed here can be contacted via phone, fax, or e-mail, and some through a Web site. Many of the Web sites provide much of the same information that is available by postal mail. Some organizations are solely Web-based and will require Internet access. Keep in mind that new Web sites appear daily while old ones expand, move, or disappear entirely. Some of the Web sites or content outlined may change. Often, a simple Internet search will point to the new Web site for a given organization. The American Cancer Society Web site provides links to outside sources of cancer information as well.

There is a vast amount of information on the Internet. This information can be quite valuable to the general public in making decisions about their health. However, since any group or individual can publish on the Internet, it is important to consider the credentials and reputation of the organization providing the information. Internet information should not be a substitute for medical advice.

The American Cancer Society does not necessarily endorse the agencies, organizations, corporations, and publications represented in this resource guide. This guide is provided for assistance in obtaining information only.

Organizations Providing Health and Cancer Information

Agency for Healthcare Research and Quality (AHRQ)

Office of Communications and Knowledge Transfer
540 Gaither Road, Suite 2000
Rockville, MD 20850
Telephone: 301-427-1364
Web site: http://www.ahrq.gov

The AHRQ, an office within the U.S. Department of Health and Human Services, provides consumers with science-based, easily understandable information that will help you make informed decisions about your own health care. They offer a number of clinical practice guidelines on common health problems in consumer versions for the public.

American College of Surgeons (ACoS) Commission on Cancer

633 North Saint Clair Street
Chicago, IL 60611-3211
Telephone: 312-202-5000; 312-202-5085
Fax: 312-202-5009
Web site: http://www.facs.org/cancer/index.html
E-mail: CoC@facs.org

The ACoS Commission on Cancer accredits cancer programs of health care organizations in the United States. This voluntary approval program includes a site visit to evaluate the program's compliance with specific standards in ten major areas—from prevention to end-of-life care.

National Cancer Data Base (NCDB)

Web site: http://www.facs.org/cancer/ncdb/index.html

The NCDB is a nationwide oncology outcomes database for close to fifteen hundred health care facilities with approved cancer programs in fifty states. It is estimated that close to 80 percent of newly diagnosed cases of cancer are submitted annually to the NCDB, which is jointly supported by the American Cancer Society and the ACoS Commission on Cancer.

American Institute for Cancer Research (AICR)

1759 R Street, NW
Washington, DC 20009
Telephone: 202-328-7744
Fax: 202-328-7226
Web site: http://www.aicr.org
E-mail: aicrweb@aicr.org

The AICR supports research into the role of diet and nutrition in the prevention and treatment of cancer. It also offers a wide range of cancer education programs and publications for health professionals and the public.

Cancer Research Institute (CRI)

National Headquarters
One Exchange Plaza
55 Broadway, Suite 1802
New York, NY 10006
Toll-free: 800-99-CANCER (800-992-2623)
Telephone: 212-688-7515
Fax: 212-832-9376
Web site: http://www.cancerresearch.org

CRI supports research aimed at developing new immunologic methods of diagnosing, treating, and preventing cancer. CRI can answer questions about cancer immunology and provide assistance in locating clinical trials studying immunotherapy.

Centers for Disease Control and Prevention (CDC)

1600 Clifton Road, NE
Atlanta, GA 30333
Toll-free: 800-CDC-INFO (800-232-4636)
TTY: 888-232-6348
Web site: http://www.cdc.gov
E-mail: cdcinfo@cdc.gov

The CDC's mission is to promote health and quality of life by preventing and controlling disease, injury, and disability. Their Web site contains information about health topics, downloadable publications, and links to related sources.

Federal Trade Commission (FTC)

Consumer Response Center
600 Pennsylvania Avenue, NW
Washington, DC 20580
Toll-free: 877-FTC-HELP (877-382-4357)
Telephone: 202-326-2222
TTY: 866-653-4261
Web site: http://www.ftc.gov

The Web site includes a Consumer Protection section (available from the home page) where information can be found on topics including health and fitness and consumer fraud.

Food and Agriculture Organization of the United Nations (FAO)

Viale delle Terme di Caracalla
0153 Rome, Italy
Telephone: +39 06 57051
Fax: +39 06 5705 3152
Web site: http://www.fao.org
E-mail: FAO-HQ@fao.org

The FAO of the United Nations was founded in 1945 with a mandate to raise levels of nutrition and standards of living, to improve agricultural productivity, and to better the condition of rural populations. Today, FAO is one of the largest specialized agencies in the United Nations system and the lead agency for agriculture, forestry, fisheries, and rural development. The FAO Web site includes information about nutrition and food safety and quality.

The Mautner Project

The National Lesbian Health Organization
1875 Connecticut Avenue, NW, Suite 710
Washington, DC 20009
Toll-free: 866-MAUTNER (866-628-8637)
Telephone: 202-332-5536
Fax: 202-332-0662
Web site: http://www.mautnerproject.org
E-mail: info@mautnerproject.org

This organization provides direct services, navigation, and support to lesbians with cancer, their families, and caregivers; education and information to the lesbian community about cancer; education to the health-providing community about the special concerns of lesbians with cancer and their families; and advocacy for lesbian health and cancer issues in national and local arenas. Some brochures are also available in Spanish.

National Cancer Institute (NCI)

NCI Public Inquiries Office
6116 Executive Boulevard, Room 3036A
Bethesda, MD 20892-8322
Toll-free: 800-4-CANCER (800-422-6237)
TTY: 800-332-8615
Web site: http://www.cancer.gov

This government agency, as part of the National Institutes of Health, provides information on cancer research, diagnosis, and treatment through several services. People with cancer, caregivers, and health care professionals may call the NCI's toll-free telephone service for cancer-related information, including information about complementary and alternative medicine and nutrition in cancer care. Spanish-speaking staff and Spanish materials are available.

Cancer Information Service (CIS)

Toll-free: 800-4-CANCER (800-422-6237)
TTY: 800-332-8615
Web site: http://cis.nci.nih.gov

The CIS provides information to consumers and health care professionals. The Web site contains a wealth of information, including pamphlets and brochures on cancer diagnosis, treatment, research, and prevention. Spanish-speaking staff is available.

Office of Cancer Complementary and Alternative Medicine (OCCAM)

National Cancer Institute (NCI)
6116 Executive Boulevard, Suite 609, MSC 8339
Bethesda, MD 20892
Toll-free: 800-4-CANCER (800-422-6237)
Telephone: 301-435-7980
Fax: 301-480-0075

Web site: http://www.cancer.gov/CAM
E-mail: ncioccam1-r@mail.gov

The OCCAM coordinates and enhances the activities of the NCI in the arena of complementary and alternative medicine. The goal of the OCCAM is to increase the amount of high-quality cancer research and information about the use of complementary and alternative therapies.

National Consumers League

1701 K Street, NW, Suite 1200
Washington, DC 20006
Telephone: 202-835-3323
Fax: 202-835-0747
Web site: http://www.nclnet.org

Experts in law, business, and labor provide consumer protection and advocacy. The National Consumers League publishes educational brochures about general health issues, including cancer-screening tests.

National Council Against Health Fraud

119 Foster Street
Peabody, MA 01960
Telephone: 978-532-9383
Web site: http://www.ncahf.org

This private, nonprofit voluntary health agency focuses on health misinformation, fraud, and quackery, and provides information on unusual methods of cancer management. It can refer people to lawyers and help those who have had negative experiences to share their story.

National Institutes of Health (NIH)

9000 Rockville Pike
Bethesda, MD 20892
Toll-free: 800-4-CANCER (800-422-6237)
Telephone: 301-496-4000
TYY: 301-402-9612
Web site: http://www.nih.gov
E-mail: NIHinfo@od.nih.gov

The NIH is one of the world's foremost medical research centers and the federal focal point for medical research in the United States. The NIH, comprises twenty-seven separate Institutes and Centers and is one of the eight health agencies of the Public Health Service, which, in turn, is part of the U.S. Department of Health and Human Services. The goal of NIH research is to acquire new knowledge to help prevent, detect, diagnose, and treat disease and disability, from the rarest genetic disorder to the common cold. The NIH mission is to uncover new knowledge that will lead to better health for everyone.

National Center for Complementary and Alternative Medicine (NCCAM)

NCCAM Clearinghouse
P. O. Box 7923
Gaithersburg, MD 20898
Toll-free: 888-644-6226
TYY: 866-464-3615
Fax: 866-464-3616
Web site: http://nccam.nih.gov
E-mail: info@nccam.nih.gov

This center provides research-based information on complementary and alternative methods being promoted to treat different diseases, including research and an up-to-date listing of clinical trials on alternative medicine.

The National Institute of Environmental Health Sciences (NIEHS)

P. O. Box 12233, MD K3-16
Research Triangle Park, NC 27709
Telephone: 919-541-3345
Fax: 919-541-4395
Web site: http://www.niehs.nih.gov

The mission of the NIEHS is to reduce the burden of human illness and dysfunction from environmental causes by understanding environmental factors, individual susceptibility, and age and how they interrelate. The NIEHS achieves its mission through multidisciplinary biomedical research programs, prevention and intervention efforts, and communication strategies that encompass training, education, technology transfer, and community outreach.

National Library of Medicine (NLM)

8600 Rockville Pike
Bethesda, MD 20894
Telephone: 301-402-1384
Fax: 301-594-5983
Web site: http://www.nlm.nih.gov
E-mail: custserv@nlm.nih.gov

The NLM collects, organizes, and makes available biomedical science information to investigators, educators, and practitioners and carries out programs designed to strengthen medical library services in the United States. Its electronic databases are used extensively throughout the world by both health professionals and the public. Materials are available in languages other than English.

MEDLINEplus

Web site: http://medlineplus.gov

MEDLINEplus is a database for consumer health information, including dictionaries; articles and journals from other organizations; textbooks, newsletters, and health news for online reading; and links to organizations that provide consumer information and clearinghouses that send health literature.

NLM Gateway

Web site: http://gateway.nlm.nih.gov/gw/Cmd

The NLM Gateway offers links to searchable databases and allows users to search simultaneously in multiple retrieval systems.

PubMed

Web site: http://www.ncbi.nlm.nih.gov/PubMed

This database provides access to millions of literature references and abstracts in MEDLINE and other databases, with links to online journals. The site is searchable by keyword.

Women's Health Initiative (WHI)

Web site: http://www.nhlbi.nih.gov/whi/index.html

The WHI, the largest clinical trial ever undertaken in the United States, addresses the most common causes of death, disability, and impaired quality of life in postmenopausal women. It is expected that the WHI will provide many answers concerning possible benefits and risks associated with use of hormone replacement therapy, dietary supplements, and other interventions in preventing cardiovascular disease, breast and colorectal cancer, and osteoporosis in postmenopausal women.

The National Heart, Lung, and Blood Institute (NHLBI)

Health Information Center
P. O. Box 30105
Bethesda, MD 20824-0105
Telephone: 301-592-8573
TTY: 240-629-3255
Fax: 301-592-8563
Web site: http://www.nhlbi.nih.gov/
E-mail: NHLBIinfo@nhlbi.nih.gov

The National Heart, Lung, and Blood Institute plans, conducts, fosters, and supports an integrated and coordinated program of basic research, clinical investigations and trials, observational studies, and demonstration and education projects. For health professionals and the public, the NHLBI conducts educational activities, including development and dissemination of materials in the above areas, with an emphasis on prevention. Since October 1997, the NHLBI has also had administrative responsibility for the NIH Woman's Health Initiative.

United States Department of Health and Human Services (HHS)

200 Independence Avenue, SW
Washington, DC 20201
Toll-free: 877-696-6775
Telephone: 202-619-0257
Web site: http://www.hhs.gov

The Department of Health and Human Services (HHS) is the U.S. government's principal agency for protecting the health of all Americans and providing essential human services, especially for those who are least able to help themselves. One of the largest federal agencies, the

HHS' responsibilities include public health (CDC, NIH, FDA, and others included), biomedical research, and more.

United States Environmental Protection Agency (EPA)

Ariel Rios Building
1200 Pennsylvania Avenue, NW
Washington, DC 20460
Telephone: 202-272-0167
TTY: 202-272-0165
Web site: http://www.epa.gov

The EPA implements the federal laws designed to promote public health by protecting our nation's air, water, and soil from harmful pollution. The Web site offers environmental news, community concerns, information about laws and other regulations, and links to other sources of information.

Office of Pesticide Programs (OPP)

Web site: http://www.epa.gov/pesticides

The mission of the OPP is to protect public health and the environment from the risks posed by pesticides and to promote safer means of pest control. The Web site provides consumer alerts, information about pesticides and their use and disposal, a kid's section, industry-related topics, and other information.

Office of Water (OW)

Safe Drinking Water Hotline: 800-426-4791
Web site: http://www.epa.gov/water

The OW is responsible for the EPA's water quality activities, including development of national programs, technical policies, and regulations relating to drinking water, water quality, ground water, pollution source standards, and the protection of wetlands, marine, and estuarine areas.

Water Quality Association (WQA)

International Headquarters and Laboratory
4151 Naperville Road
Lisle, IL 60532-3696
Telephone: 630-505-0160
Fax: 630-505-9637
Web site: http://www.wqa.org/
E-mail: info@wqa.org

The WQA is a trade association representing the household, commercial, industrial, and small community water treatment industry. WQA is a resource and information source, a voice for the industry, an educator for professionals, a laboratory for product testing, and a communicator to the public.

World Health Organization (WHO)

WHO Headquarters
Avenue Appia 20 1211
Geneva 27 Switzerland
Telephone: +41 22 791 2111
Fax: +41 22 791 3111
Web site: http://www.who.int

United States Headquarters
Regional Office for the Americas/Pan American Health Organization
525 23rd Street, NW
Washington, DC 20037
Telephone: 202-974-3000
Telephone: 202-974-3459 (Office of Public Information)
Fax: 202-974-3663

Founded in 1948, the WHO leads the world alliance for Health for All. A specialized agency of the United Nations, WHO promotes technical cooperation for health among nations, carries out programs to control and eradicate disease, and strives to improve the quality of human life.

Organizations Providing Health, Food, Diet, and Supplement Information

American Dietetic Association (ADA)

120 South Riverside Plaza, Suite 2000
Chicago, IL 60606-6995
Toll-free: 800-877-1600
Web site: http://www.eatright.org

The ADA is the world's largest organization of food and nutrition professionals. The ADA serves the public by promoting nutrition, health, and well-being. The Web site contains information on diet and nutrition, publications, and a registered dietitian locator service, including access to dietitians who specialize in oncology nutrition.

International Food Information Council (IFIC) Foundation

1100 Connecticut Avenue, NW, Suite 430
Washington, DC 20036
Telephone: 202-296-6540
Fax: 202-296-6547
Web site: http://ific.org

As the educational arm of the IFIC, the IFIC Foundation communicates science-based information on food safety and nutrition to health and nutrition professionals, educators, journalists, and others for distribution to consumers. The IFIC has established partnerships with a wide range of professional organizations and academic institutions to develop science-based information for the public.

Meals on Wheels Association of America (MOWAA)

203 S. Union Street
Alexandria, VA 22314
Telephone: 703-548-5558
Fax: 703-548-8024
Web site: http://www.mowaa.org
E-mail: mowaa@mowaa.org

Meals on Wheels is a membership association of programs that provide home-delivered and group meals. The goal of the organization is to improve the quality of life of the needy, particularly the elderly, disabled, and homebound. Some programs may provide other health and social services such as transportation, recreation, nutrition, education, information, referrals, and case management.

Memorial Sloan-Kettering Cancer Center (MSKCC)

About Herbs, Botanicals, and Other Products
http://www.mskcc.org/mskcc/html/11570.cfm

Memorial Sloan-Kettering Cancer Center's About Herbs, Botanicals, and Other Products Web site provides information for consumers about herbs, botanicals, and alternative or unproven cancer therapies, including details about adverse effects, interactions, and potential benefits or problems.

The Office of Dietary Supplements (ODS)

National Institutes of Health
6100 Executive Boulevard, Room 3B01, MSC 7517
Bethesda, MD 20892-7517
Telephone: 301-435-2920
Fax: 301-480-1845
Web site: http://ods.od.nih.gov
E-mail: ods@nih.gov

The ODS supports research and shares research results about dietary supplements. To explore the role of dietary supplements in the improvement of health care, the ODS plans, organizes, and supports conferences, workshops, and symposia on scientific topics related to dietary supplements.

Quackwatch

Web site: http://www.quackwatch.com

Quackwatch is a nonprofit corporation whose purpose is to combat health-related frauds, myths, fads, and fallacies.

United States Department of Agriculture (USDA)

1400 Independence Avenue, SW
Washington, DC 20250
Telephone: 202-720-2791
Web site: http://www.usda.gov
E-mail: AgSec@usda.gov

The USDA strives to enhance the quality of life for the American people by supporting production of agriculture. The USDA is also responsible for the food supply, managing agricultural products, forests, and rangeland, and community development.

USDA Food and Nutrition Information Center (FNIC)

National Agricultural Library
10301 Baltimore Avenue, Room 105
Beltsville, MD 20705
Telephone: 301-504-5414
Fax: 301-504-6409
Web site: http://www.nal.usda.gov/fnic

The USDA's FNIC is an information center for the National Agricultural Library. FNIC materials and services include dietitians and nutritionists available to answer inquiries, publications on food and nutrition, and resource lists and bibliographies. The FNIC Web site includes information on dietary supplements, food safety, dietary guidelines, food composition facts (including fast food), a list of available publications, and information on popular topics.

United States Food and Drug Administration (FDA)

5600 Fishers Lane
Rockville, MD 20857
Telephone: 888-INFO-FDA (888-463-6332)
Fax: 301-443-9767
Web site: http://www.fda.gov

The FDA is an agency within the U.S. Department of Health and Human Services and consists of eight centers/offices. The FDA is a public health agency charged with protecting Americans by enforcing the Federal Food, Drug, and Cosmetic Act and other laws, promoting health by helping safe and effective products reach the market in a timely manner, and monitoring products for continued safety after they are in use. The FDA regulates food, cosmetics, medicines, biologics, medical devices, and radiation-emitting consumer products, as well as feed and drugs for pets and farm animals. The Web site has extensive information about all the products the FDA regulates.

Center for Food Safety and Applied Nutrition (CFSAN) Outreach and Information Center

5100 Paint Branch Parkway (HFS-555)
College Park, MD 20740-3835
Toll-free: 888-SAFEFOOD (888-723-3366)
TYY: 800-877-8339
Web site: http://www.cfsan.fda.gov

The goal of the Outreach and Information Center is to enhance CFSAN's ability to provide and respond to the public's desire and demand for more useful, timely, and accurate information regarding its regulated products. In addition to providing food safety information, the Outreach and Information Center provides assistance with other CFSAN issues, including nutrition, dietary supplements, food labeling, cosmetics, food additives, and food biotechnology.

United States Pharmacopeia (USP)

12601 Twinbrook Parkway
Rockville, MD 20852-1790
Toll-free: 800-227-8772
Telephone: 301-881-0666
Web site: http://www.usp.org/

The U.S. Pharmacopeia (USP) is a nonprofit organization that establishes standards for medicines and dietary supplements that are recognized in U.S. federal law. Updated continuously to reflect industry and public health needs, USP standards provide specifications for strength, quality, purity, packaging, and labeling. USP also offers a Dietary Supplement Verification program through which dietary supplement manufacturers can voluntarily submit their products for laboratory testing, documentation review, and a GMP audit.

APPENDIX:
SPECIAL DIETS

Clear-Liquid Diet

What is a clear-liquid diet?

A clear-liquid diet consists of clear foods that are liquid or will become liquid at room temperature. These foods and beverages contain some electrolytes and a small amount of calories. Clear liquids are easy to digest and contain almost no residue. However, a clear-liquid diet does not supply adequate calories and protein, and for that reason, this diet should be used for short periods only. If you have diabetes, please ask your doctor whether you need to use sugar-free versions of the foods and beverages listed below. If you require insulin, talk with your doctor or registered dietitian about how to consume consistent amounts of carbohydrates while using a clear-liquid diet.

SAMPLE MENU	
Breakfast	**Lunch and Dinner**
• Clear fruit juice and/or water • Broth	• Broth • Gelatin
• Gelatin • Coffee or tea without milk and sugar	• Clear juice, water, and/or lemonade • Coffee or tea without milk and sugar

Why would I need to use a clear-liquid diet?

Your doctor or health care professional might suggest this diet before or after medical procedures such as a surgery, certain blood tests, or as a short-term solution to manage cancer symptoms or treatment side effects. For certain tests, you may be asked to avoid clear liquids that are red, such as red-colored gelatin or sports drinks.

Which foods and beverages may be included in a clear-liquid diet?
• Gelatin such as Jell-O
• Fruit ices made without milk or chunks of fruit
• Popsicles or frozen ice pops

- Clear hard candy such as lollipops, lemon drops, root beer barrels and LifeSavers
- Clear fruit juices such as apple, white grape, cranberry-apple, and cranberry
- Lemonade, limeade, and orange juice that is strained to remove all pulp
- Kool-Aid
- Clear sports drinks such as Propel, Powerade, or Gatorade
- Coffee and tea (hot or cold but without milk or creamer)
- Water
- Clear carbonated drinks such as 7-up, ginger ale, Sierra Mist, or Sprite
- Beef, poultry and vegetable broths, bouillons, or consommés (strained)
- Clear protein-containing nutritional supplements such as Enlive, or Boost Breeze
- Salt and mild seasonings such as cinnamon, paprika, lemon, lime, and vanilla
- Gummy candies are **not** allowed. While they are clear, they also contain wax and other inappropriate ingredients.

Full-Liquid Diet

What is a full-liquid diet?

A full-liquid diet contains all of the foods and beverages allowed in the clear-liquid diet and much more. It contains many foods made with and containing milk. If lactose intolerance is a problem, substitute lactose-free products for milk-containing foods and beverages. If you have diabetes, please ask your doctor whether you need to use sugar-free versions of the foods and beverages listed below. If you require insulin, talk with your doctor or registered dietitian about how to consume consistent amounts of carbohydrates while following a full-liquid diet.

SAMPLE MENU	
Breakfast	**Lunch and Dinner**
• Fruit juice • Hot cereal • Plain or vanilla yogurt • Milk • Coffee or tea with/without milk and sugar	• Broth or strained cream soup • Custard, pudding, or gelatin with whipped topping • Milk or juice • Ice cream or sherbet • Coffee or tea with/without milk and sugar

Why would I need to follow a full-liquid diet?

The full-liquid diet is often used before or after surgery, especially surgery to the gastrointestinal system. It is generally used as a transition between clear liquids to more solid foods as tolerated. A full-liquid diet might also be used to temporarily manage cancer symptoms and treatment side effects.

What foods are included in the full-liquid diet?

All foods included in the clear-liquid diet (see page 307)
• Cooked refined cereals such as Cream of Wheat, Cream of Rice, or Coco Wheats hot cereal
• Gelatin desserts, rennet desserts, sherbet and sorbet (without chunks or seeds), puddings, ice cream, and ice milk (without chunks or seeds)
• Soft custards containing eggs, pasteurized eggnog
• Fats, including butter, cream, margarine, and vegetable oils
• All fruit juices and nectars, puréed fruits

- Milk, milk shakes, yogurt (plain, vanilla, or other flavors, without food bits or seeds), sour cream, whipped toppings
- Mashed white potato used in cream soup
- Strained gravy
- Salt and mild seasonings, flavorings, chocolate syrup, cocoa powder
- Broth, bouillon, consommé, strained cream soups made from allowed foods, and tomato soups
- Honey, sugar, syrup, hard candy
- Puréed vegetables, vegetable juices
- Liquid meal replacements such as Instant Breakfast

Mechanical Soft Diet

What is a mechanical soft diet?

A mechanical soft diet includes foods that are easy to chew and swallow. The foods on this diet are changed by cooking, chopping, grinding, mashing, or puréeing and are usually moistened with sauces. By using a blender or a food processor, you can make regular foods much easier to eat and drink. Unlike the clear-liquid diet and full-liquid diet, this diet can provide adequate calories and protein for weight maintenance or weight gain and can be used for a long time.

SAMPLE MENU		
Breakfast	**Lunch**	**Dinner**
• Scrambled eggs with cheese • White bread with butter and jam • Apple juice • Coffee/tea with or without milk and sugar	• Chicken noodle soup • Cottage cheese and canned peaches • Ice cream with chocolate sauce and shortbread cookies • Water • Coffee/tea with or without milk and sugar	• Italian Wedding soup • Ravioli with tomato sauce • Creamed spinach • Sorbet • Water • Coffee/tea with or without milk and sugar

Why would I need to follow a mechanical soft diet?

Use a mechanical soft diet if you are having difficulty chewing or swallowing. If your mouth and throat are irritated, you have mouth sores, or you are recovering from oral or throat surgery, you will need foods that are soft, easy to chew, and easy to swallow. A mechanical soft diet can be used as a transition from clear liquids to solid foods and is frequently used for people recovering from long illnesses who are still weak or for people who are missing teeth.

What foods are included in a mechanical soft diet?

All food allowed on the clear-liquid and full-liquid diets (see pages 307 and 309)
• Soft bread, pancakes, and muffins (with margarine, butter, jam, or syrup added to make them easier to swallow)
• Dry breakfast cereals softened in milk
• Eggs and egg substitutes

- Fruit sauces or mashed, stewed, or canned fruit; fruit smoothies
- Soft, cooked meats and poultry with added gravies and sauces, ground meat or poultry casseroles and meatloaf
- Cottage cheese, soft cheeses such as American or Farmers, cream cheese, and cheese sauces
- Hummus, tofu, and smooth peanut butter
- Soft pasta, tortellini, or ravioli
- White rice
- Soft cakes and cookies made without nuts (consumed with milk, juice, or coffee/tea to make them easier to swallow)
- Well-cooked vegetables, and soft vegetables without skins or seeds
- Mashed or creamed white and sweet potatoes

Low-Fiber, Low-Residue Diet

What is a low-fiber, low-residue diet?

Dietary fiber is the indigestible part of plants sometimes called roughage. Residue refers to the end product that remains after the food has been digested. A low-fiber, low-residue diet limits foods that contain roughage and residue. Indigestible carbohydrate is reduced by using cooked or canned vegetables and ripe, canned, or cooked fruits from which the seeds and tough skins have been removed. Choose tender and lean cuts of meat or meat tenderized through the cooking process. Milk is generally restricted to two cups (one pint) a day since it produces bulky residue in the colon.

SAMPLE MENU		
Breakfast	**Lunch**	**Dinner**
• Cheese omelet with cooked asparagus • White English muffin with margarine and seedless jam • Orange juice (without pulp) • Coffee/tea with or without milk and sugar	• Chicken and vegetable soup (cooked soft) • Turkey and swiss cheese sandwich made with white bread • Tossed salad (iceberg lettuce) with french dressing • Orange sorbet with wafer cookies • Water • Coffee/tea with or without milk and sugar	• Cream of mushroom soup (cup) • Center-cut pork chop • Rice pilaf • Cooked green beans • Yellow cake with lemon frosting • Water • Coffee/tea with or without milk and sugar

Why would I need to follow a low-fiber, low-residue diet?

Bowel function can be altered by adding or limiting fiber- and residue-producing foods. Fiber and residue can help stimulate bowel function if you are constipated, but fiber and residue also can aggravate diarrhea or inflammatory bowel conditions such as radiation enteritis, ulcerative colitis, or diverticulitis. A low-fiber, low-residue diet can help manage these symptoms and conditions. In addition, a low-fiber, low-residue diet can be used for a short time to manage a new ileostomy or colostomy. Questions regarding individual tolerances and gradual additions to the diet (for ostomates) should be addressed with your registered dietitian or your doctor.

What foods are included in a low-fiber, low-residue diet?

- Breads, cereals, and grains: white bread; egg and potato bread; English muffins; bagels; saltine crackers; butter crackers; melba toast; pretzels; milk toast (toasted white bread softened in milk); white rice; plain pasta; refined hot cereal, such as cream of wheat, cream of rice, instant oatmeal, or grits; and refined cold cereals, such as Corn Flakes, Rice Krispies, Rice Chex, and Corn Chex
- Cottage cheese, cream cheese, mild hard cheeses (American, Cheddar, Monterey Jack), cheese sauces with pastas
- Dairy (if tolerated), including milk, ice cream, ice milk, smooth sorbets, sherbets, yogurt, pudding, and custard. Initially limit serving size to a ½ cup at a time.
- Eggs, baked, boiled, scrambled, poached, or used in soufflés
- Margarine, butter, and vegetable oils
- All fruit juices; avocado; ripe banana; canned applesauce, cherries, peaches, pears; peeled or puréed apricots
- Boiled, poached, or broiled meat, poultry or fish
- White sugar, brown sugar, clear seedless jelly/jam, honey, molasses, clear sweet dessert sauces, hard candy, gum drops, chocolate, and strawberry and caramel syrups
- All vegetable juices (unless made from strong-flavored, gassy vegetables); tender, well-cooked vegetables such as green and wax beans, carrots, beets, asparagus, mushrooms, and winter and summer squash; boiled, baked, and mashed potatoes and sweet potatoes
- Broth or milk-based soups made with allowed vegetables
- Creamy nut butters
- Salt and mild seasonings, cinnamon, paprika, lemon, vanilla

High-Fiber Diet

What is a high-fiber diet and why would I follow this diet modification?

Dietary fiber, also known as roughage, is the indigestible part of a plant. It is mainly found in fruits, vegetables, whole grains, and legumes. By definition, a high-fiber diet contains more than twenty-five grams of fiber per day. There are two types of dietary fiber: insoluble and soluble.

Insoluble fiber does not dissolve in water. When combined with plenty of water, insoluble fiber helps move food stuff through the colon. Examples of insoluble fiber include wheat bran, fruit peels/skins, nuts and many vegetables. This type of fiber not only helps relieve constipation and bowel irregularity but also has been associated with decreasing the risk for diabetes.

Soluble fiber does dissolve in water to form a gel-like material. It helps to soften the stool. Examples of soluble fiber include oat bran, peas, beans, citrus fruit, and psyllium fiber. This type of fiber is also helpful in relieving constipation and bowel irregularities; in addition, soluble fiber helps reduce blood cholesterol by interfering with the absorption in the gut.

In general, it is best to get your fiber through food. Sometimes, however, it is necessary to take fiber supplements, such as Benefiber, Metamucil, Citracel, and FiberCon. Check with your doctor or registered dietitian before starting fiber supplements or if you have additional questions about fiber.

SAMPLE MENU		
Breakfast	**Lunch**	**Dinner**
• Raisin Bran cereal (1 cup) with skim milk • Whole grain bread with margarine and raspberry jam • Orange juice (with pulp) • Coffee/tea with or without milk and sugar	• Vegetarian chili with cheese • Tossed salad (mixed greens and sliced vegetables) with oil and vinegar dressing • Oatmeal and dried cranberry cookie • Water • Coffee/tea with or without milk and sugar	• Sweet and sour soup (1 cup) • Chicken and stir-fried vegetables with brown rice • Mixed fresh fruit parfait with touch of whipping cream • Water • Coffee/tea with or without milk and sugar

Good Sources of Fiber

FOOD ITEM	FIBER CONTENT IN GRAMS*
Split peas, cooked, 1 cup	16.3
Red kidney beans, boiled, 1 cup	13.1
Raspberries, raw, 1 cup	8.0
Whole wheat or whole spaghetti, 1 cup	6.3
Oat bran muffin, medium	5.2
Pear, medium with skin	5.1
Broccoli, boiled, 1 cup	5.1
Apple, medium with skin	4.4
Oatmeal, quick, regular or instant, cooked, 1 cup	4.0
Green beans, cooked, 1 cup	4.0
Brown rice, cooked, 1 cup	3.5
Popcorn, air-popped, 2 cups	2.3
Whole wheat bread, one slice	≥1.9

* Fiber content can vary between brands. Source: USDA National Nutrient Database for Standard Reference, and www.mayoclinic.com.

GLOSSARY

Adequate Intake (AI): the average daily intake of a particular nutrient (such as a vitamin) recommended by the Food and Nutrition Board (FNB) of the United States National Academies of Sciences. AI values are based on observations of the average intake of a group of healthy people. The FNB publishes Recommended Dietary Allowances (RDA) for some nutrients but may provide an AI if there is not enough evidence to establish an RDA. *See also* Recommended Dietary Allowance.

adjuvant (AJ-uh-vunt) therapy: treatment used in addition to the main treatment. It usually refers to hormonal therapy, chemotherapy, radiation therapy, or biotherapy added after surgery to increases the chances of curing the disease or preventing recurrence.

alkaloids: organic substances in plants.

allium: a food group including garlic, shallots, and onions that may have a strong protective effect against prostate cancer.

alternative therapy (alternative medicine): an unproven medication or therapy that is recommended instead of standard (proven) therapy. Some alternative therapies have dangerous or even life-threatening side effects. With others, the main concern is that the person may lose the opportunity to benefit from standard therapy. The American Cancer Society recommends that people considering the use of any alternative or complementary therapies discuss these therapies with their conventional health care team. *Compare with* complementary therapy.

amino acid: one of several molecules that join together to form proteins. There are twenty common amino acids. *See also* protein.

androgen (AN-dro-jen): any male sex hormone. The major androgen is testosterone.

anemia (uh-NEEM-ee-uh): not having enough red blood cells. Symptoms can include shortness of breath, difficulty breathing on exertion, and fatigue. These symptoms occur because there are not enough red blood cells to carry oxygen to the body's tissues.

angiogenesis (an-jee-o-JEN-uh-sis): the formation of new blood vessels. Some cancer treatments work by blocking angiogenesis, thus preventing blood from reaching the tumor.

anorexia: loss of appetite leading to severe weight loss.

antibody: a protein produced by the body's immune system cells and released into the blood. Antibodies defend the body against foreign agents, such as bacteria. These agents contain certain substances called antigens. Each antibody works against a specific antigen. *See also* antigen, protein.

anticoagulant (an-tee-ko-AG-yuh-lunt): a drug that helps prevent blood clots from forming. Also called a blood thinner.

antiemetic (an-tie-eh-MEH-tik): a drug that prevents or relieves nausea and vomiting, which are common side effects of chemotherapy.

antiestrogen (AN-tee-ES-truh-jin): a substance (for example, the drug tamoxifen) that blocks the effects of estrogen on tumors. They are used to treat cancers that depend on estrogen for growth, such as some types of breast cancer. *See also* estrogen, tamoxifen.

anti-inflammatory: a drug that reduces pain and swelling as in arthritis.

antigen (AN-tuh-jen): a substance that causes the body's immune system to react. This reaction often involves production of antibodies, but may also involve immune system cells that attack germs or cancer cells. For example, the immune system's response to antigens that are part of bacteria and viruses helps people resist infections. Cancer cells have certain antigens that can be found by laboratory tests. Antigens are important in the diagnosis of some forms of cancer and in watching a patient's response to treatment. Other cancer cell antigens play a role in immune reactions that may help the body's resistance against cancer. *See also* antibody, immune system.

antinutrient: a substance that interferes with the use of nutrients by the body. *Compare with* nutrient.

antioxidant (an-tee-OK-sih-dent): a compound that destroys activated oxygen molecules, known as free radicals, that can damage cells. Free radicals can damage important parts of cells such as genes. Depending on how severe the damage is, the cells may die or they may become cancerous. Examples of antioxidants include vitamins C and E and beta carotene. *See also* free radical.

apoptosis (a-pop-TOE-sis): a type of cell death in which a series of molecular steps in a cell lead to its death. This is the body's normal way of getting rid of unneeded or abnormal cells and is different from the process of cell death by decay. Radiation therapy and many drugs used to treat cancer cause apoptosis. Also called programmed cell death.

ascites (uh-SY-teez): abnormal buildup of fluid in the abdomen that may cause swelling. In late-stage cancer, tumor cells may be found in the fluid in the abdomen. Ascites also occurs in people with liver disease.

aspiration (as-per-AY-shun): the accidental breathing in of food or fluid into the lungs. Also, removal of fluid or tissues through a needle.

beta carotene: a precursor of vitamin A that is found mainly in yellow and orange vegetables and fruits. It functions as an antioxidant and may play a role in cancer prevention. *See also* antioxidant.

bioactive compound: *see* phytochemical.

biologic therapy: *see* biotherapy.

biotherapy: treatments that promote or support the body's immune system response to a disease such as cancer. Also called immunotherapy or biologic therapy. *See also* immune system.

blood thinner: a drug that prevents or treats blood-clotting problems. Also called an anticoagulant.

Body Mass Index (BMI): a way to evaluate a person's weight.

botanical supplements: supplements made from plants. *See also* dietary supplements.

bran: the outer layer of a grain or seed. *See also* whole grains.

cachexia: a profound state of general poor health and malnutrition (poor dietary intake).

caffeine: a mild stimulant found in coffee, some soft drinks, and tea.

calcium: a mineral vital for biological processes in the body, found naturally in milk and other dairy products, leafy green vegetables, and other food.

calorie: a measurement of the energy your body gets from food to "fuel" all of its functions, such as breathing, circulating the blood, and physical activity.

cancer: cancer is not just one disease but a group of related diseases. In all forms of cancer, cells in the body change and grow out of control. Most types of cancer cells form a lump or mass called a tumor. The tumor can invade and destroy healthy tissue. Cells from the tumor can break away and travel to other parts of the body. There they can continue to grow. This spreading process is called metastasis. When cancer spreads, it is still named after the part of the body where it started. For example, if breast cancer spreads to the lungs, it is still called breast cancer, not lung cancer.

Some cancers, such as blood cancers, do not form a tumor. Not all tumors are cancer. A tumor that is not cancer is called benign. Benign tumors do not grow and spread the way cancer does. Benign tumors are usually not a threat to life. Another word for cancerous is malignant.

cancer vaccines: a form of biotherapy involving the use of cancer cells, parts of cells, or pure antigens. The vaccine increases the immune system's response against cancer cells in the body. *See also* biotherapy, immune system.

carbohydrates: carbohydrates supply the body with most of the calories it needs to function and create heat. Breads, pasta, grains, beans, fruits, and vegetables are all sources of carbohydrates. *See also* complex carbohydrates, simple carbohydrates.

carcinogen: a substance that causes cancer or helps cancer grow. For example, tobacco smoke contains many carcinogens that greatly increase the risk of lung cancer and several other types of cancer.

carotenoid (kuh-RAHT-in-oyd): a substance found in certain plants such as dark green, leafy vegetables and yellow and orange fruits and vegetables. Carotenoids may reduce the risk of developing cancer.

catechins: a phytochemical that has antioxidant properties. Catechin is found in green tea. *See also* phytochemical.

chemoprevention (key-mo-pre-VEN-shun): prevention or reversal of disease by using drugs, chemicals, vitamins, or minerals. Whereas this idea is not ready for widespread use, it is a very promising area of study.

chemopreventive agents: substances that prevent the development of cancer. *See* chemoprevention.

chemotherapy (key-mo-THER-uh-pee): treatment with drugs to destroy cancer cells. Chemotherapy is often used, either alone or with surgery or radiation therapy, to treat cancer that has spread or come back (recurred), or when there is a strong chance that it could recur.

cholesterol: a fat-like substance made in the liver and found in the blood and all cells of the body. Too much cholesterol in the blood can increase the risk of developing heart disease and stroke. The two main types of cholesterol are high-density lipoprotein (HDL) and low-density lipoprotein (LDL). HDL is known as the "good" cholesterol, because high levels of it seem to lower risk for heart disease, while LDL is known as the "bad" cholesterol.

clear liquid diet: a diet composed only of clear liquids. A clear liquid diet is a short-term dietary plan that includes only about five hundred calories a day and does not supply adequate nutrients for long-term health.

clinical trial: a study in which people volunteer as participants in research to test new ways of preventing, diagnosing, or treating health problems to determine their safety and effectiveness. Before a new treatment is used on people, it is studied in the laboratory. If these studies suggest the treatment will work, the next step is to test its value for participants. The main questions researchers want to answer are the following:

Does this treatment work?

Does it work better than what we're now using?

What side effects does it cause?

Do the benefits outweigh the risks?

Which patients are most likely to find this treatment helpful?

A clinical trial is done only when there is some reason to believe that the treatment being studied may be of value and is likely to be as good as the current standard of care.

The most reliable type of clinical trial is a *randomized* clinical trial, in which participants are assigned to different groups that compare treatments by chance. Randomization means that each person has an equal chance of being in the treatment (experimental) and comparison (control) groups. This helps reduce the chance of bias. *Compare with* laboratory study.

complementary therapy (complementary medicine): supportive methods that are used in addition to conventional treatments. Some complementary therapies may help relieve certain symptoms of cancer, relieve side effects of conventional cancer therapy or improve an individual's sense of well-being. Complementary methods are not intended to cure disease, rather they are provided to help control symptoms and improve quality of life. Some methods, such as massage therapy, yoga, and meditation, which are now called complementary, have been previously referred to as "supportive care." *See also* alternative therapy.

complex carbohydrates: also called starches, complex carbohydrates like vegetables, nuts, seeds, legumes, and whole grains are an important source of food energy, fiber, and key vitamins and minerals. *See also* carbohydrates. *Compare wtih* simple carbohydrates.

copper: a trace element found naturally in foods that assists in the regulation of blood pressure and heart rate and the absorption of iron in the body. *See also* iron.

corticosteroids: steroid substances from the adrenal glands, sometimes used as an anti-cancer treatment or to reduce persistent nausea.

cruciferous vegetable: a plant, such as broccoli or cauliflower, that has four flowers resembling a cross and contains certain chemicals that may reduce the risk of cancer.

cytotoxicity: cell-destroying ability.

Daily Values (DV): numbers on current nutrition labels that show the percentage of a nutrient a person gets by eating one serving of the labeled food. DV are based on U.S. Recommended Dietary Allowances for people eating two thousand calories per day. *See also* Recommended Dietary Allowance and Adequate Intake.

dehydration: when the body loses too much water to function well. Severe diarrhea or vomiting can cause dehydration.

Dietary Reference Intakes (DRI): recommendations developed by U.S. and Canadian scientists about the amounts of nutrients to be eaten each day to meet the needs of most healthy people. Dietary Reference Intakes are replacing the previous system of recommendations, called the Recommended Daily Allowances. *See also* Adequate Intake, Recommended Dietary Allowance, Estimated Average Requirement, and Tolerable Upper Intake Level.

Dietary Supplement Health and Safety Act (DSHEA): a law passed in 1994 giving legal definition to dietary supplements and giving the Federal Drug Administration permission to stop production of a dietary supplement if it is proved that the product poses a significant risk to the health of Americans. *See also* dietary supplement.

dietary supplement: legally defined as "…a product (other than tobacco) that is intended to supplement the diet that bears or contains one or more of the following dietary ingredients: a vitamin, a mineral, an herb or other botanical, an amino acid [the individual building blocks of protein], a dietary substance for use by man to supplement the diet by increasing the total daily intake, or a concentrate, metabolite, constituent, extract, or combinations of these ingredients." This definition includes ordinary multivitamins that help increase intake of essential substances that are part of a usual diet, as well as products like shark cartilage extract or echinacea, which are not ordinarily considered essential nutrients or part of a usual diet.

dietitian: *see* registered dietitian.

digestive tract: the parts of the body involved with eating, digesting, and excreting food, including the mouth, esophagus, stomach, intestines, rectum, and anus. Also called the gastrointestinal tract or GI tract.

distillation: a water treatment process that turns water into a vapor. Since minerals are too heavy to vaporize, they are left behind, and the vapors are condensed into water again.

diuretic: a chemical that increases urination.

edema: buildup of fluid in the tissues, causing swelling. Edema of the arm or leg can develop after surgery or radiation. Arm edema can also develop after radical mastectomy or axillary dissection of lymph nodes. Leg edema can develop if lymph nodes in the groin are removed. *See also* lymphedema, lymph nodes.

electrolyte: a substance that can conduct electrical current when it is dissolved in body fluids or water. Some examples of electrolytes are sodium, potassium, chloride, and calcium. Electrolytes are important in the normal functioning of cells and in metabolic activities.

endosperm: a seed's source of energy. *See also* whole grains.

enteral nutrition: a method of feeding in which a small, thin flexible tube is placed into the nose and threaded into the stomach to provide liquid nutrients when a person cannot eat enough.

enzyme: a protein that speeds up chemical reactions in the body. *See also* protein.

epidemiologic study: the study of diseases in populations by collecting and analyzing statistical data. In the field of cancer, epidemiologists look at how many people have cancer, who gets specific types of cancer, and what factors (such as environment or personal habits) play a part in the development of cancer. The two main types of epidemiologic research are observational studies (such as ecologic, case control, and cohort studies) and intervention studies (clinical trials). In typical usage, when people refer to epidemiologic studies, they are usually thinking of observational studies. *See also* clinical trial, observational study, intervention study.

essential nutrient: a substance that must be obtained from the diet because the body cannot make enough of it to meet its needs. *See also* nutrient.

Estimated Average Requirement (EAR): the amount of a nutrient that is estimated to meet the requirement of half of all healthy individuals in the population. *See also* nutrient.

estrogen (ES-truh-jin): a female sex hormone produced mainly by the ovaries, and in smaller amounts by the adrenal glands. In women, estrogen regulates the development of secondary sex characteristics, including breasts; regulates the monthly cycle of menstruation; and prepares the body for pregnancy. In breast cancer, estrogen may promote the growth of cancer cells.

estrogen receptors (ES-truh-jin rih-SEP-ters): proteins found in certain normal tissues as well as in some cancer cells. The hormone estrogen binds to these receptors and may cause the cells to grow. The tissues affected by estrogen normally contain estrogen receptors; other organs and tissues in the body do not. Therefore, when estrogen circulates in the blood, it only affects cells that contain estrogen receptors. *See also* estrogen.

fat soluble: able to be stored by the body in its fat stores. Fat-soluble nutrients include vitamins A, D, E, and K. *Compare with* water soluble. *See also* fats.

fats: nutrients that provide the body with fatty acids and calories for heat and for physical activity. *See also* fatty acid.

fatty acid: an important component of fats that is used by the body for energy and tissue development. There are two general categories of fat: saturated fat (saturated fatty acids) and unsaturated fat (unsaturated fatty acids). Saturated fatty acids are mostly found in fatty meats, animal fats such as lard and tallow, fat-containing dairy products, chocolate, and coconut oil, cottonseed oil, and palm kernel oil. Unsaturated fatty acids can be classified as monounsaturated fat (monounsaturated fatty acids), polyunsaturated fat (polyunsaturated fatty acids), omega-3 fatty acids, omega-6 fatty acids, and trans fat.

fiber: a wide variety of plant carbohydrates that are not digested by humans. Fibers are classified as "soluble" (like oat bran) and "insoluble" (like wheat bran). Soluble fiber helps reduce blood cholesterol, thereby lowering the risk of heart disease. Good sources of fiber are beans, vegetables, whole grains, and fruits. Links between fiber and cancer risk are inconclusive. Eating these foods is still recommended because they have other health benefits and contain other substances that can help prevent cancer. *See also* fat soluble, water soluble.

flavonoids: plant chemicals that are found in a broad range of grains, vegetables, and fruits, some of which may mimic the actions of estrogen. *See also* estrogen.

folate: *see* folic acid.

folic acid: a vitamin (also called vitamin B9) that influences growth, reproduction, blood cell production, and the nervous system. Green leafy vegetables, liver, citrus fruits, mushrooms, nuts, peas, dried beans, and wheat bread contain vitamin B9.

food additive: any substance used in the production, processing, treatment, packaging, transportation, or storage of food. *See also* indirect food additive.

free radical: a highly reactive chemical that has an unpaired electron. Free radicals often contain oxygen and can damage important cellular molecules such as DNA, lipids, or other parts of the cell, and this damage can lead to cancer. Free radicals can also be produced when cells are exposed to radiation and chemotherapy and are an important way in which these treatments kill cancer cells.

functional foods: foods bred or bioengineered to offer liberal doses of nutrients. Also called nutraceuticals. *See also* nutrients.

genetically modified food: food changed in a laboratory to make it resistant to pests and disease or to increase its concentration of nutrients. *See also* nutrients.

germ: the sprout of a new plant. *See also* whole grains.

glucosinolate: a type of phytochemical found in cabbage and other foods. *See also* phytochemical.

glycemic index: a way of classifying carbohydrates that measures how quickly and how highly a person's blood sugar level rises after eating a carbohydrate. *See also* high-glycemic foods, insulin, low-glycemic foods, carbohydrates.

Good Manufacturing Practices (GMPs): the set of standards developed by the Department of Health and Human Services for the manufacture of dietary supplements to prevent their contamination. *See also* dietary supplement.

herbal supplements: an entire plant or combination of plants or leaves, roots, or other parts that are sold dried, finely chopped, powdered, in capsule or liquid form. Herbal supplements contain many chemical ingredients, some helpful and others dangerous.

herbicide: a chemical that kills weeds.

high-glycemic foods: foods (such as highly processed carbohydrates, in which the bran and germ layers are removed) that cause fast, significant increases in a person's blood sugar levels. *See also* glycemic index, carbohydrates. *Compare with* low-glycemic foods.

hormone: a chemical substance released into the body by the endocrine glands such as the thyroid, adrenal, or ovaries. Hormones travel through the bloodstream and set in motion various body functions. Testosterone and estrogen are examples of male and female hormones.

hormonal therapy: treatment with hormones, with drugs that interfere with hormone production or hormone action, or the surgical removal of hormone-producing glands. Hormonal therapy may kill cancer cells or slow their growth. *See also* hormone.

hyperalimentation: giving liquid nutrition into a vein. Also called parenteral nutrition, total parenteral nutrition, or TPN.

immune system: the complex system by which the body resists infection by germs such as bacteria or viruses and rejects transplanted tissues or organs. The immune system may also help the body fight some cancers.

immunosuppression: weakening of the immune system. *See also* immune system.

immunotherapy (im-yoo-no-THER-uh-pee): *see* biotherapy.

indirect food additive: a substance that becomes part of food in trace amounts because of packaging, storage, or other handling. *Compare with* food additive.

insoluble fiber: dietary fiber not digested by humans, such as wheat bran and cellulose. *See also* fiber. *Compare with* soluble fiber.

insulin: a hormone made by the pancreas. Insulin controls the amount of sugar in the blood by moving it into cells, where it can be used by the body for energy. *See also* hormone.

insulin-like growth factor (IGF): a hormone-like substance. High levels of IGF in the blood have been linked to prostate and breast cancer risk.

intervention study: a human study in which researchers intentionally change at least one factor they believe is related to the risk of a disease. A clinical trial is a type of intervention study. *See also* clinical trial, observational study. *Compare with* laboratory study.

investigational treatments: therapies being studied in a clinical trial. Also called research treatments. *See also* clinical trial.

iron: an essential mineral and an important component of proteins involved in oxygen transport and metabolism. Iron is found in meat, fish, and poultry and in plants such as lentils, beans, as well as in products enriched or fortified with iron. *See also* protein.

irradiated food: food in which harmful organisms are killed by radiation in order to slow spoilage.

isoflavones: sometimes called phytoestrogens, or plant estrogens, these compounds act like weak forms of estrogens but are not produced by the body. They are found in soy and other foods. Genistein and daidzein are soy isoflavones thought to be the main factors responsible for the protective effects of soy. *See also* estrogen.

laboratory study: early-stage research in which scientists test substances on bacteria, animal, or human cells grown in laboratory dishes or test tubes. They are sometimes called test tube studies. *Compare with* clinical trial, observational study, intervention study.

lactase: an enzyme that breaks down the milk sugar lactose. *See also* lactose intolerance.

lactose: milk sugar. *See also* lactose intolerance.

lactose intolerance: a state in which the body does not produce enough lactase to break down lactose, which remains in the intestine. The body directs water to try to dilute lactose, and bacteria ferment it. This fluid retention and fermentation can cause diarrhea, gas, and cramping. *See also* lactase.

leukocytes: the medical term for white blood cells.

leukopenia: a decreased number of white blood cells.

lignans: compounds that can act as antiestrogens or as weak estrogens, which may play a role in preventing estrogen-dependent cancers such as breast cancer and other cancers. *See also* estrogen, antiestrogen.

low-glycemic foods: foods such as whole grains that contain unrefined or complex carbohydrates, take longer to digest, and raise blood levels more slowly and less than processed foods. *See also* glycemic index, carbohydrates. *Compare with* high-glycemic foods.

lutein: an antioxidant that is abundant in green, leafy vegetables such as collard greens, spinach, and kale. *See also* antioxidant.

lycopene: the compound that gives tomatoes their color and may also have anticancer effects.

lymphedema (limf-uh-DEE-muh): swelling due to a collection of excess fluid in the arms or legs. Swelling may happen after the lymph nodes and vessels are removed or are injured by radiation, or it can happen many years after treatment. It may also happen when a tumor disrupts normal fluid drainage. Lymphedema can persist and interfere with activities of daily living. *See also* lymph nodes.

lymph nodes: small, bean-shaped collections of immune system tissue such as lymphocytes, found along lymphatic vessels. They remove cell waste, germs, and other harmful substances from lymph. They help fight infections and also have a role in fighting cancer, although cancers sometimes spread through lymph nodes. Also called lymph glands. *See also* immune system.

macrobiotic diet: a dietary regimen that involves eating whole grains, vegetables and fruits, soups, occasional fish, and tea. Macrobiotic diets often involve cooking with specific materials or without using electricity.

macronutrients: nutrients the body uses in relatively large amount: carbohydrates, protein, and fats. *See also* nutrients, protein, carbohydrates, fats. *Compare with* micronutrients.

magnesium: a mineral found in fish, whole grains, nuts, and leafy green vegetables that helps bones form and reduces the risk of osteoporosis, builds protein, and converts food to energy.

meal replacements: substances that boost or support nutrition when you cannot eat enough calories or nutrients but are not a substitute for food. They can include liquid nutritional supplements, such as Instant Breakfast, Ensure, or Boost.

megadosing: the practice of using large doses of vitamins to attack disease.

metabolic therapy: an alternative dietary therapy that involves using a combination of special diets and other elements in an attempt to remove toxins from the body and strengthen the body's defenses against disease. It is based on the theory that disease is caused by toxic substances that have accumulated in the body.

metabolism: the total of all physical and chemical changes that take place in a cell or organism. The changes produce the energy and materials needed for important life processes.

micronutrients: substances the body needs in very small amounts, such as vitamins and minerals. *See also* vitamins, mineral. *Compare with* macronutrients.

mineral: inorganic elements consumed as nutrients and required to maintain health. Some minerals like calcium are needed in relatively large amounts; others like iodine are required in smaller amounts.

molybdenum: a mineral involved in many important biological processes. Common sources include legumes, cereals, leafy vegetables, liver, and milk. *See also* mineral.

monoclonal antibody (mah-no-KLO-nuhl an-tih-BAH-dee): a man-made version of immune system proteins called antibodies. Several monoclonal antibodies (MAbs) are approved for use as drugs for treating cancer and other diseases. Others are used in laboratory tests to help detect cancer cells and to diagnose many other health problems. *See also* antibody, immune system.

monounsaturated fatty acids: omega-3 and omega-6 fatty acids are mostly found in plant foods like vegetables and grains, as well as in some seafood. Monounsaturated fats do not lead to the formation of artery-clogging fatty deposits the way saturated fats do.

mucositis: ulcerations or swelling in the mouth.

myelosuppression: insufficient production of blood cells.

natural killer cell: a type of white blood cell that contains enzymes that can kill tumor cells or viral cells. *See also* enzyme.

nitrites: sodium nitrites are salts added to many meats to maintain color and to prevent contamination with bacteria. Nitrites may be converted in the stomach to carcinogenic nitrosamines, which may increase the risk of stomach cancer.

neutropenia: a reduction in the number of neutrophils, a type of white blood cell.

neutrophil: a type of white blood cell.

nutraceutical: *see* functional food.

nutrient: chemical compounds, such as water, protein, fat, carbohydrate, vitamins, and minerals, that make up foods.

Nutrition Facts panel: a label on the side or back of labels of frozen, packaged, and canned items specifying nutrient content. *See also* Percent Daily Value.

nutritionist: someone who counsels others about food and nutrition. There are no educational requirements associated with the title. *Compare with* registered dietitian.

obesity: a condition marked by an abnormally high, unhealthy amount of body fat. Adults with a body mass index (BMI) greater than 25 but less than 30 are considered overweight. Adults with a BMI greater than 30 are considered obese. Anyone more than 100 pounds overweight or with a BMI greater than 40 is considered morbidly obese.

observational study: a type of study in which individuals are observed or certain outcomes (such as survival, presence of various symptoms, or quality of life) are measured. The researchers look for a statistical link between outcomes and factors such as diet, exercise, use of various complementary or alternative methods. No attempt is made by the researchers to affect the outcome (for example, no treatment is given or recommended). *See also* clinical trial. *Compare with* intervention study, laboratory study.

omega-3 fatty acids: important nutrients involved in many body processes that must be obtained from dietary sources like fish or from supplements. *See also* fatty acid, omega-6 fatty acids.

omega-6 fatty acids: fatty acids found in many vegetable oils (corn, safflower, and sunflower), cereals, snack foods, and baked goods. *See also* fatty acid, omega-3 fatty acids.

organic food: plant foods grown without pesticides or genetic modifications and meat, poultry, eggs, and dairy raised without antibiotics or growth hormones.

parenteral nutrition: a form of nutrition that is delivered into a vein. Parenteral nutrition does not use the digestive system. A person can receive all necessary protein, calories, and nutrients through parenteral nutrition. Also called hyperalimentation, total parenteral nutrition, or TPN.

Percent Daily Value: *see* Daily Values.

pesticides: substances applied to many commercially grown fruit and vegetable crops to help protect them from insects, diseases, weeds, and mold.

phytochemicals: compounds found in fruits, vegetables, beans, grains, and other plants that seem to benefit the body and may even fight cancer. Thousands of phytochemicals have been identified, including beta carotene, ascorbic acid (vitamin C), folic acid, and vitamin E. Some phytochemicals have either antioxidant or estrogen-like actions. Polyphenols and flavonoids are phytochemicals. Also called bioactive food compounds or bioactive compounds.

phytoestrogen: an estrogen-like substance that is found in some plants and plant products. Phytoestrogens may have anticancer effects. *See also* estrogen.

polyphenols: chemicals including flavonoids that have antioxidant properties. *See also* antioxidant, flavonoids.

polyunsaturated fatty acids: a type of unsaturated fatty acid. Polyunsaturated fats do not lead to the formation of artery-clogging fatty deposits the way saturated fats do. *See also* fatty acid.

potassium: a mineral that helps regulate major body functions. The body cannot manufacture potassium and must obtain it from foods including apricots, potatoes, bananas, whole grains, beans, and lean meat. *See also* mineral.

progesterone: a female sex hormone. *See also* estrogen.

prostate-specific antigen (PSA): a substance produced by the prostate that may be found in an increased amount in the blood of men who have prostate cancer. *See also* antigen.

protein: a nutrient that provides the body with amino acids, which ensure growth, repair body tissue, maintain a healthy immune system, and aid in other body functions. Without enough protein, the body takes longer to recover from illness and lowers its resistance to infection. *See also* amino acid.

proven treatment: evidence-based, or mainstream medical treatments that have been tested following a strict set of guidelines and found to be safe and effective.

psyllium: a plant that has seeds that can be used as a mild laxative.

Recommended Dietary Allowance (RDA): intake level for a particular nutrient sufficient to meet the nutrient requirement of nearly all (97 to 98 percent) healthy individuals. RDAs are established by the Food and Nutrition Board (FNB) of the United States National Academies of Sciences. *See also* Adequate Intake.

recurrence: cancer that has come back after treatment. *Local recurrence* means that the cancer has come back at the same place as the original cancer. *Regional recurrence* means that the cancer has come back in the lymph nodes near the first site. *Distant recurrence* is when cancer metastasizes after treatment to organs or tissues (such as the lungs, liver, bone marrow, or brain) farther from the original site than the regional lymph nodes.

refined grains: grains stripped of the bran and germ during processing that are therefore low in fiber and in the protective substances that accompany fiber. *Compare with* whole grains.

registered dietitian (RD): an expert in food and diet required to have at least a bachelor's degree and who has passed a national competency exam. RDs can help people with cancer through dietary counseling and education. *Compare with* nutritionist.

saturated fatty acids: mostly found in meats and whole-milk products, saturated fatty acids (also called saturated fat) lead to the formation of artery-clogging fatty deposits. The role of fat in cancer risk is controversial and continues to be studied. *See also* fatty acid.

selenium: researchers think this mineral is an antioxidant. Selenium may also play a role in normal growth, development, and fertility. The best nutritional sources of selenium are meat, whole grains, and Brazil nuts. *See also* antioxidant, mineral.

simple carbohydrate: a type of sugar, such as sugar and honey, which lacks the vitamins, minerals, proteins, and fiber that are generally found in complex carbohydrates. Also called simple sugar. *See also* carbohydrate. *Compare with* complex carbohydrate.

simple sugar: *see* simple carbohydrate.

slurry: a thin paste of water and flour stirred into hot dishes as a thickener that can make foods moist and easier to swallow.

sodium: a mineral required to keep body fluids in balance. Sodium is found in table salt. Too much sodium can cause you to retain water. *See also* mineral.

soluble fiber: dietary fiber like oat bran not digested by humans that helps reduce blood cholesterol, lowering the risk of coronary heart disease. *See also* fiber. *Compare with* insoluble fiber.

sulfides: a group of phytochemicals found in garlic and onions. *See also* phytochemicals.

systemic treatment (systemic therapy): treatment that reaches and affects cells throughout the entire body; for example, chemotherapy.

tamoxifen (tuh-MOK-si-fin): (brand name Nolvadex) a drug used to treat breast cancer that has estrogen receptors (is estrogen–receptor positive). After starting the drug, some women who have breast cancer with bone metastases may notice a temporary flare (increase in bone pain), which usually indicates the cancer is responding to treatment.

Tolerable Upper Intake Level (UL): highest average daily intake level of a particular nutrient as likely to pose no health risk for nearly all individuals. ULs are established by the Food and Nutrition Board (FNB) of the United States National Academies of Sciences. As intake increases above the UL, the potential risk of adverse health affects increases.

total parenteral nutrition (TPN): delivery of nutrients directly into the bloodstream through a needle inserted into a vein.

trace element: a chemical element, such as copper or zinc, found in small amounts in the human body that is necessary for bodily processes.

trans fatty acids: fats found in margarines, vegetable shortenings, and packaged breads, cakes, cookies, and crackers. They are similar to saturated fat in that they form artery-clogging deposits. Also called trans fats and trans-saturated fats. *See also* fatty acid.

tube feeding: *see* enteral nutrition.

UL: *see* Tolerable Upper Intake Level.

vegetarianism: a dietary regimen that involves eating food from plant sources such as vegetables and fruits, grains, legumes, seeds, and nuts. Some vegetarian diets include no animal products (vegan), while others include dairy products (lactovegetarian), dairy and eggs (lacto-ovo-vegetarian), and fish (semivegetarian).

vitamin A: a vitamin essential for normal growth, bone development, reproduction, and vision taken in directly as vitamin A from animal sources and taken in indirectly from many fruits and vegetables as beta carotene, which the body converts to vitamin A.

vitamin B1: a vitamin (also called thiamine) that regulates enzymes that influence the functions of the muscles, nerves, and heart and found in cereals and whole grains, as well as potatoes, pork, seafood, liver, and kidney beans.

vitamin B2: a vitamin (also called riboflavin) that influences the production of energy in cells and health of the skin and mucous membranes of the digestive and respiratory systems and is found in enriched bread, dairy products, liver, and green leafy vegetables.

vitamin B3: a vitamin (also called niacin) that has a role in production of energy in cells and in maintaining health of the skin, nervous system, and digestive system. It is found in liver, fish, chicken, lean red meat, nuts, whole grains, and dried beans.

vitamin B5: a vitamin (also called pantothenic acid) that influences normal growth and development and is found in almost all foods.

vitamin B6: a vitamin (also called pyridoxine) with an effect on protein, carbohydrate, and fat metabolism, and on maintaining health of red blood cells, skin, the nervous system, and the digestive system. Fish, liver, pork, chicken, potatoes, wheat germ, bananas, and dried beans are good sources of vitamin B6.

vitamin B12: a vitamin (also called cobalamin) that plays a role in growth, development, the production of blood cells, the functions of the nervous system, and how the body uses folic acid and carbohydrates. It is found in meats, fish, eggs, and dairy products. *See also* folic acid, carbohydrates.

vitamin C: an essential vitamin that must be obtained from the diet, in citrus fruits like oranges, grapefruit, and lemons, and in green leafy vegetables, potatoes, strawberries, bell peppers, and cantaloupe. Vitamin C helps bones and teeth form, helps resist infection, helps wounds heal, and is needed for blood clotting. It is also an antioxidant. *See also* antioxidant.

vitamin D: a vitamin that maintains normal blood levels of calcium and phosphorus. It aids in the absorption of calcium, helping to form and maintain strong bones. Only a few foods naturally contain significant amounts of vitamin D, including fatty fish and fish oils. In the United States, milk is fortified with vitamin D.

vitamin E: an essential nutrient that helps build normal cells and form red blood cells. The main sources of vitamin E in the diet are vegetable oils (especially safflower oil, sunflower oil, and cottonseed oil), green leafy vegetables, nuts, cereals, meats, egg yolks, wheat germ, and whole wheat products.

vitamin K: an essential nutrient the liver needs to form substances that promote blood clotting and prevent abnormal bleeding. The human body obtains vitamin K from certain foods and bacteria that normally live in the intestines. Dietary sources of vitamin K include leafy greens, as well as cereals, dairy products, some fruits, liver, and pork.

vitamins: key nutrients, such as vitamins A, C, and E, that the body needs in small amounts to grow and stay strong.

water soluble: a term used to describe nutrients that are unable to be stored in the body. Humans need to take in water soluble nutrients such as vitamins B and C every day. *See also* fat soluble.

whole grains: grains such as barley, brown rice, whole wheat, or bulgur that contain the germ, endosperm, and bran of a grain or seed. Different whole grain foods differ in nutrient content, but they provide more vitamins, minerals, fiber, and other protective substances than refined grains. *See also* germ, endosperm, bran. *Compare with* refined grains.

zinc: a trace element that plays a key role in many body processes, including the building of DNA, energy production, cell metabolism, and regulation of the immune system. Zinc is found in lean meat, seafood, soybeans, nuts, pumpkin and sunflower seeds, eggs, cheese, and wheat bran.

INDEX

About the Authors

Barbara L. Grant, MS, RD, CSO, LD, is the outpatient clinical oncology dietitian at the Saint Alphonsus Cancer Care Center, in Boise, Idaho. She is a board certified specialist in oncology nutrition. She received her Master of Science in Adult Education from the University of Idaho, her Bachelor of Science in Foods and Nutrition from Washington State University, and completed her Dietetic Internship at the University of Minnesota Hospitals and Clinics. She is a published author and has presented to professional and community organizations on a variety of diet, nutrition, and cancer-related topics. She has served on local and national boards, committees, and workgroups of the American Cancer Society, the National Cancer Institute, the Susan G. Komen for the Cure Foundation, the American College of Surgeon's Commission on Cancer, the Commission on Dietetic Registration, and the American Dietetic Association. She resides in Boise, Idaho.

Abby S. Bloch, PhD, RD, is executive director of programs and research for The Robert C. and Veronica Atkins Foundation. Previously, she was the director of the Clinical Nutrition Support Unit at Memorial Sloan-Kettering Cancer Center. She earned her Bachelor of Science from Cornell University, her Master of Science from Columbia University, and her PhD from New York University. Dr. Bloch was the chairperson for the American Cancer Society Advisory Committee on Nutrition and Physical Activity for five years, in addition to many years served as part of the committee. She has published numerous books, chapters in textbooks, articles in peer-reviewed journals, and other publications relating to nutrition and cancer prevention, cancer management, and clinical aspects of nutrition and diet. She resides in New York, New York.

Kathryn K. Hamilton, MA, RD, CSO, CSO, is an outpatient clinical oncology dietitian with the Carol G. Simon Cancer Center at the Morristown Memorial Hospital in Morristown, New Jersey. She also serves as an assistant professor at College of St. Elizabeth in Morristown and is an annual guest lecturer in clinical nutrition. She is a board certified specialist in oncology nutrition. She has published numerous articles in peer-reviewed journals, chapters in textbooks, and booklets on the subject of nutrition and cancer. She resides in Upper Saddle River, New Jersey.

Cynthia A. Thomson, PhD, RD, CSO, is an associate professor at the University of Arizona's Department of Nutritional Sciences. She is a faculty member at the University of Arizona Comprehensive Cancer Center. She is a board certified specialist in oncology nutrition. Most recently, Dr. Thomson was a nominee for the Sidney Salmon Memorial Award for Cancer

Research in 2009, and she has received numerous awards for excellence in nutrition education. She received her Doctorate and her Master of Science in Nutritional Sciences from the University of Arizona and her Bachelor of Science in Nutrition and Dietetics from West Virginia University. She is a consultant for a number of health organizations, including the Fred Hutchinson Cancer Research Center in Seattle, Washington. She has published more than eighty articles in peer-reviewed journals, in addition to more than twenty chapters in textbooks. Dr. Thomson's areas of research interest include diet and cancer prevention and dietary methodology. She resides in Tucson, Arizona.

Other Books Published by the American Cancer Society

Available everywhere books are sold and online at **cancer.org/bookstore**

TOOLS FOR THE HEALTH CONSCIOUS

American Cancer Society's Healthy Eating Cookbook, Third Edition
Celebrate! Healthy Entertaining for Any Occasion
Good for You! Reducing Your Risk of Developing Cancer
The Great American Eat-Right Cookbook
Kicking Butts: Quit Smoking and Take Charge of Your Health
What to Eat During Cancer Treatment: 100 Great-Tasting, Family-Friendly Recipes to Help You Cope

INFORMATION FOR PEOPLE WITH CANCER

American Cancer Society Complete Guide to Complementary and Alternative Cancer Therapies, Second Edition
American Cancer Society's Guide to Pain Control, Revised Edition
Lymphedema: Understanding and Managing Lymphedema After Cancer Treatment

SUPPORT FOR FAMILIES AND CAREGIVERS

Cancer Caregiving A to Z: An At-Home Guide for Patients and Families
The Survivorship Net: A Parable for the Family, Friends, and Caregivers of People with Cancer
What Helped Get Me Through: Cancer Survivors Share Wisdom and Hope

BOOKS FOR CHILDREN

Healthy Me: A Read-Along Coloring & Activity Book
Kids' First Cookbook: Delicious-Nutritious Treats to Make Yourself!
Nana, What's Cancer?
Our Dad Is Getting Better
Our Mom Has Cancer (available in hard cover and paperback)
Our Mom Is Getting Better